Modern Management of Uterine Fibroids

Modern Management of Uterine Fibroids

Edited by

Mostafa Metwally
The University of Sheffield and Sheffield Teaching Hospitals

Tin-Chiu Li
The Chinese University of Hong Kong

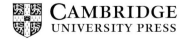

CAMBRIDGE
UNIVERSITY PRESS

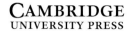

CAMBRIDGE
UNIVERSITY PRESS

University Printing House, Cambridge CB2 8BS, United Kingdom

One Liberty Plaza, 20th Floor, New York, NY 10006, USA

477 Williamstown Road, Port Melbourne, VIC 3207, Australia

314–321, 3rd Floor, Plot 3, Splendor Forum, Jasola District Centre, New Delhi – 110025, India

79 Anson Road, #06–04/06, Singapore 079906

Cambridge University Press is part of the University of Cambridge.

It furthers the University's mission by disseminating knowledge in the pursuit of education, learning, and research at the highest international levels of excellence.

www.cambridge.org
Information on this title: www.cambridge.org/9781108420174
DOI: 10.1017/9781108332798

First published 2020

Printed in Singapore by Markono Print Media Pte Ltd

A catalogue record for this publication is available from the British Library.

Library of Congress Cataloging-in-Publication Data
Names: Metwally, Mostafa, editor. | Li, Tin-Chiu, editor.
Title: Modern management of uterine fibroids / edited by Mostafa Metwally, Tin-Chiu Li.
Description: Cambridge, United Kingdom ; New York, NY : Cambridge University Press, 2020. | Includes bibliographical references and index.
Identifiers: LCCN 2019042617 (print) | LCCN 2019042618 (ebook) | ISBN 9781108420174 (hardback) | ISBN 9781108332798 (epub)
Subjects: MESH: Leiomyoma–surgery | Leiomyoma–diagnostic imaging | Uterine Myomectomy–methods | Hysterectomy–methods | Laparoscopy–methods
Classification: LCC RG391 (print) | LCC RG391 (ebook) | NLM WP 459 | DDC 618.1/453–dc23
LC record available at https://lccn.loc.gov/2019042617
LC ebook record available at https://lccn.loc.gov/2019042618

ISBN 978-1-108-42017-4 Hardback

Additional resources for this publication at www.cambridge.org/metwally

Cambridge University Press has no responsibility for the persistence or accuracy of URLs for external or third-party internet websites referred to in this publication and does not guarantee that any content on such websites is, or will remain, accurate or appropriate.

....

Contents

Contributors

Shahram Abdi
Consultant Radiologist, Department of Radiology,
The Royal Hallamshire Hospital, Sheffield Teaching
Hospitals, Sheffield, England, UK

Ayman Al-Hendy
Professor of Obstetrics and Gynaecology, Department
of Obstetrics and Gynaecology, University of Illinois,
Chicago, USA

Mohamed Ali
Department of Obstetrics and Gynaecology,
Medical College of Georgia, Augusta University,
Augusta, GA, USA; Clinical Pharmacy Department,
Faculty of Pharmacy, Ain Shams University,
Cairo, Egypt

Jimena B. Alvarez
Department of Obstetrics and Gynecology, Saint
Anthony Hospital, Chicago, IL USA

Rudi Campo
Life Expert Centre, Leuven, Belgium; European
Academy for Gynaecological Surgery, Leuven,
Belgium

Zunir Tayyeb Chaudhry
Saint James School of Medicine, St. Vincent,
Caribbean

Jacqueline P. W. Chung
Department of Obstetrics and Gynaecology, Prince of
Wales Hospital, The Chinese University of Hong
Kong, Shatin, New Territories, Hong Kong, Special
Administrative Region of China

Trevor J. Cleveland
Consultant Vascular Interventional Radiologist,
Sheffield Vascular Institute, Northern General
Hospital, Sheffield Teaching Hospitals, Sheffield,
England, UK

Mary E. Connor
Consultant Gynaecologist, Department of Obstetrics
and Gynaecology, The Royal Hallamshire Hospital,
Sheffield Teaching Hospitals, Sheffield, England, UK

Hilary O. D. Critchley
Professor of Reproductive Medicine, Centre for
Reproductive Health, University of Edinburgh and
Edinburgh Royal Infirmary, Edinburgh, UK

Cristine Di Cesare
Department of Obstetrics and Gynaecology,
Fondazione Policlinico Universitario Agostino
Gemelli, Catholic University of Sacred Heart, Rome,
Italy; European Academy for Gynaecological Surgery,
Leuven, Belgium

Krit Dwivedi
Specialist Trainee and Academic Clinical Fellow in
Radiology, Sheffield Teaching Hospital, Sheffield,
England, UK

Ahmed M. El-Minawi
Professor of Obstetrics and Gynaecology, Kasr Al
Aini School of Medicine, Cairo University,
Cairo, Egypt

Alpha K. Gebeh
Consultant in Reproductive Medicine and Surgery,
East and North Hertfordshire NHS Trust,
Stevenage, UK

Jessica Gelman
Obstetrics and Gynaecology Resident Physician,
Advocate Lutheran General Hospital, Park Ridge,
IL, USA

S. Gordts
Life Expert Centre, Leuven, Belgium; European
Academy for Gynaecological Surgery, Leuven,
Belgium

Swati Jha
Consultant Urogynaecologist, The Royal Hallamshire Hospital, Sheffield Teaching Hospitals and Sheffield University, Sheffield, England, UK

Tülay Karasu
Consultant in Reproductive Medicine and Surgery, Cambridge University Hospitals, Cambridge, UK

Tin-Chiu Li
Department of Obstetrics and Gynaecology, Prince of Wales Hospital, UK; The Chinese University of Hong Kong, Shatin, New Territories, Hong Kong, Special Administrative Region of China; Fuxing Hospital, Capital Medical University, Beijing, China

Mostafa Metwally
Consultant in Reproductive Medicine and Surgery, The Royal Hallamshire Hospital, Sheffield Teaching Hospitals and The University of Sheffield, Sheffield, England, UK

Charles E. Miller
The Advanced Gynaecologic Surgery Institute, Naperville, IL, USA; Director, Minimally Invasive Gynaecologic Surgery, Advocate Lutheran General Hospital, Park Ridge, IL, USA

Mohamed Otify
Centre for Reproductive Health, University of Edinburgh and Edinburgh Royal Infirmary, Edinburgh, UK

Elizabeth A. Pritts
Wisconsin Fertility Institute, Middleton, WI, USA

John Mark Regi
Consultant Vascular Interventional Radiologist, Sheffield Vascular Institute, Northern General Hospital, Sheffield Teaching Hospitals, Sheffield, England, UK

Sotirios H. Saravelos
Subspecialty Fellow in Reproductive Medicine and Surgery, Hammersmith Hospital, Imperial College, London, England, UK

Ertan Saridogan
Consultant in Gynaecology and Minimal Access Surgery, University College London Hospitals, Women's Health Division, London, England, UK

Lisa Shannon
Consultant Radiologist, Barnsley General Hospital, Barnsley, UK

Enlan Xia
Fuxing Hospital, Capital Medical University, Beijing, China

Ephia Yasmin
Consultant in Reproductive Medicine and Surgery, University College London Hospitals, Women's Health Division, London, England, UK

Dan Yu
Fuxing Hospital, Capital Medical University, Beijing, China

Foreword

This new volume on fibroids covers a broad range of information, as there have been many recent advances in the understanding of the pathology of fibroids and the medical and surgical modalities and techniques of treatment. Published data do not provide this information succinctly, in sufficient technical detail, or in a readily accessible manner. These 19 chapters cover developments in biochemistry and genetics, and the role of imaging, extending to 3D ultrasound and MRI scanning, leading to different classifications. The impact of these benign tumours on fertility and aspects of obstetrics in both the untreated and treated states is described. The variety of medical treatments and pretreatments prior to other interventions has expanded, and surgery now provides many options.

The classical open surgery with an emphasis on microsurgical technique, laparoscopic procedures ranging from myomectomy to hysterectomy, and the use of vaginal hysterectomy, are all described in their complexity. The location of the fibroid determines the approach, so hysteroscopic removal also provides many options, both as inpatient and as outpatient, again with technical definition of procedures and instruments. Illustrations of methods with examples are generously featured.

Much confusion has attended the question of the prevalence of leiomyosarcoma and the role played by morcellation in its spread. These issues are forensically analysed to provide clarity and guidance to the current situation. Finally, the technique of embolization has come of age, and its role and outcomes are described together with the early work on developing MRI ultrasound-guided lysis, which is developing apace. Even a description of residual fibroids after menopause, and how they might react, finds a place.

This is a comprehensive account of the current approach to the commonest benign tumour in women. Although there are many self-help books directed at patient comprehension of this area, there are no recent books covering such a broad spectrum of information for professionals. It should stimulate interest and close study of a rapidly developing area of benign gynaecology. The editors, Mostafa Metwally and Tin-Chiu Li, have achieved their aim of providing an up-to-date, well-referenced volume to assist reproductive medicine specialists in this increasingly complex field.

Ian Cooke
Emeritus Professor
Academic Unit of Reproductive and
Developmental Medicine
Department of Human Metabolism
University of Sheffield

Pathophysiology of Uterine Fibroids

Mohamed Otify and Hilary O. D. Critchley

1.1 Introduction

Uterine fibroids are a major cause of morbidity in women [1]. Fibroids have variable clinical presentations, depending on size and location. These include pelvic pain (20–40% of patients), bleeding (30% of patients), and anaemia. Fibroids are the leading cause of hysterectomy in the United States [2]. Bleeding from fibroids generally presents as abnormal uterine bleeding (AUB) and often prolonged or heavy menstrual bleeding (HMB) [3]. Fibroids that bleed are more frequently submucosal or extend into the endometrial cavity. Other problems related to fibroids include problems with implantation [1], preterm labour, recurrent loss of pregnancy, obstruction of labour, and urinary incontinence [4]. Medical costs for patients with fibroids in the United States were estimated as 4.1–9.4 billion US dollars in 2010 [2].

The self-reported prevalence of uterine fibroids in women from France, Germany, Italy, the United Kingdom, the United States, Canada, Brazil, and South Korea has ranged from 4.5% in the United Kingdom to 9.8% in Italy [5]. The highest prevalence was seen in women aged 40–49 years in the United Kingdom (9.4%) and Italy (17.8%). The worldwide mortality from fibroids in developed countries has remained about 0.01/100,000 women over the last 25 years [6].

There is a variable risk of developing fibroids in women, depending on race, hormone exposure, age, diet, and other factors. Some factors may be modified and, if altered, have the potential to reduce the impact of fibroid-related morbidity. Herein, we review these factors and the associated genetic changes that have been described to date.

1.2 Aetiology

1.2.1 Definition

Uterine leiomyomas, or fibroids, are common, benign, smooth muscle tumours of the uterus.

Fibroid growth involves clonal uterine smooth muscle cell expansion along with production of a large amount of extracellular matrix. Uterine fibroids are commonly found presenting after puberty and diminishing after menarche [7]. Uterine fibroids usually become symptomatic in women during their fourth and fifth decades, and 20–40% of women develop symptoms related to their fibroids [8].

1.2.2 Epidemiology

A number of factors have been linked to the development of fibroids and the different patterns in which they become clinically evident. Some factors are modifiable and may be useful in promoting preventive health care. Numerous risk factors for fibroid development have been described, several of which may be affected by changes in diet or lifestyle (Table 1.1).

1.2.2.1 Fibroid Growth Rates

The Fibroid Growth Study followed 262 fibroids in 38 black and 34 white premenopausal women over a 12-month period [9]. Black women 35 years of age or older had a 2.8-fold increased risk of rapid fibroid growth (>20% increase in volume over 6 months) when compared to similar white women [10]. Fibroids from women more than 45 years of age grew more rapidly in black women (increase in volume of 15% over 6 months) than in white women (increase in volume of 2% over 6 months) [9]. White women, but not black women, had a decrease in growth rate with age. Rapid growth was seen more frequently in young white women than in older white women. The frequency of fibroids with rapid growth did not vary by age in black women. Fibroid volume changes in a 6-month period ranged from −89% to +138%. Both black and white women had a median increase in volume of 9% over 6 months. About 34% of fibroids increased in volume by 20%, and 7% experienced a 20% decrease in volume over 6 months. Fibroid shrinkage was generally

Table 1.1 Risk factors for fibroid development have been described, several of which may be influenced by changes in diet or lifestyle

	Effect	May be modified with
Race		
Black women have		
• ↓ urinary 2-HE/16α-HE metabolite excretion	↑ oestrogen exposure	Diet: high-fibre, low-fat diet
• ↓ vitamin D blood levels	↑ fibroid risk	↑ sun exposure, oral vitamin D
• ↑ aromatase blood levels	↑ oestrogen exposure	Diet: high-fibre, low-fat diet
Oestrogen		
Early age of menarche	↑ oestrogen exposure associated with	Diet: high-fibre, low-fat diet
	↑ cellular proliferation	
	↑ risk of genetic mutation	
	↑ expression of progesterone receptors	
Progesterone		
	Associated with suppressed apoptosis (↑ bcl-2 expression)	
	↑ TGF-β expression	
	↑ cellular proliferation	
	↑ extracellular matrix formation	

associated with loss of arterial blood supply as indicated by contrast enhancement. Women often had fibroids with varying growth and shrinkage [7].

Fibroid growth rates were faster in women with a single fibroid than in women with multiple fibroids [9]. Fibroid growth rates did not differ by patient BMI, parity, size, or location. About 62% of women undergoing surgical resections of fibroids without hysterectomy have been reported to have a recurrence of a fibroid at least 2 cm in diameter within 5 years, and 9% required surgery for this recurrence [11].

1.2.2.2 Age

Fibroids are often diagnosed in older premenopausal women. Most fibroids occur in women in their thirties or forties, associated with chronic exposure to oestrogen and progesterone throughout the reproductive life course [12]. The Seveso Women's Health Study found fibroids in 21.4% of Italian women aged 30–60 who were screened by ultrasound [11]. Most fibroids diagnosed by fibroid screening are symptomatic. Ultrasound identified fibroids in 3.3% of Swedish women aged 25–32 years and 7.8% of women aged 33–40 years. A woman's age at birth of the last child was inversely related to risk of fibroids [13]. Fibroids have not been described in prepubertal girls [12].

1.2.2.3 Race

Most studies evaluating race-related risk of developing fibroids were performed in the United States. The incidence of fibroids by age 50 was estimated as 70% for white women and 80% for African-American or black women [7]. Black women had a lower urinary 2-hydroxyoestrone/16α-hydroxyoestrone metabolite ratio than white women [14]. 2-hydroxyoestrone metabolites have less oestrogenic activity than 16α-hydroxyoestrone metabolites, possibly leading to greater oestrogen exposure in black women. Black women had a three times greater risk of clinically symptomatic fibroids, and were younger at first diagnosis, had more severe disease, and underwent hysterectomy more frequently than white women [12]. Fibroids were detected about 10 years earlier in black women than in white women [15, 16].

A random selection of adult women in an American health plan found that 35% of premenopausal women had a previous diagnosis of fibroids and that 51% of the premenopausal women with no clinical diagnosis had ultrasound-detectable fibroids [7]. Black women had fibroids more frequently than white women (cumulative incidence by age 50, >80% vs. 70%, OR = 2.9). There was little change in risk after adjustment for parity or body mass index (BMI). White women appeared to have an increasing risk with increasing age, while black women had a constant higher risk. Parity was not a risk factor in black women, and about two-thirds of white women were nulliparous. Black women were diagnosed at a younger age than white women (33 vs. 36 years). Black women were more likely to have multiple fibroid tumours than white women (73% vs. 45%). This difference was greatest in younger women (35–39 years, 74% vs. 31%). Clinically relevant premenopausal fibroids were present in about half of black women and 25% of white women [7]. A much lower incidence was reported in 334 Swedish women screened with ultrasound [17]. Only about 5% of all Swedish women were affected and only 8% of women 33–40 years of age. Pathologic study of 2-mm sectioned hysterectomy specimens obtained from adult American women demonstrated fibroids in 77% [18]; 84% of these women had multiple fibroids.

The Study of Environment, Lifestyle and Fibroids evaluated 1,696 black American women with ultrasound and found 22% had at least one fibroid 0.5 cm in diameter [15]. Prevalence increased with age: 10% for women 23–25 years of age and 32% for women 32–35 years of age.

The incidence of newly diagnosed fibroids has been reported to be about 3% per year in reproductive-age black women [11]. It has been reported that 73% of black women and 45% of white women have multiple fibroids [7]. Hispanic women have been reported to have a similar incidence of fibroids as white women [4].

1.2.2.4 Obesity

BMI is inversely associated with sex hormone-binding globulin level and these levels are higher in obese patients [19]. Thus women with increased BMI may have more bioavailable circulating oestrogens and androgens. Obesity has been associated with a modest increased risk of fibroids in several, but not all, international studies [13, 19]. Each 10 kg increase in weight in adults was associated with an 18% increase in the development of fibroids [11]. BMI during adolescence has not to date been associated with an increased risk of fibroids.

1.2.2.5 Diet and Exercise

Several studies have suggested an association between diet and the development of fibroids. Increased

consumption of red meat (RR = 1.7) and decreased consumption of green vegetables (RR = 2.0) have been associated with an increased risk of fibroids [11, 12]. A double-blinded randomized study showed that intake of green tea extract was associated with a reduction in uterine fibroid size and clinical severity, and an improvement in quality of life, compared to placebo control [20].

The dietary habits of 22,583 premenopausal black women were evaluated for their association with the development of fibroids [21]. Fruit and vegetable intake were each inversely associated with the risk of fibroids (2 servings/day vs. 2 servings/week). Citrus fruit had the highest inverse association (3 servings/week vs. 1 serving/month). Increasing fruit and vegetable consumption was observed with increasing patient age and multivitamin use. Risk was not associated with intake of vitamins C or E, folate, or carotenoids.

The National Institute of Environmental Health Sciences Uterine Fibroid Study correlated plasma vitamin D levels with the ultrasound diagnosis of fibroids in randomly selected 35- to 49-year-old women [22]. Moreover, 50% of white women and 10% of black women had normal plasma levels of 25-hydroxy vitamin D (>20 ng/mL). Women with normal levels of 25-hydroxy vitamin D had a 32% lower risk of having fibroids. Sun exposure for more than 1 hour per day was also associated with reduction in risk of having fibroids (adjusted OR = 0.6). Vitamin D deficiency is more common among black women, as their pigment inhibits sunlight-related stimulation of vitamin D production in the skin [23].

Premenopausal vegetarian women excreted three times more faecal oestrogen, had less urinary oestrogen excretion, and had 15–20% lower plasma oestrogen levels than non-vegetarian women [14]. Increased faecal excretion of oestrogen was linked to decreased deconjugation of faecal oestrogen that is needed for its reabsorption. Postmenopausal women placed on a low-fat diet experienced a 17% decrease in plasma oestradiol concentrations.

The effect of exercise on fibroid pathophysiology is not clear. While former college athletes were less likely than non-athletes (RR = 0.72) to develop fibroids, other differences such as diet and weight were not accounted for [14].

1.2.2.6 Caffeine

The Black Women's Health Study found an increased risk of fibroids in the subgroup of women less than

35 years of age who drank over three cups of coffee a day or consumed more than 500 mg caffeine a day [19]. This association was not found when women of all ages were included in the evaluation.

1.2.2.7 Alcohol

Alcohol intake has been associated with the development of fibroids in most studies [19]. A report on Japanese women found fibroids, diagnosed by ultrasound, more frequently in those in the highest third of alcohol intake, compared to those in the lowest third (OR = 2.8, about 1 drink/day vs. non-drinkers). Current drinkers in the Black Women's Health Study also had a higher risk than non-drinkers. The highest risk, a 60% increase, was with women drinking beer (7+ drinks/week vs. non-drinkers).

1.2.2.8 Smoking

Smoking is historically associated with a decreased risk of fibroid formation [12]. Smoking two packs of cigarettes a day was associated with an 18% increase in the development of fibroids [11]. More recent studies, including the National Institute of Environmental Health Sciences Uterine Fibroid Study, showed no association between risk of fibroids and smoking [19]. Protective effects found in earlier studies have been attributed to bias introduced by improper selection of the control groups.

1.2.2.9 Menarche

Early age of menarche increases a woman's overall lifetime exposure to oestrogen and is associated with a higher risk for fibroids [13]. Women who are ≤10 years at menarche have a higher risk of fibroids than women who were 12 years of age or more at menarche (RR = 1.24) [14].

1.2.2.10 Menopause

Uteri evaluated pathologically using 2 mm sections were found to have similar numbers of fibroids whether they were obtained from pre- or postmenopausal women. However, the fibroids were smaller in postmenopausal women. Postmenopausal women have a decrease in circulating oestrogen and progesterone levels, and this has been attributed to fibroid shrinkage [14]. These findings could however be affected by selection bias, as postmenopausal women were often treated more conservatively and did not undergo hysterectomy.

1.2.2.11 Parity

High concentrations of oestrogen and progesterone are found in pregnancy and with oral contraceptive (OC) use, two conditions associated with a decreased risk of fibroids [12]. Pregnancy longer than 20 weeks in duration has been associated with decreased risk of fibroid formation. Women undergoing childbirth had a lower risk of fibroids than women who never had children (RR = 0.5) [14]. A progressive decrease in risk was seen with increasing number of births. Pregnancy has been associated with a five-fold reduction in the incidence of fibroids [11]. This number may be biased, as women with fibroids are less likely to become pregnant or deliver at term.

1.2.2.12 Oral Contraceptives (OCs)

The use of OCs in adult women is associated with a decrease in clinically evident fibroids [12, 24]. Women taking oral contraceptives for more than 12 years had 50% fewer fibroids than similarly aged women who did not take oral contraceptives [11]. This study may have been biased because women with fibroids tend to have more trouble with conception and take oral contraceptives for shorter periods than women without fibroids. Nevertheless, the relative risk of developing fibroids was shown to decrease in a dose-dependent fashion with the duration of oral contraceptive use. The Nurses' Health Study II, a study of 95,061 American women, found that oral contraceptive use between the ages of 13 and 16 years was associated with an increased risk of clinically symptomatic fibroids [24].

1.2.2.13 Hormone Replacement Therapy

Symptoms related to fibroid growth often decrease after menopause, when circulating oestrogen and progesterone levels decline. It has been reported in several studies that women who take hormones after menopause may experience renewal of these symptoms [12].

Postmenopausal women with small asymptomatic uterine fibroids were randomly treated with either transdermal oestradiol (E2) plus medroxyprogesterone acetate (MPA) or conjugated equine oestrogen (CEE) plus MPA [25]. Women treated with transdermal E2 plus MPA had larger fibroids after 1 year, while women treated with conjugated equine oestrogen plus MPA had no change in fibroid size. In a separate study, 70 postmenopausal women with fibroids were treated with either transdermal 17β-oestradiol patches plus MPA or calcium carbonate for about 11 months [26]. No change in fibroid size was observed in either treatment group. Post-menopausal women with solitary uterine fibroids that were taking CEE and MPA for 3 years were evaluated for fibroid growth [27]. This hormone replacement combination increased fibroid size, although the main effect was observed during the first 2 years.

1.2.2.14 Tamoxifen

Animal studies have shown that tamoxifen inhibits the growth of fibroids [28]. These findings have not been reproduced in women, where results have been mixed. A randomized trial evaluating the effect of tamoxifen on fibroid growth is not available.

1.2.2.15 Xeno-oestrogens

Xeno-oestrogens have been hypothesized to antagonize fibroid growth. Xeno-oestrogens are synthetic or natural chemicals with oestrogenic activity. Synthetic xeno-oestrogens include polychlorinated biphenyls, bisphenol A, the pesticide DDT, and phthalates. Natural xeno-oestrogens are generally plant-derived chemicals called phyto-oestrogens. Phyto-oestrogens are converted into oestrogenic substances by bacterial degradation during digestion and absorbed [14]. Soy and flax contain the greatest quantities of these compounds. The anti-oestrogenic effects sometimes reported with phyto-oestrogens may be due to their ability to compete with natural oestrogens such as oestradiol at the oestrogen receptor (ER).

1.2.3 Theories of Fibroid Growth

Historically, the development of cancer has been modelled into four stages, these being initiation, promotion, progression, and malignant transformation. Initiation introduces changes in the normal cellular machinery and is thought to be caused by mutagens in the local tissue environment. Promoters introduce additional changes in the cellular machinery that selectively enhance the growth of initiated cells. Promotion is considered reversible. Removal of the promoter results in reversion of cells into the previous phenotype. Tumour progression is a permanent change in cellular function and can lead to malignant transformation [14, 29, 30]. Complete carcinogens are able to promote cellular change through all four stages, while incomplete carcinogens cannot.

Promotion and progression are not well defined in fibroids and are considered together here.

More recently, malignant transformation has been explained by loss of function or gain of function mutations in tumour suppressor genes and oncogenes [29, 30]. The formation and growth of some benign tumours appears to have some characteristics of all these models, while not progressing to an invasive or metastatic phenotype. Factors related to the formation and growth of uterine leiomyomas are illustrated in Figure 1.1.

1.2.3.1 Initiation

While many genetic events have been described in fibroids, the initiating events are not clear [14]. Hypothesized initiating events include chronic exposure to high levels of oestrogen and progesterone, leading to increased cellular proliferation and an associated introduction of genetic mutations through errors during gene copying. Increased levels of ERs are found in fibroids and may be a contributing factor. Genetic findings in fibroids similar to those found in scars have led to the 'injury' hypothesis [31]. Here, vasoconstrictive factors secreted during menses are thought to lead to ischaemia and local uterine muscle injury [14]. Another potential initiating factor may be activation of genes associated with the familial or inherited occurrence of fibroids [14, 32, 33].

1.2.3.2 Promotion and Progression

Oestrogen is more generally accepted as the principal promoter of fibroid growth [14]. Several observations suggest oestrogens contribute to fibroid development and growth. Oestradiol binds to oestrogen receptor α (ERα), activating transcription of multiple genes, including the progesterone receptor (PR) [28]. Fibroids have been observed to increase in size after exposure to exogenous oestrogen, the increased levels of oestrogen found in pregnancy, or hormone replacement therapy. They have been observed to decrease in size after menopause or gonadotrophin-releasing hormone (GnRH) agonist treatment [8]. Leiomyoma (fibroid) cells transfected with an inactive ERα mutant suppressed both ERα- and PR-related gene expression [28]. Expression of IGF-I, a growth factor related to cellular proliferation, is not found in leiomyoma samples obtained from women with decreased oestrogen levels [34].

Fibroids have been observed to have a greater number of PRs (both A and B forms) than normal

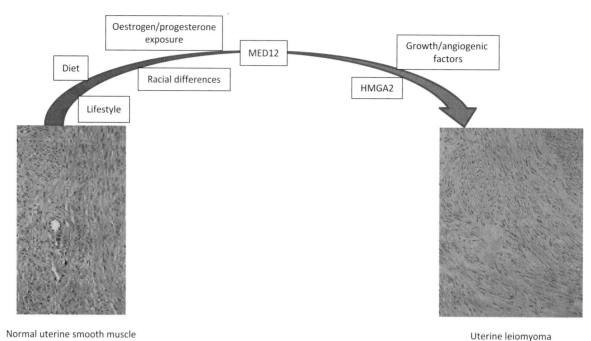

Normal uterine smooth muscle

Uterine leiomyoma

Figure 1.1 Factors related to the formation and growth of uterine leiomyomas. Normal uterine smooth muscle tissue is thought to transform into a uterine leiomyoma under the influence of multiple forces (see Tables 1.1–1.3). Altered expression of MED12 appears to play a major role in the development of uterine leiomyomas.

uterine muscle [8]. Animal studies have shown that PR-A is linked to ovulation and the anti-proliferative effects of progesterone in the uterus, and that PR-B is associated with mammary gland development [28].

Progesterone is also thought to contribute to tumour promotion [14]. Progesterone binds to the PR, activating genes related to suppression of apoptosis, cellular proliferation, and extracellular matrix formation [28]. Anti-progestins will block these effects. The mitotic index of fibroids increases during the progesterone-rich luteal phase of the menstrual cycle. Leiomyoma proliferative activity in post-menopausal women has been shown to increase after administration of oestrogen plus progestin, but not with oestrogen alone [28]. The administration of progestins with GnRH antagonists is associated with an inhibition of the GnRH antagonist effect on uterine shrinkage [8].

Progesterone has been shown to increase the expression of the growth factor, epidermal growth factor (EGF), and the anti-apoptotic protein bcl-2 by binding to progesterone response elements found on these genes. EGF activates c-Myc, a transcription factor that increases cellular proliferation and decreases apoptosis by down-regulating Bcl-2 expression [28].

IGF-I, IGF-II, and IGF-II receptor, but not IGF-I receptor type, are more highly expressed in fibroid tissues than in normal uterine muscle cells [34]. In vitro studies have shown that IGF-I stimulates the proliferation of leiomyoma cells. In vitro treatment with the selective progesterone receptor modulator (SPRM) asoprisnil decreases the expression of IGF-I in fibroids, but not in normal uterine smooth muscle cells [34].

The SPRMs mifepristone, asoprisnil, ulipristal acetate, and telapristone acetate have been reported in clinical trials to suppress uterine bleeding and decrease leiomyoma size [28, 34]. Ulipristal acetate (UPA) is an SPRM that has been shown to initiate apoptosis in uterine fibroids and to decrease fibroid size [35]. Treatment with UPA did not alter GnRH blood levels and maintained oestradiol levels above 1.05×10^{-3} pm/L [35]. Use of Depo-MPA, an injectable progestin contraceptive, has been associated with a reduced risk of fibroid development [19]. Both progestins and anti-progestins may diminish ER signalling and leiomyoma cell growth, suggesting crosstalk occurs between ER and PR signalling [13]. Risk factors for fibroid formation that frequently affect the expression of cellular factors are listed in Table 1.2.

Table 1.2 Risk factors for fibroid formation that frequently affect the expression of cellular factors that control cell growth

	Associated Findings
Increased expression in fibroids	
• Oestrogen receptors	↑ leiomyoma cell proliferation
• Progesterone A and progesterone B receptors	↑ leiomyoma cell proliferation
• IGF-I, IGF-II, and IGF-II receptors	↑ leiomyoma cell proliferation
• EGF	↑ cellular transcription ↓ apoptosis (↓ bcl-2)
• TGF-β3	↑ leiomyoma cell proliferation
• bFGF	↑ leiomyoma cell proliferation
Increased expression in fibroid extracellular matrix:	
• Greater volume of matrix than that found in normal uterus	
• bFGF	↑ angiogenesis
• Decorin	Organizes type I and II collagen
• TGF-β3	↑ ECM formation

1.2.3.3 Effectors

Oestrogen and progesterone mediate their effects through transcriptional activation or suppression of growth factors and their receptors, and by direct activation or suppression of growth factor pathways.

Aromatase

Most endogenous oestrogen is thought to originate from the ovary [28]. Oestrogen is also produced by ovarian aromatization of androgens released from the adrenal glands and ovaries [28]. Aromatase P450 in the ovary converts androstenedione, testosterone, and 16α-hydroxyandrostenedione to oestrone (E1), oestradiol-17β (E2), and oestriol (E3), respectively [36]. Aromatase P450 is expressed 1.5–25 fold more in leiomyomas than in normal uterine smooth muscle cells. The high level of aromatase activity results in higher local oestrogen levels, contributing to fibroid growth. Blocking this activity with aromatase inhibitors results in fibroid shrinkage similar to that reported with GnRH antagonists, even if peripheral oestrogen levels are elevated.

Black women have higher levels of aromatase activity in their fibroids than white women [37]. Increased fibroid aromatase activity has been associated with an increased prevalence of uterine fibroids and clinical presentation at a younger age.

Growth Factors

Basic fibroblast growth factor (bFGF) stimulates uterine fibroid cell growth. Fibroids have increased cellular expression of basic fibroblast growth factor (bFGF), and a large pool of bFGF is found in the abundant extracellular matrix (ECM) that is present in fibroids [12]. Growth factors secreted by uterine muscle cells act to promote angiogenesis [13]. These factors include bFGF (angiogenesis), parathyroid-hormone-related protein (PTH-RP) (a potent vasorelaxant), prolactin (angiogenesis), and prolactin cleaved by cathepsin D (inhibits angiogenesis). Matrix components that promote angiogenesis include bFGF, heparin-binding EGF, and PDGF.

Expressions of TGF-β, IGF 1 and 2, PDGF, and EGF also contribute to fibroid cell growth and the formation of ECM, and increased expression is demonstrated in fibroids [13, 38]. TGF-β3 appears most consistently elevated in fibroids, compared to normal uterine smooth muscle cells [34]. The highest expression of TGF-β3 was observed during the progesterone-rich secretory phase. Asoprisnil, an SPRM, decreases TGF-β3 expression [39].

Dermatopontin (DPT) is an extracellular matrix protein that has been hypothesized to regulate TGF-β activity [10]. The expression of DPT is lower in fibroids than in normal uterine muscle and also lower in fibroids from older black women than in those from older white women. Expression of fibulin 1, the calcium-related migratory and endocytotic molecules netrin 1 and stoning 1, and pyruvate dehydrogenase kinase isoenzyme IV was similarly downregulated [10]. Fibroids share cellular changes found in fibrotic pathologies including expression of type I and III collagen and TGF-β [12].

DNA samples from fibroid and normal uterine muscle obtained from women participating in the Fibroid Growth Study have been analysed using Affymetrix Gene Chip expression arrays [10]. A key finding in fibroid samples was down-regulation of receptor tyrosine-protein kinase erbB-2 (ERBB2) expression. Down-regulation of ERBB2 appeared linked to down-regulation of dermatopontin. SNAIL2, a mediator of epithelial–mesenchymal transition

(EMT), and cyclin B2 were over-expressed in fibroid tissue. The von Hippel-Lindau (VHL) gene, a normally expressed hypoxia-induced gene and a tumour suppressor gene, and PARP1 were frequently over-expressed in fibroids, while expression of EGFR was frequently down-regulated [10]. PARP1 expression was frequently associated with over-expression of PRKDC, catenin-β1, and MED12 [10].

Bcl-2 inhibits apoptosis and is over-expressed in fibroids, especially in the secretory phase [28]. Oestrogen and progesterone may have an impact on expression of these growth factors. The cell proliferation marker Ki67, proliferating cell nuclear antigen (PCNA) expression, and mitotic counts in human fibroids are highest during the luteal and secretory phases [28].

Hormone Receptors

Oestrogen and progesterone receptors (ER and PR) appear to contribute to fibroid growth. Increased expression of ER and PR-A and PR-B are reported in fibroids, compared to normal uterine muscle [13, 28]. Leiomyoma cells transfected with an inactive ERα mutant suppresses both ERα- and PR-related gene expression [28]. The selective ER modulator (SERM) raloxifene has been shown to decrease leiomyoma cell proliferation in vitro and cause uterine fibroid regression in animal models [28]. A randomized study of raloxifene in postmenopausal women also demonstrated a significant decrease in fibroid size. These findings were not reproduced in premenopausal women where the higher levels of circulating oestrogen were thought to counteract the inhibitory effects of raloxifene. In another study, premenopausal women randomized to raloxifene plus GnRH had a greater decrease in fibroid size than women treated with GnRH alone, supporting the above hypothesis.

Fibroids have increased cellular expression of the bFGF receptor [40], and fibroids that bleed have higher expression of the type I bFGF receptor. Expression of TGF receptors is increased in fibroids, a finding similar to fibrotic disease states [12].

1.2.3.4 Genetic Findings
Inheritance

Several types of familial expression of fibroids have been observed [12]. Increased expression of fibroids has been found in women with Reed's syndrome (with subcutaneous myomas), Bannayan-Zonana syndrome (with other benign tumours including lipomas

and haemangiomas), Alport's syndrome, cutaneous leiomyomatosis, intravenous leiomyomatosis, and gastrointestinal stromal tumours [12, 16, 33]. Hereditary defects in hereditary leiomyomatosis and renal cell cancer (HLRCC – fumarate hydratase, FH), tuberous sclerosis (TSC2), Birt-Hogg-Dubé (folliculin – FLCN), and the high-mobility group protein 2a (HMG2a) have also been associated with the development of fibroids [13, 33].

Cytogenetics

About 60% of fibroids have normal cytogenetic studies [16]. Patients with cytogenetic abnormalities most frequently have a 12:14 translocation, trisomy 12, a 6:10 translocation, or deletions of chromosome 3 and 7. The most common finding is the 12:14 translocation, occurring in about 20% of women with cytogenetic abnormalities [16]. Fibroids with a chromosome 12:14 translocation have increased expression of high-mobility group DNA-binding protein (HMGA2) compared to normal uterine smooth muscle. In vitro studies blocking fibroid HMGA2 activity led to cell senescence. Fibroids with abnormal cytogenetic findings are generally larger than fibroids with no cytogenetic abnormalities [32].

Microarray Studies

Microarray studies of fibroids and matched normal uterine smooth muscle demonstrate increased expression of cellular retinoic acid-binding protein II, the inotropic glutamate receptor GluR2, insulin-like growth factor II, TGF-β, and CD24 [16]. TGF-β3 expression in fibroids is three times greater than that of normal adjacent uterine smooth muscle. Decreased expression of alcohol dehydrogenase, prostaglandin E receptor, EP3 subtype, ATP-binding cassette subfamily A, activating transcription factor 3, and dermatopontin is observed. These genes are associated with uterine muscle growth, development, and differentiation, and the development of extracellular matrix. About a quarter of all differentially expressed genes were related to extracellular matrix formation [16].

The genetic features found in fibroids are similar to those found in keloid scar formation [31]. Pirfenidone blocks TGF-β expression and has been administered to block collagen formation in disease states characterized by fibrosis. A pilot study of eight women demonstrated a 32–56% reduction in fibroid size after 3 months of pirfenidone treatment. It is interesting that microarray studies did not detect alterations in ER and PR isoforms or any nuclear receptor cofactor expression that augments transcription of steroid hormones [16].

Genomic Screening

In a study, 457,044 single nucleotide polymorphisms (SNPs) were evaluated in a series of over 9,600 fibroids and normal uterine muscle controls [41]. Three loci were associated with fibroid development, chromosome 10q24.33, 22q13.1, and 11p15.5. The associated SNPs were rs7913069 (OR = 1.47), rs12484776 (OR = 1.23), and rs2280543 (OR = 1.39), respectively. Genes of interest on chromosome 10q24.33 included SLK (STE20-like kinase) and AKAP13 (A-kinase anchor protein-13). SLK is found in proliferating myoblasts and has a role in cellular differentiation and motility. AKAP13 is found to be associated with cytoskeletal filaments in leiomyoma cells and facilitates cellular responses to mechanical stress, such as that found with abnormal excessive extracellular matrix deposition.

Genetic Findings

In one study, 7.8% of fibroids had rearrangement of chromosome 12q14–15, 69.9% had a mutation in the transcription factor MED12, and 22.3% had a different or no genetic abnormality identified [42]. MED12 mutations are thus the most common mutation found in fibroids [28, 32]. MED12 regulates transcription and binds with ERα and ERβ. Loss of function of MED12 through physiologic changes or mutation has been associated with increased expression of the TGF-β receptor, increasing the influence of TGF-β on fibroid metabolism [37]. Specific genetic mutations have been associated with the development or growth of leiomyoma as listed in Table 1.3.

Leiomyoma stem/progenitor cells have been identified as the leiomyoma-derived side population (SP) cells [43, 44]. These cells can be divided into three groups based on CD34 and CD49b expression. It has been estimated that about 6% of fibroids are leiomyoma stem cells. These cells are CD34⁺/CD49b⁺ and have low expression of ERα and PR. Fibroid stem cells contain a MED12 mutation, while normal uterine stem cells do not [44, 45].

Mutations in MED12 may be an early change in uterine smooth muscle transformation. The pattern of tumour growth is demonstrated in animal models where CD34⁺/CD49b⁺ cells form leiomyoma-like

Table 1.3 Specific genetic mutations have been associated with the development or growth of leiomyoma

Mediator of RNA polymerase II transcription, subunit 12 homolog (MED12)
MED12 mutations are frequently found in leiomyoma
MED12 mutations are found in fibroid stem cells, not normal uterine stem cells

MED12:
- Binds to oestrogen receptors α and β
- ↑ cellular transcription
- ↑ progesterone-related responses
- Can activate Wnt/β-catenin signalling in normal uterine smooth muscle

  · MED12-Wnt/β-catenin signalling:

    ↑ cellular proliferation
    ↑ TGF-β3 expression

High-Mobility Group AT-Hook 2 (HMGA2)
HMGA2:
- ↑ expression is found in a smaller subset of leiomyoma
- Mutations in HMGA2 are associated with

  · Larger fibroids
  · Solitary fibroids

- Normally will ↓ expression of the cellular senescence factors p16INK4a and p16Arf
- A nearby HPV-binding site has been hypothesized to affect HMGA expression

tumours with progesterone treatment and CD34⁻/CD49b⁻ cells form flat fibrotic lesions. CD34⁺/CD49b⁺ cells are characterized by the greatest expression of the stem cell markers KLF4, NANOG, SOX2, and OCT4. These cells can proliferate to maintain their lineage or to give rise to CD34⁺/CD49b⁻ leiomyoma intermediate cells. These cells comprise about 7% of cells and have high expression of ERα and PR. Leiomyoma intermediate cells appear to differentiate into leiomyoma differentiated cells, which comprise about 87% of cells. These cells are CD34⁻/CD49b⁻ and have the highest expression of ERα and PR.

While leiomyoma stem cells have the lowest expression of ERα and PR, they demonstrate marked proliferation in response to oestrogen and progesterone. This proliferation is dependent on the local presence of leiomyoma or normal uterine smooth muscle cells, suggesting the presence of an oestrogen- and progesterone-mediated paracrine loop. The wingless-type (Wnt)/β-catenin pathway may be involved in this paracrine signalling [28]. Human normal uterine smooth muscle cells treated with oestrogen and progesterone secrete Wnt ligands which stimulate nuclear translocation of β-catenin co-cultured leiomyoma stem cells, activating genes related to cell growth and proliferation [46]. β-catenin binds to MED12 in normal uterine smooth muscle cells, activating transcription. Mutations in MED12 have been shown to activate Wnt/β-catenin signalling in normal human uterine smooth muscle cells [46]. Selective inhibition of Wnt/β-catenin activity abrogated cell growth and proliferation in vitro and decreased tumour growth in animal models. The activated Wnt/β-catenin pathway also stimulates TGF-β3 expression, a stimulator of cellular proliferation and extracellular matrix formation [37]. TGF-β3 is also thought to inhibit clotting locally, leading to increased uterine bleeding [47].

In a study, 58.8% of fibroids analysed had a mutation in MED12, all of which occurred in bp 130 or 131 [45]. Codon 44 mutations were observed in 95.8% of fibroids with mutations; 41.7% of these were bp 131 mutations G to A, 18.8% were bp 130 G to A mutations, 16.7% were bp 130 G to C mutations, and other mutations occurred less frequently. MED12 mutations were found in 80% of fibroids with a normal karyotype and in no fibroids with chromosome 12q14–15 rearrangements. Fibroids with a MED12 mutation and a normal karyotype were smaller tumours than those with HMGA2 rearrangements. Fibroids with bp 130 or 131 G to A mutations were larger than fibroids with other mutations in this area.

HMGA2 expression in patients with chromosome 12q14–15 rearrangements are known to be strongly up-regulated [48]. HMGA2 down-regulates the expression of p16INK4a and p14Arf, which both have cellular senescence promoting activity [48]. Fibroids with mutations in HMGA2 were larger than those without a mutation [37]. In 70.0% of fibroids, HMGA2 mutations presented clinically as solitary nodules, and 85.5% of fibroids with a MED12 mutation presented clinically with multiple, clonally individual, fibroids [42]. These findings suggest that (1) different genetic forces may drive fibroid formation and that (2) forces exist to form different MED12 mutations in an individual patient. It is noteworthy that the herpes papilloma virus (HPV) insertion site is 50–100 kbp from the HMGA2 gene [19]. The effect of HPV infection on fibroid growth is not known.

The abundant ECM found in fibroids contains enzymes to break down the matrix and allow endothelial cell migration as well as collagens I and III, and bFGF, which stimulates angiogenesis [38]. Decorin, a proteoglycan that helps organize type I and II collagen, is present in ECM in greater amounts. Decorin modulates the activity of TGF-β1 in ECM and has been shown to inhibit angiogenesis. A higher than normal molecular late form of decorin is found in an abnormal distribution pattern in fibroid ECM. ECM found in fibroids consists primarily of collagen, fibronectin and proteoglycans [20]. Collagen in ECM has an abnormal fibril structure and orientation compared to that found in normal uterine tissue [49]. Large amounts of the glycosaminoglycan dermatan sulfate are found in fibroid ECM.

1.2.4 Fibroid Classification Systems

Fibroid classification systems are meant to convey the risk of fibroid-associated morbidity. There is currently no internationally fully accepted staging system for the categorization of fibroids. Bleeding is a common feature of clinically relevant fibroids. Uterine fibroids may be classified according to the International Federation of Gynecology and Obstetrics (FIGO) PALM-COEIN system [50]. Fibroids in this system are classified and assigned a numerical description according to their submucosal (0 – pedunculated intracavitary, 1 – <50% intramural, 2 – ≥50% intramural) or other location (3 – contacts endometrium 100% intramural, 4 – intramural, 5 – subserosal ≥50% intramural, 6 – subserosal <50% intramural, 7 – subserosal pedunculated, 8 – other). Number and size of fibroids are not included in this system.

The FIGO classification system complements that of the European Society of Hysteroscopy that has classified fibroids according to luminal extension [51]. Type 0 fibroids are pedunculated, submucosal, tumours without intramural extension. Type I fibroids are submucosal, sessile tumours with less than 50% intramural extension. Type II fibroids are submucosal, sessile tumours with 50% or more intramural extension [51]. This classification indicates which tumours are more easily resected for the treatment of fibroid-associated uterine bleeding.

1.2.5 Uterine Sarcoma

The uterus is the most common anatomical subsite and leiomyosarcomas are the most common histological subtype. The published literature exposes a wide variation in the incidence of undiagnosed leiomyosarcoma. Age and menopausal status are very important factors. The peak age of incidence of uterine sarcoma is between 50 and 55 [52]. Risk is stratified by age and recognized risk factors include history of tamoxifen use and a history of pelvic irradiation [53, 54].

Alterations in hormonal levels or treatment using hormonal agents are not associated with increased risk. The hereditary condition, hereditary leiomyomatosis and renal cell cancer (HLRCC), is characterized by skin leiomyomas and papillary renal cell carcinoma, uterine leiomyomas, and an increased risk of uterine sarcomas [1]. Patients most frequently present with local symptoms including vaginal bleeding (56%), palpable pelvic mass (54%), or pelvic pain (22%) [53, 54]. Leiomyosarcomas of the uterus have different genetic changes from fibroids and appear to originate through a different pathologic process [12]. Currently there are no specific biomarkers for uterine sarcoma [52]. Imaging (MRI, CT) may be useful in assisting with the identification of uterine sarcomas but to date there is no single pathognomonic feature with 'imaging' indicating the presence of a leiomyosarcoma.

1.3 Summary

Uterine fibroids are a common finding in premenopausal women and are frequently symptomatic. Clinical presentation varies with patient, race and age. The costs of fibroid management to the health care system are staggering. Some modifiable factors have been linked to fibroid growth. Several somatic genetic changes have been observed in fibroids, mutations associated with different risks of having several or single fibroids, and faster or slower growing fibroids. A globally accepted, standardized fibroid classification system is not currently available. Factors influencing such a system would ideally include genetic information related to growth, related symptoms, and method of diagnosis.

Acknowledgements

We thank Mrs Sheila Milne for her assistance with manuscript preparation.

References

1. Laughlin SK, Stewart EA. Uterine leiomyomas: individualizing the approach to a heterogeneous condition. *Obstet Gynecol* 2011;**117**:396–403.

2. Cardozo ER, Clark AD, Banks NK, et al. The estimated annual cost of uterine leiomyomata in the United States. *Am J Obstet Gynecol* 2012;**206**:211.e1–9.

3. Whitaker L, Critchley HO. Abnormal uterine bleeding. *Best Pract Res Clin Obstet Gynaecol* 2016;**34**:54–65.

4. Cook H, Ezzati M, Segars JH, McCarthy K. The impact of uterine leiomyomas on reproductive outcomes. *Minerva Ginecol* 2010;**62**:225–36.

5. Zimmermann A, Bernuit D, Gerlinger C, Schaefers M, Geppert K. Prevalence, symptoms and management of uterine fibroids: an international internet-based survey of 21,746 women. *BMC Womens Health* 2012;**12**:6.

6. Graphiq. Uterine fibroids. International Statistics on Mortality and Affected Populations [Internet]. Available from: http://global-diseases .healthgrove.com/l/208/Uterine-Fibroids

7. Baird DD, Dunson DB, Hill MC, Cousins D, Schectman JM. High cumulative incidence of uterine leiomyoma in black and white women: ultrasound evidence. *Am J Obstet Gynecol* 2003;**188**:100–7.

8. Chavez NF, Stewart EA. Medical treatment of uterine fibroids. *Clin Obstet Gynecol* 2001;**44**:372–84.

9. Peddada SD, Laughlin SK, Miner K, et al. Growth of uterine leiomyomata among premenopausal black and white women. *Proc Natl Acad Sci USA* 2008;**105**:19887–92.

10. Davis BJ, Risinger JI, Chandramouli GV, et al. Gene expression in uterine leiomyoma from tumors likely to be growing (from black women over 35) and tumors likely to be non-growing (from white women over 35). *PLoS One* 2013;**8**:e63909.

11. Payson M, Leppert P, Segars J. Epidemiology of myomas. *Obstet Gynecol Clin North Am* 2006;**33**:1–11.

12. Stewart EA. Uterine fibroids. *Lancet* 2001;**357**:293–8.

13. Walker CL, Stewart EA. Uterine fibroids: the elephant in the room. *Science* 2005;**308**:1589–92.

14. Flake GP, Andersen J, Dixon D. Etiology and pathogenesis of uterine leiomyomas: a review. *Environ Health Perspect* 2003;**111**:1037–54.

15. Baird DD, Harmon QE, Upson K, et al. A prospective, ultrasound-based study to evaluate risk factors for uterine fibroid incidence and growth: methods and results of recruitment. *J Womens Health (Larchmt)* 2015;**24**:907–15.

16. Catherino W, Salama A, Potlog-Nahari C, et al. Gene expression studies in leiomyomata: new

directions for research. *Semin Reprod Med* 2004;**22**:83–90.

17. Borgfeldt C, Andolf E. Transvaginal ultrasonographic findings in the uterus and the endometrium: low prevalence of leiomyoma in a random sample of women age 25–40 years. *Acta Obstet Gynecol Scand* 2000;**79**:202–7.

18. Cramer SF, Patel A. The frequency of uterine leiomyomas. *Am J Clin Pathol* 1990;**94**:435–8.

19. Laughlin SK, Schroeder JC, Baird DD. New directions in the epidemiology of uterine fibroids. *Semin Reprod Med* 2010;**28**:204–17.

20. Islam MS, Akhtar MM, Ciavattini A, et al. Use of dietary phytochemicals to target inflammation, fibrosis, proliferation, and angiogenesis in uterine tissues: promising options for prevention and treatment of uterine fibroids? *Mol Nutr Food Res* 2014;**58**:1667–84.

21. Wise LA, Radin RG, Palmer JR, et al. Intake of fruit, vegetables, and carotenoids in relation to risk of uterine leiomyomata. *Am J Clin Nutr* 2011;**94**:1620–31.

22. Baird DD, Hill MC, Schectman JM, Hollis BW. Vitamin D and the risk of uterine fibroids. *Epidemiology* 2013;**24**:447–53.

23. Harris SS. Vitamin D and African Americans. *J Nutr* 2006;**136**:1126–9.

24. Marshall LM, Spiegelman D, Goldman MB, et al. A prospective study of reproductive factors and oral contraceptive use in relation to the risk of uterine leiomyomata. *Fertil Steril* 1998;**70**:432–9.

25. Sener AB, Seckin NC, Ozmen S, et al. The effects of hormone replacement therapy on uterine fibroids in postmenopausal women. *Fertil Steril* 1996;**65**:354–7.

26. Palomba S, Sena T, Noia R, et al. Transdermal hormone

replacement therapy in postmenopausal women with uterine leiomyomas. *Obstet Gynecol* 2001;**98**:1053–8.

27. Yang CH, Lee JN, Hsu SC, et al. Effect of hormone replacement therapy on uterine fibroids in postmenopausal women – a 3-year study. *Maturitas* 2002;**43**:35–9.

28. Marsh EE, Bulun SE. Steroid hormones and leiomyomas. *Obstet Gynecol Clin North Am* 2006;**33**:59–67.

29. Ruddon RW. What makes a cancer cell a cancer cell? In: Kufe DW, Pollock RE, Weichselbaum RR, et al., editors. *Holland-Frei Cancer Medicine*, 6th ed. Hamilton, ON: B. C. Decker; 2003. Available from: www.ncbi.nlm.nih.gov/books/NBK12516/

30. Wong E. Introduction to neoplasia. 2016. Available from: www.pathophys.org/introneoplasia/

31. Leppert PC, Catherino WH, Segars JH. A new hypothesis about the origin of uterine fibroids based on gene expression profiling with microarrays. *Am J Obstet Gynecol* 2006;**195**:415–20.

32. Levy G, Hill MJ, Beall S, et al. Leiomyoma: genetics, assisted reproduction, pregnancy and therapeutic advances. *J Assist Reprod Genet* 2012;**29**:703–12.

33. Stewart EA, Morton CC. The genetics of uterine leiomyomata: what clinicians need to know. *Obstet Gynecol* 2006;**107**:917–21.

34. Kim JJ, Sefton EC, Bulun SE. Progesterone receptor action in leiomyoma and endometrial cancer. *Prog Mol Biol Transl Sci* 2009;**87**:53–85.

35. Taylor DK, Holthouser K, Segars JH, Leppert PC. Recent scientific advances in leiomyoma (uterine fibroids) research facilitates better understanding and management. *F1000Research* 2015;**4**:183.

36. Bulun SE, Noble LS, Takayama K, et al. Endocrine disorders

associated with inappropriately high aromatase expression. *J Steroid Biochem Mol Biol* 1997;**61**:133–9.

37. Bulun SE. Uterine fibroids. *N Engl J Med* 2013;**369**:1344–55.

38. Stewart EA, Nowak RA. Leiomyoma-related bleeding: a classic hypothesis updated for the molecular era. *Hum Reprod Update* 1996;**2**:295–306.

39. Wang J, Ohara N, Wang Z, et al. A novel selective progesterone receptor modulator asoprisnil (J867) down-regulates the expression of EGF, IGF-I, TGFbeta3 and their receptors in cultured uterine leiomyoma cells. *Hum Reprod* 2006;**21**:1869–77.

40. Anania CA, Stewart EA, Quade BJ, Hill JA, Nowak RA. Expression of the fibroblast growth factor receptor in women with leiomyomas and abnormal uterine bleeding. *Mol Hum Reprod* 1997;**3**:685–91.

41. Cha PC, Takahashi A, Hosono N, et al. A genome-wide association study identifies three loci associated with susceptibility to uterine fibroids. *Nat Genet* 2011;**43**:447–50.

42. Markowski DN, Helmke BM, Bartnitzke S, Loning T, Bullerdiek J. Uterine fibroids: do we deal with more than one disease? *Int J Gynecol Pathol* 2014;**33**:568–72.

43. Bulun SE, Moravek MB, Yin P, et al. Uterine leiomyoma stem cells: linking progesterone to growth. *Semin Reprod Med* 2015;**33**:357–65.

44. Ono M, Qiang W, Serna VA, et al. Role of stem cells in human uterine leiomyoma growth. *PLoS One* 2012;**7**:e36935.

45. Markowski DN, Bartnitzke S, Loning T, et al. MED12 mutations in uterine fibroids – their relationship to cytogenetic subgroups. *Int J Cancer* 2012;**131**:1528–36.

46. Halder SK, Elam LA, Laknaur A, Diamond MP, Al-Hendy A.

Introduction of exon 2 mutant MED12 gene triggers activation of Wnt/β-catenin signaling in normal human uterine smooth muscle cells. *Fertil Steril* 2015;**104**(Suppl.):e30.

47. Sinclair DC, Mastroyannis A, Taylor HS. Leiomyoma simultaneously impair endometrial BMP-2-mediated decidualization and anticoagulant expression through secretion of TGF-beta3. *J Clin Endocrinol Metab* 2011;**96**:412–21.

48. Moravek MB, Bulun SE. Endocrinology of uterine fibroids: steroid hormones, stem cells, and genetic contribution. *Curr Opin Obstet Gynecol* 2015;**27**:276–83.

49. Jorge S, Chang S, Barzilai JJ, Leppert P, Segars JH. Mechanical signaling in reproductive tissues: mechanisms and importance. *Reprod Sci* 2014;**21**:1093–107.

50. Munro MG, Critchley HO, Broder MS, Fraser IS. FIGO classification system (PALM-COEIN) for causes of abnormal uterine bleeding in nongravid women of reproductive age. *Int J Gynaecol Obstet* 2011;**113**:3–13.

51. Wamsteker K, Emanuel MH, de Kruif JH. Transcervical hysteroscopic resection of submucous fibroids for abnormal uterine bleeding: results regarding the degree of intramural extension. *Obstet Gynecol* 1993;**82**:736–40.

52. Morcellation for Myomectomy or Hysterectomy; RCOG Consent Advice No. 13 October 2019.

53. D'Angelo E, Prat J. Uterine sarcomas: a review. *Gynecol Oncol* 2010;**116**:131–9.

54. Kobayashi H, Uekuri C, Akasaka J, et al. The biology of uterine sarcomas: a review and update. *Mol Clin Oncol* 2013;**1**:599–609.

Evaluation of Uterine Fibroids Using Two-Dimensional and Three-Dimensional Ultrasonography

Sotirios H. Saravelos

2.1 Introduction

Uterine fibroids are perhaps the commonest benign tumours a gynaecologist will encounter, with an estimated lifetime prevalence of approximately 30%; however, approximately three-quarters of cases are thought to be asymptomatic [1]. Given that the majority of fibroids are asymptomatic, they are likely to be encountered for the first time within the context of infertility investigations, assuming that couples will undergo a baseline screening which will invariably include an ultrasound scan of the female pelvis.

The question therefore arises: do fibroids require intervention, and if so, in which cases? In women with symptomatology, such as pressure symptoms and menorrhagia, the accurate diagnosis of fibroids is of utmost importance since it will determine whether indeed the symptoms can be attributed to the fibroid detected. For example, a 2 cm subserosal fibroid is not likely to be the culprit in significant menorrhagia, whereas a 2 cm submucosal fibroid may well be. Even more subtle differences become of increasing importance in women with infertility, where meta-analyses have shown that submucosal, intramural and subserosal fibroids affect fertility in reducing order of significance [2]. In such cases, further characterization of – for example – intramural fibroids (i.e. size, exact location, distance from the endometrium/junctional zone) may determine whether a woman may benefit from intervention or not.

It therefore becomes apparent that the correct evaluation (i.e. diagnosis and characterization) of fibroids is pivotal in the modern management of these tumours. This depends wholly on the classification models that are available, but also on the correct use and interpretation of diagnostic methodology, both of which will be examined in the present chapter.

2.2 Classifications

The traditional classification of fibroids is dependent on where the fibroids are located with respect to two anatomical planes: the uterine endometrium and the uterine serosa. The terms submucosal, intramural and subserosal have therefore been coined for several decades. Historically, however, there was no consensus as to what precisely constituted each category, and this was proving to be particularly confusing in borderline cases. A classification was therefore suggested by Bajekal and Li in 2000 which helped distinguish three diagnostic categories [3]:

1. Submucosal: A fibroid that distorts the uterine cavity. Subdivisions included type 0 (pedunculated fibroid with no intramural extension); type 1 (with intramural extension of <50%); type 2 (with intramural extension of >50%).
2. Intramural: A fibroid that does not distort the uterine cavity and with <50% extension beyond the serosal surface.
3. Subserosal: A fibroid that extends >50% beyond the serosal surface and can be either sessile or pedunculated.

This classification was later expanded by the International Federation of Gynecology and Obstetrics (FIGO) Menstrual Disorders Working Group, which devised the classification of causes of abnormal uterine bleeding in the reproductive years, otherwise known as the PALM-COEIN (Polyp, Adenomyosis, Leiomyoma, Malignancy and Hyperplasia, Coagulopathy, Ovulatory Disorders, Endometrial Disorders, Iatrogenic Causes, and Not Classified) classification system [4]. It included a total of nine types of myomas (types 0–8) with a view to being able to further characterize the

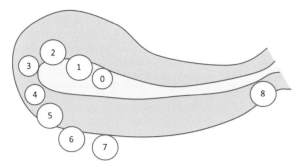

Figure 2.1 A schematic representation of the different types of fibroids in accordance with the FIGO classification (Munro et al. [4]). Small fibroids have been used here to facilitate the representation of the classification in a single uterine image.

intramural and subserosal types. Therefore, in this classification, fibroids are classified as follows (schematically presented in Figure 2.1):

1. Type 0: Pedunculated intracavitary (i.e. submucosal) fibroid.
2. Type 1: Intracavitary fibroid with intramural extension of <50%.
3. Type 2: Intracavitary fibroid with intramural extension of >50%.
4. Type 3: Intramural fibroid in contact with the endometrium but with no extension into the uterine cavity or serosal surface.
5. Type 4: Intramural fibroid not in contact with the endometrium and with no extension into the uterine cavity or serosal surface.
6. Type 5: Fibroid of which >50% is intramural and <50% is subserosal (intramural in the previous classification)
7. Type 6: Fibroid of which <50% is intramural and >50% is subserosal (subserosal in the previous classification)
8. Type 7: Pedunculated subserosal fibroid
9. Type 8: Other types of fibroids (e.g. cervical, parasitic)
10. Hybrid type [2–5]: Combined submucosal–subserosal with <50% indentation into the cavity and also into the serosal surface.

By devising this classification, the working group hoped to create a system that would be universally accepted and would allow for both effective and accurate communication between clinicians and patients, and also aid in the conduction of appropriately designed trials.

2.3 Diagnosis

2.3.1 Two-Dimensional Ultrasound

The next logical step after the acceptance of an appropriate classification is ascertaining an accurate diagnostic modality to apply the given classification. Indeed most classifications, systematic reviews and international consensuses advocate the use of two-dimensional (2D) ultrasound (US) as an accurate means of diagnosing and characterizing uterine fibroids [3–7]. This has been consistently supported by data from the last few decades that has shown 2D US to have sensitivities of 90–100%, specificities of 87–98%, positive predictive values (PPV) of 81–93% and negative predictive values (NPV) of 98–100% [5, 8–11]

Interestingly, irrespective of the FIGO anatomical classification, until recently, there was no universally accepted consensus on how specifically to scan, characterize and report uterine fibroids. This is something the MUSA (Morphological Uterus Sonographic Assessment) group attempted to achieve with the publication of their long and comprehensive consensus [7]. This suggested a systematic approach to assessing and reporting the myometrium and associated fibroids, including the following parameters (examples shown in Figure 2.2):

1. *Uterine corpus*: Measurement of length, anteroposterior diameter, transverse diameter and volume
2. *Serosal contour*: Regular versus lobulated
3. *Myometrial walls*: Symmetrical versus asymmetrical
4. *Myometrial echogenicity*: Homogeneous versus heterogeneous
5. *Myometrial lesions*:
   a. Well-defined versus ill-defined
   b. Number
   c. Location (anterior, posterior, fundal, right or left lateral, global)
   d. Site (type according to FIGO classification)
   e. Size (three perpendicular diameters)
   f. Outer lesion-free margin (distance from the serosal surface)
   g. Inner lesion-free margin (distance from the endometrial surface)
   h. Echogenicity (homogeneous versus heterogeneous; hypo-, iso-, hyper-echogenic)

15

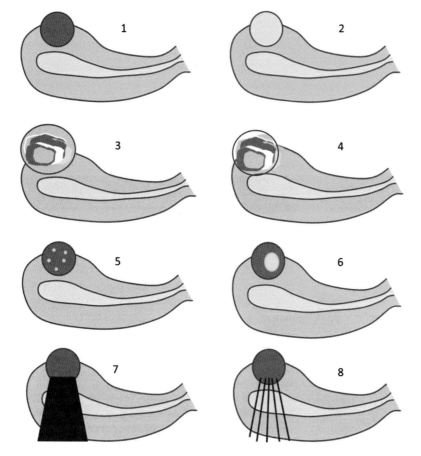

Figure 2.2 Schematic representation of the commonest fibroid characteristics as described by the MUSA group (Van den Bosch et al., [7]): (1) hypoechogenic; (2) hyperechogenic; (3) heterogeneous echogenicity; (4) ill-defined outline; (5) echogenic areas; (6) cystic area; (7) internal shadowing; (8) fan-shaped shadowing.

i.   Shadowing (edge, internal, fan-shaped)
j.   Myometrial cysts (size, number, echogenicity)
k.   Hyperechogenic islands (outline, number, size)
l.   Subendometrial echogenic lines/buds

Indeed, for the majority of fibroids, the MUSA consensus for characterizing and reporting fibroids can be applied via use of 2D transvaginal ultrasound. However, for large-volume uteri this may require complementation using transabdominal 2D ultrasound, where the penetration achieved may be higher [12]. Furthermore, for fibroids in which the anatomical relations to the endometrial cavity and tubal ostia cannot be adequately ascertained, three-dimensional (3D) US and saline-infusion (SI) US may have a role, as described below.

2.3.2 Three-Dimensional Ultrasound

Assessment of fibroids using 3D ultrasound appears to be an upcoming and promising prospect [13]. To date, however, the data with regards to 3D ultrasound and the diagnosis of fibroids are relatively sparse. Two well-designed prospective studies compared 3D versus 2D ultrasound and found the former to be superior [14, 15]. In particular, it was thought that 3D ultrasound could provide a clearer visualization of the endometrial cavity and an overall better estimation of the size, outline and fibroid characteristics. The authors of the first study considered this to be of benefit in terms of preoperative planning [14]. The authors of the second study reported that 3D ultrasound corrected the diagnosis in many cases where 2D ultrasound had suggested that a fibroid was distorting the endometrial cavity. In fact, they reported that the rate of normal endometrial cavity examinations increased from 7.2% to 30.1% when 3D ultrasound was employed compared with 2D ultrasound alone [15]. Despite the lack of robust evidence to date, these advantages of 3D US in the assessment of uterine fibroids have been supported by subsequent expert authors in their systematic reviews [16, 17].

(a)   (b)

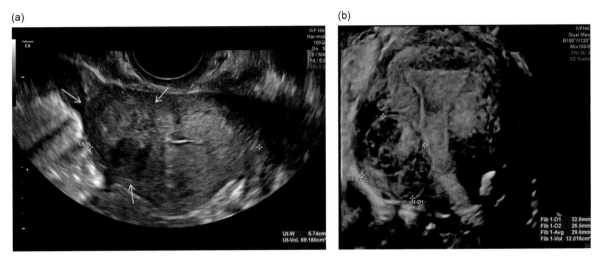

Figure 2.3 Example of a FIGO type 2–5 fibroid (i.e. intramural fibroid with <50% extension into the endometrial cavity and <50% extension beyond the serosal surface). The precise relation between the fibroid and the endometrial cavity is not so apparent on 2D US alone (a). However, with 3D US mapping, this becomes very clear as the fibroid can be seen protruding beyond the serosal surface by approximately 25% and abutting to the right lower third of the uterine cavity with a minor indentation of approximately 5%. The arrows (a) and callipers (b) are used to denote the fibroid.

(a)   (b)

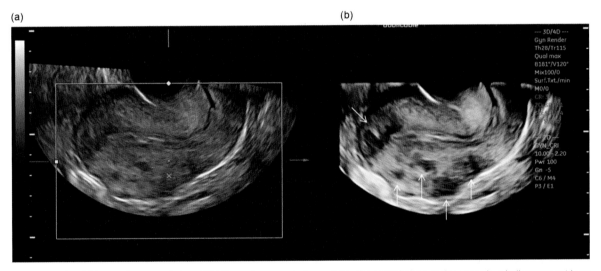

Figure 2.4 In addition to the coronal plane, 3D US can also prove to be useful in the sagittal plane. In this example, a bulky uterus with no distinct fibroids was seen on 2D US (a); when applying 3D US rendering on the same sagittal plane, it is possible to see clearly a number of hypoechogenic intramural fibroids (as indicated by the arrows) (b).

Most characteristically, Salim et al. commented that 3D ultrasound enables the assessment of the uterus from any angle and in any arbitrary plane, making it possible to assess both the size and the extent of cavity indentation of each individual fibroid perpendicularly to the endometrium, in a way which cannot be achieved with any other conventional diagnostic technique [18]. Examples of such fibroid mapping with 3D ultrasound are shown in Figures 2.3–2.6.

2.3.3 Saline-Infusion Ultrasound (SI US)

Saline-infusion ultrasound (SI US) has long been thought to enhance the diagnostic accuracy of ultrasound due to the ability to clearly delineate the uterine cavity [9, 11]. This claim has now been substantiated by a recent systematic review and meta-analysis that has demonstrated a pooled sensitivity and specificity for diagnosing submucosal fibroids of 82%

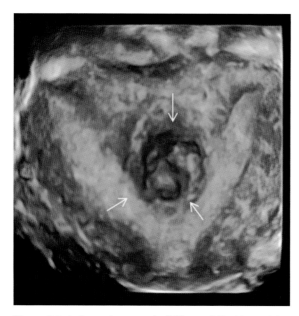

Figure 2.5 An interesting case of a FIGO type 2 fibroid co-existing with a complete septate uterus. Surgical treatment may involve a two-step procedure consisting of an initial resection of the fibroid followed by resection of the residual septate tissue.

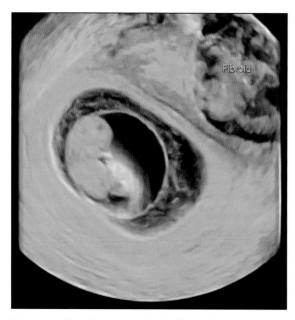

Figure 2.6 Fibroid mapping with 3D US can also be used during early pregnancy, particularly in those with known uterine fibroids. In this particular case, an intramural fibroid can be seen millimetres away from the implantation site. The fibroid did not distort the gestational sac and the outcome of this case was good.

(95% CI: 69–92) and 100% (98–100), respectively, with positive and negative likelihood ratios of 44.14 (95% CI: 17.77–109.64) and 0.26 (95% CI: 0.15–0.45), respectively [19]. The authors concluded that SI US is a highly sensitive investigative modality and comparable to the gold-standard tool, hysteroscopy, in the detection of intrauterine abnormalities, including submucosal fibroids. With regards to 3D SI US, the authors concluded that 3D SI US may replace 2D SI US altogether owing to improved accuracy rates for preliminary studies. Furthermore, they went on to comment that 3D SI US may become a confirmatory test rather than a screening tool and may overtake diagnostic hysteroscopy as the gold-standard imaging method of choice [19]. Examples of fibroid mapping with 3D SI US are shown in Figures 2.7 and 2.8.

2.3.4 Magnetic Resonance Imaging

Although not within the remit of the present chapter, MRI is becoming increasingly available, with an increasing role in the assessment of uterine fibroids. The pertinent question is: when is MRI evaluation of uterine fibroids required? Overall, authors appear to support that US is as efficient as MRI in the diagnosis and evaluation of fibroids in the majority of cases, particularly when they are fewer than five in number and they measure less than 375 mL in volume [20]. However, in larger and more numerous fibroids (i.e. >4 in number of >375 mL in volume), MRI appears to have an advantage, as it is not limited by acoustic shadowing and reduced penetration, and appears to suffer less inter-observer variability [21].

2.4 Special Considerations

2.4.1 Adenomyosis

Although adenomyosis is outside the remit of the present chapter, in clinical practice there can occasionally be a discrepancy or difficulty in distinguishing adenomyosis from fibroids when performing US. Therefore, it is important to distinguish both the histological and the US features of adenomyosis from those of fibroids. Adenomyosis is defined as the benign invasion of ectopic endometrial glands within the myometrium, either diffusely (adenomyosis) or in a localized manner (adenomyoma) [22, 23]. Conversely, fibroids consist of a collection of disorganized proliferated smooth muscle cells, commonly surrounded by an extracellular matrix and presenting

(a)   (b)   (c)

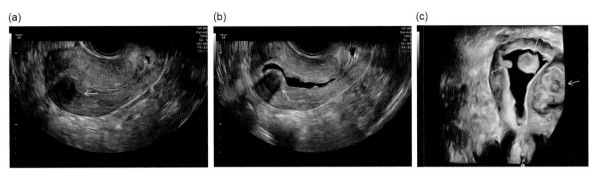

Figure 2.7 An example of a presumed intramural fibroid that was detected on 2D US (a). As the relation to the endometrial cavity could not be clearly delineated, 2D SI US was performed, which demonstrated a significant extension into the cavity and therefore a type 2 submucosal fibroid (b). Subsequently, 3D SI US was performed to further map out the location of the fibroid. Incidentally, and within a single coronal plane, an additional small polyp was identified near the right ostium, while a further intramural fibroid (type 4) was found to be adjacent to the left lateral cavity wall outline (c).

(a)   (b)   (c)

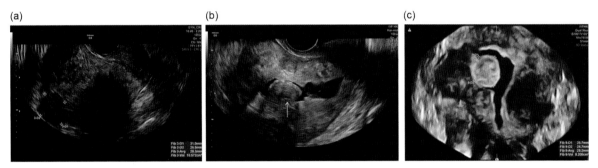

Figure 2.8 A case of multiple fibroids in which 2D US could not delineate the uterine cavity (a). 2D SI US demonstrated FIGO type 1 fibroid on the posterior wall of the uterine cavity (b). 3D SI US mapping demonstrated that the fibroid of 8.2 mL volume was occupying the entire right mid to ostial region of the uterine cavity while the remaining cavity was surrounded by type 2–3 fibroids (c).

in varying shapes, sizes, numbers and forms [24]. As the implications and management of each condition are different, the correct US differentiation and diagnosis is pivotal. The distinguishing appearances of each entity are therefore presented clearly in this chapter in Table 2.1.

2.4.2 Leiomyosarcomas

In contrast to the high prevalence of benign fibroids, leiomyosarcomas occur with an approximate annual incidence of 0.64/100,000 women. In women with myometrial lesions without any evidence of sarcomatous change, the risk of leiomyosarcomas is thought to be in the region of 1 in 700 [25]. Unfortunately, there are no pathognomonic features to distinguish between a leiomyosarcoma and a fibroid. Rapid growth may be a cardinal feature of leiomyosarcomas;

however, this can also occur with fibroids. One insightful study, however, reported that leiomyosarcomas appeared to be solitary and significantly larger than other smooth muscle tumours, commonly with a diameter of >8 cm, and occasionally with irregular cystic changes (owing to necrosis) and increased peripheral and central vascularity [26]. In this respect, MRI may also play a potential role in distinguishing between leiomyosarcomas and fibroids via assessing some of the characteristics mentioned above. Another interesting preliminary study demonstrated that contrast enhancement after administration of gadolinium occurred in 10/10 (100%) leiomyosarcoma cases, but only in 4/32 (12.5%) degenerated fibroid cases, possibly indicating that MRI may play an important role in the assessment of these tumours in the near future [27].

Table 2.1 Features that aid the differentiation of fibroids versus adenomyosis

Features	Fibroids	Adenomyosis
Contour of uterus	Lobulated or regular	Globular
Symmetry of uterine walls	Dependent on lesions	Anteroposterior asymmetry
Junctional zone	Regular and/or thin	Irregular and/or thickened
Outline of lesion	Well-defined	Ill-defined
Shape of lesion	Round, oval, lobulated	Ill-defined
Contour of lesion	Smooth	Ill-defined
Rim of lesion	Hypo-, hyper-echogenic	Ill-defined
Shadowing of lesion	Edge, internal, fan-shaped	Mostly fan-shaped
Echogenicity of lesion	Uniform or mixed echogenicity	Mixed echogenicity
Vascularity	Circumferential flow	Translesional flow

Source: Adapted from Van der Bosch [7].

2.5 Conclusion

In conclusion, there are currently clear classifications and consensuses available in the literature for the diagnosis, evaluation and reporting of uterine fibroids. Two-dimensional ultrasound (with saline infusion where necessary) is the mainstay of diagnosis, with interesting and exciting prospects arising with the development of 3D ultrasound. MRI can be used as a complementary method in cases of multiple or enlarged fibroids. However, to date, the pre-histological imaging differentiation between certain fibroids, adenomyosis and even leiomyosarcomas remains an important challenge.

References

1. Younas A, Hadoura E, Majoko F, Bunkheila A. A review of evidence-based management of uterine fibroids. *Obstet Gynaecol* 2016;**18**:33–42.

2. Pritts EA, Parker WH, Olive DL. Fibroids and infertility: an updated systematic review of the evidence. *Fertil Steril* 2009;**91**:1215–23.

3. Bajekal N, Li T-C. Fibroids, infertility and pregnancy wastage. *Hum Reprod Update* 2000;**6**:614–20.

4. Munro MG, Critchley HO, Fraser IS, Group FMDW. The FIGO classification of causes of abnormal uterine bleeding in the reproductive years. *Fertil Steril* 2011;**95**:2204–8, 8.e1–3.

5. Somigliana E, Vercellini P, Daguati R, et al. Fibroids and female reproduction: a critical analysis of the evidence. *Hum Reprod Update* 2007;**13**:465–76.

6. Leone FP, Timmerman D, Bourne T, et al. Terms, definitions and measurements to describe the sonographic features of the endometrium and intrauterine lesions: a consensus opinion from the International Endometrial Tumor Analysis (IETA) group. *Ultrasound Obstet Gynecol Off J Int Soc Ultrasound Obstet Gynecol* 2010;**35**:103–12.

7. Van den Bosch T, Dueholm M, Leone FP, et al. Terms, definitions and measurements to describe sonographic features of myometrium and uterine masses: a consensus opinion from the Morphological Uterus Sonographic Assessment (MUSA) group. *Ultrasound Obstet Gynecol Off J Int Soc Ultrasound Obstet Gynecol* 2015;**46**:284–98.

8. Fedele L, Bianchi S, Dorta M, et al. Transvaginal ultrasonography versus hysteroscopy in the diagnosis of uterine submucous myomas. *Obstet Gynecol* 1991;**77**:745–8.

9. Cicinelli E, Romano F, Anastasio PS, et al. Transabdominal sonohysterography, transvaginal sonography, and hysteroscopy in the evaluation of submucous myomas. *Obstet Gynecol* 1995;**85**:42–7.

10. Indman PD. Abnormal uterine bleeding. Accuracy of vaginal probe ultrasound in predicting abnormal hysteroscopic findings. *J Reprod Med* 1995;**40**:545–8.

11. Becker E, Jr., Lev-Toaff AS, Kaufman EP, et al. The added value of transvaginal sonohysterography over

transvaginal sonography alone in women with known or suspected leiomyoma. *J Ultrasound Med Off J Am Inst Ultrasound Med* 2002;**21**:237–47.

12. Vitiello D, McCarthy S. Diagnostic imaging of myomas. *Obstet Gynecol Clin North Am* 2006;**33**:85–95.

13. Saravelos SH, Jayaprakasan K, Ojha K, Li T-C. Assessment of the uterus with three-dimensional ultrasound in women undergoing ART. *Hum Reprod Update* 2017;**23**:188–210.

14. Kupesic S, Kurjak A, Skenderovic S, Bjelos D. Screening for uterine abnormalities by three-dimensional ultrasound improves perinatal outcome. *J Perinat Med* 2002;**30**:9–17.

15. Sylvestre C, Child TJ, Tulandi T, Tan SL. A prospective study to evaluate the efficacy of two- and three-dimensional sonohysterography in women with intrauterine lesions. *Fertil Steril* 2003;**79**:1222–5.

16. Armstrong L, Fleischer A, Andreotti R. Three-dimensional volumetric sonography in gynecology: an overview of clinical applications. *Radiol Clin North Am* 2013;**51**:1035–47.

17. Groszmann YS, Benacerraf BR. Complete evaluation of anatomy and morphology of the infertile patient in a single visit: the modern infertility pelvic ultrasound examination. *Fertil Steril* 2016.

18. Salim R, Lee C, Davies A, et al. A comparative study of three-dimensional saline infusion sonohysterography and diagnostic hysteroscopy for the classification of submucous fibroids. *Hum Reprod* 2005;**20**:253–7.

19. Seshadri S, El-Toukhy T, Douiri A, Jayaprakasan K, Khalaf Y. Diagnostic accuracy of saline infusion sonography in the evaluation of uterine cavity abnormalities prior to assisted reproductive techniques: a systematic review and meta-analyses. *Hum Reprod Update* 2015;**21**:262–74.

20. Dueholm M, Lundorf E, Hansen ES, Ledertoug S, Olesen F. Accuracy of magnetic resonance imaging and transvaginal ultrasonography in the diagnosis, mapping, and measurement of uterine myomas. *Am J Obstet Gynecol* 2002;**186**:409–15.

21. Dueholm M, Lundorf E, Sorensen JS, et al. Reproducibility of evaluation of the uterus by transvaginal sonography, hysterosonographic examination, hysteroscopy and magnetic resonance imaging. *Hum Reprod* 2002;**17**:195–200.

22. Campo S, Campo V, Benagiano G. Adenomyosis and infertility. *Reprod Biomed Online* 2012;**24**:35–46.

23. de Ziegler D, Pirtea P, Galliano D, Cicinelli E, Meldrum D. Optimal uterine anatomy and physiology necessary for normal implantation and placentation. *Fertil Steril* 2016;**105**:844–54.

24. Galliano D, Bellver J, Diaz-Garcia C, Simon C, Pellicer A. ART and uterine pathology: how relevant is the maternal side for implantation? *Hum Reprod Update* 2015;**21**:13–38.

25. Brolmann H, Tanos V, Grimbizis G, et al. Options on fibroid morcellation: a literature review. *Gynecol Surg* 2015;**12**:3–15.

26. Exacoustos C, Romanini ME, Amadio A, et al. Can gray-scale and color Doppler sonography differentiate between uterine leiomyosarcoma and leiomyoma? *J Clin Ultrasound (JCU)* 2007;**35**:449–57.

27. Goto A, Takeuchi S, Sugimura K, Maruo T. Usefulness of Gd-DTPA contrast-enhanced dynamic MRI and serum determination of LDH and its isozymes in the differential diagnosis of leiomyosarcoma from degenerated leiomyoma of the uterus. *Int J Gynecol Cancer* 2002;**12**:354–61.

Chapter 3

Ulipristal and Other Medical Interventions for Treatment of Uterine Fibroids

Mohamed Ali, Zunir Tayyeb Chaudhry and Ayman Al-Hendy

3.1 Introduction

3.1.1 Uterine Fibroids

Uterine fibroids (UFs) are the most common non-malignant neoplasms affecting women of reproductive age. Some estimates suspect nearly 70–80% of all women will develop at least one fibroid during their lifetime [1]. Women suffering from UFs can present with heavy or prolonged vaginal bleeding, pain or pressure in pelvic region, dysmenorrhoea, dyspareunia, bladder problems, constipation, subfertility, and even loss of pregnancy [2]. Many women with fibroids experience heavy menstrual bleeding (HMB), thereby making them more prone to developing iron deficiency anaemia [3]. Many women suffering from severe symptomatic fibroids choose to have a hysterectomy, making it the second most commonly performed procedure in the United States [4]. Unfortunately the risks involved with surgery, in conjunction with the possibility of eradicating any hope of future pregnancies, make it a less favourable option for women. Thus understanding the pathogenesis behind fibroid formation is paramount for the development of novel therapeutic strategies.

3.1.2 Role of Female Sex Hormones

The current perspective on the development and maintenance of fibroids portrays a critical role of ovarian steroid hormones [5]. Fibroids have been shown to have an increased expression of oestrogen receptors (ERs) and progesterone receptors (PRs) when compared to adjacent tissue [6]. Interestingly, the female sex hormones oestrogen (E2) and progesterone (P4) have been implicated as having a critical role in the regulation of various pathways involved in fibroid growth and progression. Clinically, fibroids have been shown to increase in size during the first part of pregnancy, which is thought to be due to an increase in circulating E2 and P4 [7]. Conversely, fibroids are

expected to shrink once patients become post-menopausal due to a decline in ovarian hormone production. Subsequently, common therapeutic approaches targeting hormonal regulation have become a prime focus of research efforts.

3.2 Pharmacologic Treatment

3.2.1 Role of Pharmacologic Treatment

Uterine fibroids are difficult to treat, as there is currently no long-term cure, barring surgical intervention. Primary treatment goals of non-surgical intervention include improvement of patients' quality of life, a marked reduction in symptoms, and preservation of fertility. Many of these medical interventions exploit fibroid dependence on hormonal regulation. These therapies seek to alleviate symptoms until surgical intervention is necessary or there is a natural regression of fibroids.

3.2.2 Selective Progesterone Receptor Modulators (SPRMs)

Once the role of progesterone in promoting growth and maintenance of fibroids was established, therapeutic avenues emerged targeting progesterone and its respective receptors. Consequently, selective progesterone receptor modulators (SPRMs) were developed. SPRMs are a class of agents with mixed agonistic and antagonistic activities targeting tissue-specific progesterone receptors (PRs) [8]. Currently, the principal indication for SPRMs is emergency contraception and pregnancy termination [9]. Research avenues are, however, exploring the use of SPRMs in a multitude of other conditions such as UFs, endometriosis and breast cancer [10]. The number of drugs in this family has expanded considerably since the advent of mifepristone (RU-486) to include ulipristal acetate (UPA), asoprisnil, onapristone, lonaprisan, vilaprisan and telapristone. Five agents in particular – UPA, mifepristone, asoprisnil, vilaprisan and telapristone acetate – have shown the ability to reduce fibroid size and/or control uterine bleeding [11, 12].

3.2.2.1 Ulipristal Acetate (UPA)

Within the family of SPRMs, ulipristal has become the most promising agent for non-surgical management of UFs. UPA has already been approved for the management of UFs in Europe, Canada and several other countries. Recently, the pharmaceutical company Allergan announced that the US Food and Drug Administration (FDA) had accepted Allergan's New Drug Application (NDA) for the use of UPA in the treatment of abnormal uterine bleeding in women with UFs. Excitingly, if approved, UPA will become the first oral agent to be FDA-approved for the treatment of UFs in the United States.

The European Medicines Agency (EMA) and Canada have approved the use of UPA in the management of fibroids. Meanwhile, in the United States, UPA is currently the only FDA-approved drug for emergency contraception, due to its ability to inhibit ovulation and its immediate effects on the endometrium preventing implantation.

To date, the only pharmacologic agent approved by the FDA for use in fibroids is leuprolide, a gonadotrophin-releasing hormone (GnRH) agonist. However, GnRH agonists come with adverse effects that are not present with UPA, such as vasomotor symptoms and loss of bone mineral density [13]. A randomized double-blind study published data citing that a daily dose of 5 or 10 mg of UPA was non-inferior to once-a-month leuprolide in symptomatic control of UFs and had better compliance [14].

UPA is a synthetic steroid with tissue-specific mixed agonistic and antagonistic activity targeting particularly the uterus, cervix, ovaries and hypothalamus [15]. At the molecular level, UPA has been shown to increase apoptosis, decrease proliferation, decrease angiogenesis and reduce collagen synthesis [13]. It does so by regulating several factors involved in molecular pathways including caspase 3, B-cell lymphoma 2 (BCL2), tumour necrosis factor-alpha (TNF-α), vascular endothelial growth factor (VEGF), as well as many others [13, 16]. Additionally, UPA alters the ratio between two isoforms of the progesterone receptor, PR-A and PR-B, both of which have increased expression within fibroid tissue [13, 16]. Alteration of this ratio giving preference towards

one isoform versus the other can lead to anti-proliferative and pro-apoptotic effects [16].

Fibroids contain large deposits of ECM which increase over time [11]. UPA shrinks extracellular matrix (ECM) volume by reducing collagen deposition within the fibroids [17]. One study found that UPA-treated fibroids had a decreased fraction of ECM volume when compared to untreated fibroids [18].

A pivotal series of well-designed trials called the PEARL studies (PEARL I/II/III/IV) demonstrated that UPA use resulted in significant control of symptomatic fibroids with rapid control of bleeding, thereby improving anaemia, and showed a reduction in fibroid volumes [14, 19]. It was shown that over 90% of patients experienced relief from uterine bleeding after 5–7 days of UPA use [14, 20]. Additionally, the PEARL III trial assessed the safety profile of UPA. The results showed that emergent adverse events occurred in 120 women (57.4%); however, only 8 women (3.8%) described severe adverse events such as headache (16.3%) and abdominal pain (5.3%) [14, 20].

Another important trial assessed long-term use of UPA by administering four 12-week treatment cycles of UPA 5 and 10 mg. The study found that long-term use was well tolerated by patients, with high compliance [21]. At the end of the treatment, patients reported better quality of life (QoL), decreased bleeding and pain, and no increase in fibroid size [21].

The safety profile after extended use of UPA was assessed by a study published in 2017 which showed that after extended repeats of 3 months of treatment with UPA 10 mg/day, there were no major adverse events to contraindicate its use [22]. Interestingly, in all trials involving UPA, patients did not experience fibroid regrowth after discontinuation of UPA, in contrast with GnRH agonists which have shown regrowth after cessation [14, 20, 21].

It is worth noting that UPA's teratogenicity has not been assessed; however, it should be avoided in pregnant women as it is also used as an emergency contraceptive agent. Additionally, hormonal contraceptive options may interfere with UPA's therapeutic effect; thus, it is suggested that patients use barrier methods for contraception as opposed to oral or injection methods.

Of note, there is concern about endometrial morphological change with SPRM use. This histologic change is known as progesterone receptor modulator-associated endometrial changes (PAECs). Fortunately, these changes have been proven to be benign and are reversible within a few weeks to 6 months after cessation of the agent [13, 15].

3.2.2.2 Mifepristone (RU-486)

Mifepristone (RU-486), considered the pioneer agent in the SPRM family, acts predominantly through almost pure antagonistic activity on PRs. It is currently used as an abortifacient. A large meta-analysis of mifepristone used to treat symptomatic fibroids found that a dose of 2.5 mg/day for 3–6 months improved fibroid-related quality of life and bleeding, and showed a reduction in fibroid volume [23]. Contrastingly, another systematic review found there was no reduction of fibroid volume after mifepristone use [19]. Several initial studies were discontinued after there was fear of endometrial hyperplasia; however, there has been a recent resurgence of studies focusing on mifepristone.

3.2.2.3 Telapristone Acetate

Telapristone acetate, also branded as Proellex, is a newer SPRM being evaluated for use in UFs and endometriosis. Unfortunately, phase III trials were terminated early due to safety concerns over significantly elevating liver enzyme levels [24]. At present, there is an ongoing phase II clinical trial started in 2014 aiming to evaluate both safety and efficacy of lower oral as well as vaginal doses of telapristone acetate.

3.2.2.4 Asoprisnil (J867)

Asoprisnil has been studied in the treatment of UFs, endometriosis, and dysfunctional uterine bleeding. A large study found that a 12-week regimen of asoprisnil resulted in a reduction in fibroid size and control of uterine bleeding [25]. However, further studies have been discontinued due to the agent failing a phase III trial showing unsafe changes in the endometrial lining [25].

3.2.2.5 Vilaprisan

Vilaprisan is a novel SPRM which recently passed a 12-week phase I clinical trial successfully, in which most of the women who took the medication, at a daily dose of 1–5 mg, reported absence of menstrual bleeding. These results supported the initiation of advanced clinical trials to evaluate vilaprisan in women with symptomatic UFs [26]

3.2.3 Gonadotrophin-Releasing Hormone Agonists

To date, leuprolide acetate, a GnRH agonist, is the only FDA-approved non-surgical treatment modality for uterine fibroids. Leuprolide targets the pituitary gland, down-regulating GnRH receptors by continuous stimulation. Leuprolide is an analogue and thus it has an initial 'flare' effect in which hormone levels rise before they are suppressed after continuous stimulation. The result is a decrease in follicle-stimulating hormone (FSH) and luteinizing hormone (LH), and consequently suppression of ovarian steroid hormone production [27]. This creates an iatrogenic reversible menopause-like state. The downstream effect is a reduction in both bleeding and bulk-related symptoms, and a reduction in fibroid volume [27].

Unfortunately, GnRH analogues have a side-effect profile that includes hypo-oestrogenic symptoms such as hot flashes, vaginal dryness, headaches, and loss of bone mineral density [28]. Due to these adverse effects, therapy is limited to 6 months or less without the addition of add-back therapy [29]. Add-back therapy is an approach to alleviate hypo-oestrogenic side effects by concomitant use of a second agent. Hormonal regimens have explored the use of progestins, oestrogens, a combination of progestin/oestrogen, tibolone and raloxifene as add-back therapies [29]. Accordingly, alleviating hypo-oestrogenic symptoms through add-back therapy improves compliance to therapy.

However, in addition to the adverse effects from GnRH analogue therapy, fibroids regrow rapidly after discontinuing therapy [29]. Accordingly, leuprolide is only approved for preoperative shrinkage of fibroids rather than a long-term management option.

3.2.4 Gonadotrophin-Releasing Hormone Antagonists

GnRH antagonists competitively block GnRH receptors resulting in an immediate suppression of FSH, LH and ovarian steroid hormones. The immediate suppression is an advantage GnRH antagonists enjoy as opposed to GnRH agonists, which have an initial 'flare' effect of increasing hormones before suppression [30]. Agents in this category include cetrorelix, ganirelix, degarelix, abarelix and the new orally administered ones elagolix, relugolix and OBE2109.

Elagolix is a short-acting non-peptide GnRH antagonist with oral dosing. Elagolix has shown promise in the treatment of endometriosis and UFs due to its ability to suppress LH and FSH in a dose-dependent manner. A recent trial published data stating that a 300 mg twice-daily dose of elagolix showed a 36% reduction in fibroid and fibroid uterus volume as well as significantly reducing heavy menstrual bleeding, yet an add-back therapy is needed to avoid postmenopausal-like symptoms [31].

Relugolix (TAK-385) is a highly selective orally active GnRH antagonist. It is an investigational drug that completed a small phase III trial for the treatment of pain symptoms associated with UFs in May of 2017. It is currently being researched for UFs, endometriosis, and as an androgen-castration agent in prostate cancer [32]. Time will tell whether relugolix will be successfully added to the list of medications for controlling symptomatic fibroids.

Another GnRH antagonist of note is the orally active OBE2109, which is currently undergoing clinical trials for heavy menstrual bleeding associated with UFs.

3.2.5 Aromatase Inhibitors

Uterine fibroids generate high levels of local oestrogen relative to adjacent myometrium, possibly due to elevated expression of the enzyme aromatase [33]. This mechanism allows for targeting of fibroids through in-situ aromatase inhibition. Agents within this category include anastrozole, letrozole and fadrozole. Studies on postmenopausal women lacking natural ovarian oestrogen production have been successful in inhibiting fibroid-associated aromatase [33]. Unfortunately, long-term use may necessitate concomitant add-back therapy because of an increased association with bone loss [34]. Additionally, fibroids are more prevalent in obese patients. Adipose tissue is known to have an increased expression of aromatase, thereby contributing to elevated circulating oestrogen levels. This mechanism can theoretically be targeted by an aromatase inhibitor to decrease circulating oestrogen's impact on fibroid growth. Aromatase inhibitors may have potential in short-term preoperative management of fibroids; however, better trials are needed before their use can be recommended.

3.2.6 Selective Oestrogen Receptor Modulators (SERMs)

Selective oestrogen receptor modulators (SERMs) are non-steroidal oestrogen receptor ligands that act through mixed agonist and antagonist activity [35]. SERMs exert their actions through tissue-specific receptor targets. The two major agents in this family are tamoxifen and raloxifene, both of which are commonly used in the treatment of breast cancer. Tamoxifen has an agonistic effect on the endometrium, thus making its use in UF treatment unwarranted. Raloxifene, commonly used for breast cancer and osteoporosis, however, does not target the endometrium. A trial conducted on raloxifene 180 mg daily in women with symptomatic fibroids found a reduction in fibroid size by 22.2% after 3 months when compared to a placebo [35]. However, literature on the use of raloxifene in UFs is scarce and more research is required with larger controlled trials.

3.3 Conclusion

The management of uterine fibroids is heading in an exciting new direction with several pharmacologic agents emerging that will change daily medical practice. What was once a condition that could only be treated with surgical intervention may now become one that clinicians can manage medically. Women wanting to preserve their fertility will have more options to consider before deciding on a treatment. As researchers continue to explore the efficacy and safety of pharmacologic agents, to date, surgery remains the only cure for symptomatic fibroids. Shrinking fibroids preoperatively has been shown to be effective in creating better surgical outcomes. As of now, however, leuprolide acetate, a gonadotrophin-releasing hormone analogue, remains the only FDA-approved agent to shrink fibroids before surgery. Yet, it seems ulipristal acetate (UPA), a selective progesterone receptor modulator (SPRM) with oral dosing, may become the next agent approved in the United States for UF management. SPRMs have been successful in controlling fibroid-related symptoms while shrinking fibroid size. However, clinicians should be wary of possible endometrial changes associated with progesterone antagonism. Nevertheless, it remains apparent that larger and better controlled trials are needed to demonstrate short-term and long-term potential of agents in the medical management of uterine fibroids.

References

1. Baird DD, Dunson DB, Hill MC, Cousins D, Schectman JM. High cumulative incidence of uterine leiomyoma in black and white women: ultrasound evidence. *Am J Obstet Gynecol* 2003;**188** (1):100–7.

2. Stewart EA. Uterine fibroids. *Nat Rev Dis Primers* 2016;**2**:16043.

3. Pritts EA, Parker WH, Olive DL. Fibroids and infertility: an updated systematic review of the evidence. *Fertil Steril* 2009;**91** (4):1215–23.

4. Cardozo ER, Clark AD, Banks NK, et al. The estimated annual cost of uterine leiomyomata in the United States. *Am J Obstet Gynecol* 2012;**206**(3):211.e1–9.

5. Bulun SE. Uterine fibroids. *N Engl J Med* 2013;**369**(14):1344–55.

6. Borahay MA, Asoglu MR, Mas A, et al. Estrogen receptors and signaling in fibroids: role in pathobiology and therapeutic implications. *Reprod Sci* 2017;**24** (9):1235–44.

7. Ciavattini A, Di Giuseppe J, Stortoni P, et al. Uterine fibroids: pathogenesis and interactions with endometrium and endomyometrial junction. *Obstet Gynecol Int* 2013;**2013**:173184.

8. Lusher SJ, Raaijmakers HC, Vu-Pham D, et al. Structural basis for agonism and antagonism for a set of chemically related progesterone receptor modulators. *J Biol Chem* 2011;**286**(40):35079–86.

9. Bouchard P. Selective progesterone receptor modulators: a class with multiple actions and applications in reproductive endocrinology, and gynecology. *Gynecol Endocrinol* 2014;**30**(10):683–4.

10. Wagenfeld A, Saunders PT, Whitaker L, Critchley HO. Selective progesterone receptor modulators (SPRMs): progesterone receptor action, mode of action on the endometrium and treatment options in gynecological therapies. *Expert Opin Ther Targets* 2016;**20** (9):1045–54.

11. Donnez J, Donnez O, Dolmans MM. The current place of medical therapy in uterine fibroid management. *Best Pract Res Clin Obstet Gynaecol* 2017.

12. Reis FM, Bloise E, Ortiga-Carvalho TM. Hormones and pathogenesis of uterine fibroids. *Best Pract Res Clin Obstet Gynaecol* 2016;**34**:13–24.

13. Ali M, Al-Hendy A. Selective progesterone receptor modulators for fertility preservation in women with symptomatic uterine fibroids. *Biol Reprod* 2017;**97** (3):337–52.

14. Donnez, J, Tomaszewski J, Vázquez F, et al. Ulipristal acetate versus leuprolide acetate for uterine fibroids. *N Engl J Med* 2012;**366**(5):421–32.

15. Donnez J, Donnez O, Courtoy GE, Dolmans MM. The place of selective progesterone receptor modulators in myoma therapy. *Minerva Ginecol* 2016;**68** (3):313–20.

16. Yoshida S, Ohara N, Xu Q, et al. Cell-type specific actions of progesterone receptor modulators in the regulation of uterine leiomyoma growth. *Semin Reprod Med* 2010;**28**(3):260–73.

17. Xu Q, Ohara N, Liu J, et al. Progesterone receptor modulator CDB-2914 induces extracellular matrix metalloproteinase inducer in cultured human uterine leiomyoma cells. *Mol Hum Reprod* 2008;**14**(3):181–91.

18. Courtoy GE, Donnez J, Marbaix E, Dolmans MM. In vivo mechanisms of uterine myoma volume reduction with ulipristal acetate treatment. *Fertil Steril* 2015;**104**(2):426–34.e1.

19. Murji A, Whitaker L, Chow TL, Sobel ML. Selective progesterone receptor modulators (SPRMs) for uterine fibroids. *Cochrane Database Syst Rev* 2017;**4**: CD010770.

20. Donnez J, Tatarchuk TF, Bouchard P, et al. Ulipristal acetate versus placebo for fibroid treatment before surgery. *N Engl J Med* 2012;**366**(5):409–20.

21. Donnez J, Donnez O, Matule D, et al. Long-term medical management of uterine fibroids with ulipristal acetate. *Fertil Steril* 2016;**105**(1):165–73.e4.

22. Fauser BC, Donnez J, Bouchard P, et al. Safety after extended repeated use of ulipristal acetate for uterine fibroids. *PLoS One* 2017;**12**(3):e0173523.

23. Shen Q, Hua Y, Jiang W, et al. Effects of mifepristone on uterine leiomyoma in premenopausal women: a meta-analysis. *Fertil Steril* 2013;**100**(6):1722–6.e1–10.

24. Luo X, Yin P, Coon V JS et al. The selective progesterone receptor modulator CDB4124 inhibits proliferation and induces apoptosis in uterine leiomyoma cells. *Fertil Steril* 2010;**93** (8):2668–73.

25. Wilkens J, Chwalisz K, Han C, et al. Effects of the selective progesterone receptor modulator asoprisnil on uterine artery blood flow, ovarian activity and clinical symptoms in patients with uterine leiomyomata scheduled for hysterectomy. *J Clin Endocrinol Metab* 2008;**93**(12):4664–71.

26. Schutt B, Kaiser A, Schultze-Mosgau MH, et al. Pharmacodynamics and safety of the novel selective progesterone receptor modulator vilaprisan: a double-blind, randomized, placebo-controlled phase 1 trial in healthy women. *Hum Reprod* 2016;**31**(8):1703–12.

27. Lethaby A, Vollenhoven B, Sowter M. Efficacy of preoperative gonadotrophin hormone releasing analogues for women with uterine fibroids undergoing hysterectomy or myomectomy: a systematic

review. *BJOG* 2002;**109** (10):1097–108.

28. Lee MJ, Yun BS, Seong SJ, et al. Uterine fibroid shrinkage after short-term use of selective progesterone receptor modulator or gonadotropin-releasing hormone agonist. *Obstet Gynecol Sci* 2017;**60**(1):69–73.

29. Moroni R, Vieira CS, Ferriani RA, Candido-dos-Reis FJ, Brito LGO. Pharmacological treatment of uterine fibroids. *Ann Med Health Sci Res* 2014;**4**(Suppl 3): S185–92.

30. Struthers RS, Nicholls AJ, Grundy J, et al. Suppression of gonadotropins and estradiol in premenopausal women by oral administration of the nonpeptide gonadotropin-releasing hormone antagonist elagolix. *J Clin Endocrinol Metab* 2009;**94** (2):545–51.

31. Archer DF, Stewart EA, Jain RI, et al. Elagolix for the management of heavy menstrual bleeding associated with uterine fibroids: results from a phase 2a proof-of-concept study. *Fertil Steril* 2017;**108**(1):152–60.e4.

32. MacLean DB, Shi H, Faessel HM, Saad F. Medical castration using the investigational oral GnRH antagonist TAK-385 (relugolix): phase 1 study in healthy males. *J Clin Endocrinol Metab* 2015;**100** (12):4579–87.

33. Sumitani H, Shozu M, Segawa T, et al. In situ oestrogen synthesized by aromatase P450 in uterine leiomyoma cells promotes cell growth probably via an autocrine/ intracrine mechanism. *Endocrinology* 2000;**141** (10):3852–61.

34. Hadji P, Body JJ, Aapro MS, et al. Practical guidance for the management of aromatase inhibitor-associated bone loss. *Ann Oncol* 2008;**19**(8):1407–16.

35. Deng L, Wu T, Chen XY, Xie L, Yang J. Selective oestrogen receptor modulators (SERMs) for uterine leiomyomas. *Cochrane Database Syst Rev* 2012;**10**: CD005287.

The Role of Magnetic Resonance Imaging in the Management of Fibroids

Lisa Shannon and Shahram Abdi

4.1 Introduction and Overview

Ultrasound is the investigation of choice for the initial assessment of fibroids. However, the density, number, size or location of the fibroids can degrade the image quality due to the attenuation of the sound waves. Magnetic resonance imaging (MRI) does not suffer the same limitations and is not operator-dependent; it provides detailed and consistent assessment, making it the ideal tool to evaluate fibroid characteristics over time, such as change in size or amount of necrosis following treatment.

In this chapter, the basic MRI technique and features of the various types of fibroids will be discussed with the aid of illustrations.

4.2 MRI Technique

The physics of MRI is complex and beyond the scope of this book. This section covers the basic principles of how an image is produced [1].

MRI takes advantage of the properties of hydrogen atoms in the body. As a spinning charged particle, each hydrogen proton produces a small magnetic field known as the magnetic moment that aligns with the stronger magnetic field of the MRI scanner. The majority of the protons' magnetic moments form north–south pairs, creating a net magnetism of zero. However, a small excess of protons are unpaired, making their magnetic moments detectable.

A radiofrequency (RF) pulse excites the protons to a higher energy state. On termination of the pulse, the protons return to their original state and the excess energy is released as a radiofrequency signal. The signal from the unpaired protons is detected, amplified, and transformed into an image.

Various parameters are used to manipulate the initial RF pulse and the returning signal; this creates the variety of tissue contrast in the different MRI sequences. The commonest MRI sequences are T1 and T2. Tissues with inherently high signal intensity (bright) on T1 include fat, blood and protein. Fluid and fat have inherently high signal intensity on T2. Gadolinium is used as a contrast agent for MRI and returns high signal intensity on T1 sequences.

The magnetic field produced by a typical MRI scanner (1.5 tesla) is 30,000 times stronger than the Earth's magnetic field strength. Any ferromagnetic object is a potential projectile that could cause significant harm to the patient or scanner. The strong magnetic field can also have an adverse effect on medical equipment, notably pacemakers; therefore, safety is paramount.

4.3 Features of Fibroids

The typical features of a fibroid on MRI are isodense signal intensity (similar to the skeletal muscle) on T1, low signal intensity (dark) on T2, and a well-defined capsule (usually with a smooth border). The position of a fibroid is assessed by examining the scans in the sagittal, axial and coronal planes (Figures 4.1 and 4.2).

The pattern of enhancement of a fibroid following the MRI contrast medium varies greatly depending on the vascular supply. This particular feature can be used to assess the therapeutic effect of an embolization procedure (Figure 4.3).

The type of degeneration in a fibroid determines its appearance on the MRI sequences [2]. Necrosis of a fibroid may produce disconcerting features that can be misleading. An intact smooth capsule with no other features of invasion or spread, such as lymphadenopathy, is reassuring and points to a benign necrotic process (Figure 4.4).

The main MRI feature of a fibroid undergoing haemorrhagic degeneration (also known as red degeneration) is the presence of blood products of various ages within a well-encapsulated fibroid. The form of haemoglobin within the haemorrhage

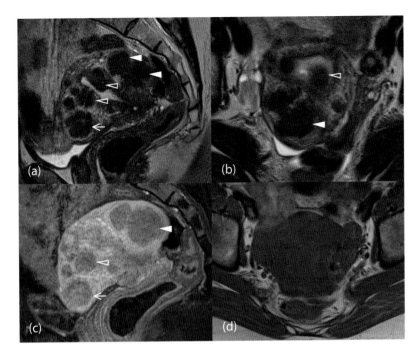

Figure 4.1 Multiple fibroids. (a) Sagittal T2. (b) Axial T2. (c) Sagittal T1 fat-saturated post-contrast. (d) Axial T1. Subserosal (arrow), intramural (solid arrowheads), submucosal (arrowheads). Typical fibroids are of low signal intensity on T2 and inconspicuous on T1. Fibroids have variable degrees of enhancement following gadolinium administration.

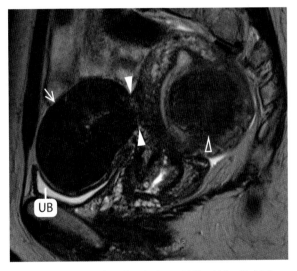

Figure 4.2 Large pedunculated subserosal fibroid (sagittal T2). The fibroid (arrow) is of low T2 signal intensity and indents the urinary bladder (UB). It has a narrow pedicle (solid arrowheads). There is also a posterior intramural fibroid (arrowhead) distorting the endometrial cavity.

determines how it appears on T1 and T2 sequences, and varies according to the age of the blood products. For example, a predominance of the methaemoglobin form in the intracellular space leads to high signal intensity on T1 and intermediate to low signal intensity on T2 scans. Haemosiderin is of low signal intensity on both T1 and T2 sequences and surrounds the haemorrhagic area (Figure 4.5).

Fatty degeneration of a fibroid behaves like any other fat-containing structure; it has high signal intensity on T1 and T2 images. The use of fat suppression techniques, usually when obtaining a T1 sequence, is the confirmatory test for the presence of fat (Figure 4.6).

4.4 Uterine Fibroids and Sarcomas

Differentiating a necrotic fibroid from a uterine (myometrial) sarcoma can be challenging in any form of imaging. The features of a malignant uterine mass on MRI are breach of the capsule, invasion of the surrounding tissues, lymphadenopathy, and the presence of metastatic deposits (Figure 4.7) [3, 4]. However, the absence of any or all of these features on MRI does not rule out a uterine sarcoma. Diffusion-weighted imaging (DWI) can improve the accuracy of the diagnosis [5].

4.5 Mimickers of a Fibroid

An adenomyoma can be indistinguishable from a fibroid on ultrasound as they both arise from the

29

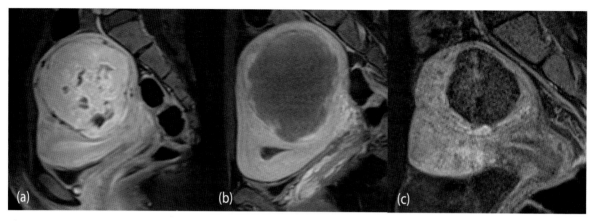

Figure 4.3 Posterior intramural fibroid before and after embolization (sagittal T1 post-contrast). (a) Pre-embolization. (b) 3 months post-embolization. (c) 2 years post-embolization.
Note the diminishing enhancement and size of the fibroid after embolization.

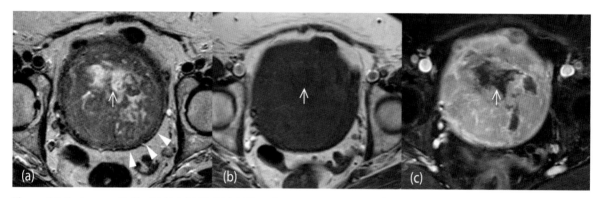

Figure 4.4 Benign necrotic fibroid. (a) Axial T2. (b) Axial T1 without contrast. (c) Axial T1 fat-saturated post-contrast.
10 cm fibroid with an irregular central area of necrosis (arrow) that is of high signal intensity on T2, low signal intensity on T1 and does not enhance. The fibroid has a smooth intact capsule (solid arrowheads), best seen on T2 and post-contrast sequences.

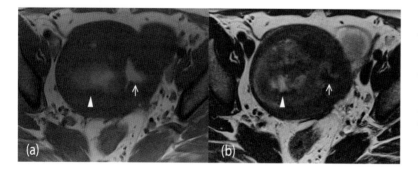

Figure 4.5 Benign haemorrhagic degeneration. (a) Axial T1. (b) Axial T2.
The central necrotic area contains blood products of different ages. The areas of high signal intensity on T1 and low signal intensity on T2 represent the products with the highest concentration of methaemoglobin (arrow). The haemosiderin rim is of low signal intensity on T1 and T2 (solid arrowhead).

myometrium; however, adenomyomas exhibit specific features on MRI that are usually diagnostic: small islands of blood on T1 and T2 sequences, expansion of the junctional zone of the myometrium, and an ill-defined endometrium–myometrium interface. The endometrium may be difficult to delineate as large crypts open into the adenomyoma (Figure 4.8) [6].

An ovarian fibroma or fibrothecoma can be misdiagnosed as a fibroid when it is in contact with the uterus; multiplanar MRI imaging can aid

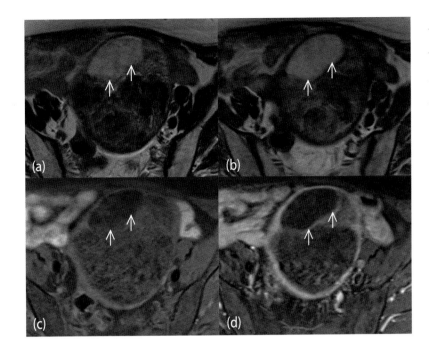

Figure 4.6 Fatty degeneration. (a) Axial T2. (b) Axial T1. (c) Axial T1 fat-saturated. (d) Axial T1 fat-saturated post-contrast. The fatty component of the fibroid (arrows) is of high signal intensity on T2 and T1, and characteristically loses signal on fat-saturated sequences. There is no enhancement following contrast administration.

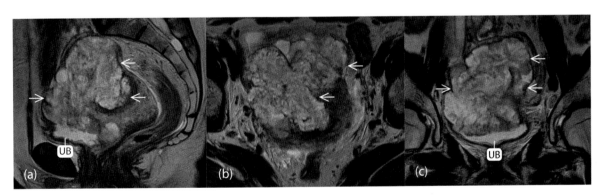

Figure 4.7 Myometrial sarcoma. (a) Sagittal T2. (b) Axial T2. (c) Coronal T2.
Large heterogeneous irregular mass replacing the normal uterine anatomy (arrows). It breaches the uterine serosa and invades the urinary bladder (UB).

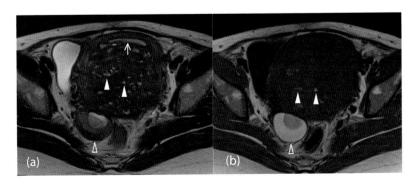

Figure 4.8 Adenomyoma. (a) Axial T2. (b) Axial T1.
Focal mass in the posterior myometrium displacing the endometrial cavity (arrow). Multiple cystic areas of high signal intensity on T2 and T1 (solid arrowheads) demonstrate small islands of blood within the myometrium. Incidental right ovarian endometrioma (arrowhead).

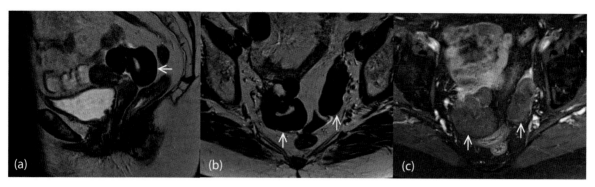

Figure 4.9 Bilateral ovarian fibromas. (a) Sagittal T2. (b) Axial T1. (c) Axial T1 fat-saturated post-contrast. Note the low signal intensity of the ovarian masses on both T1 and T2 sequences (arrows). There is minimal enhancement on the post-contrast image.

identification of the origin of the mass (Figure 4.9) [7]. If there is uncertainty following the MRI, an ultrasound scan may be helpful as it enables real-time dynamic imaging.

References

1. Allisy-Roberts P, William J. *Farr's Physics for Medical Imaging*. 2nd ed. Edinburgh: Saunders; 2007.

2. Arleo EK, Schwartz PE, Hui P, McCarthy S. Review of leiomyoma variants. *Am J Roentgenol* 2015;**205**(40):912–21.

3. Amant F, Coosemans A, Debiec-Rychter M, Timmerman D, Vergote I. Clinical management of uterine sarcomas. *Lancet Oncol* 2009;**10**(12):1188–98.

4. Benson C, Miah AB. Uterine sarcoma – current perspectives. *Int J Women's Health* 2017;**9**:597–606.

5. Li HM, Liu J, Qiang JW, et al. Diffusion-weighted imaging for differentiating uterine leiomyosarcoma from degenerated leiomyoma. *J Comput Assist Tomogr* 2017;**41** (4):599–606.

6. Novellas S, Chassang M, Delotte J et al. MRI characteristics of the uterine junctional zone: from normal to the diagnosis of adenomyosis. *Am J Roentgenol* 2011;**196**(5): 1206–13.

7. Shinagare AB, Meylaerts LJ, Laury AR, Mortele KJ. MRI features of ovarian fibroma and fibrothecoma with histopathologic correlation. *Am J Roentgenol* 2012;**198**(3): W296–303. doi: 10.2214/AJR.11.7221.

Chapter 5

Fibroids and Fertility

Tülay Karasu and Mostafa Metwally

5.1 Introduction

Uterine fibroids (also known as leiomyomas or myomas) are the most common benign uterine tumours in women, with an estimated incidence of 50–60% [1]. They are smooth muscle tumours originating from the myometrium [2]. The majority of uterine fibroids are asymptomatic but 30–40% are symptomatic, depending on the location and size, and can present with abnormal uterine bleeding, pressure symptoms, pelvic pain and infertility [3]. Additional symptoms include urinary problems and constipation. Uterine fibroids can also lead to reproductive problems like infertility, miscarriage, preterm labour, fetal malpresentation, increased risk of caesarean section, low birth weight and postpartum haemorrhage [4].

Race, genetic, epigenetic and environmental factors, such as age, early menarche and nulliparity, play an important role in the development of uterine fibroids [5]. The incidence of uterine fibroids increases with advancing age and the cumulative lifetime incidence is estimated between 70% and 84% [1, 6]. There is a current trend of women delaying childbirth, and therefore women who wish to conceive are more likely to present with uterine fibroids. Uterine fibroids may be associated with 5–10% of infertility cases [7].

Black women have a greater incidence of uterine fibroids when compared to white Caucasian women; the fibroids also tend to be larger and found in multiple locations, and to lead to severe symptoms [8].

5.2 Fibroids and Infertility

Uterine fibroids may be associated with 5–10% of women presenting with infertility [7], and they are the sole abnormal finding in 1–2.4% of infertile women [3]. The impact of uterine fibroids on fertility is determined by location and size. However, there has been a debate whether uterine fibroids cause infertility or are associated with infertility [9], and whether removal of the fibroids in asymptomatic women improves fertility and pregnancy outcome.

There are a few explanations of how fibroids can impair fertility:

1. Anatomic distortion of the uterine cavity [10]
2. Increased uterine contractility and changes to the endometrial blood supply [3]
3. Changes to the hormonal milieu within the uterine cavity that may have an effect on implantation [11, 12].

Fibroid location and fertility have been investigated in many studies. Unfortunately, most of them are only observational studies, with few well-designed randomized controlled trials. However, there is agreement that the greater the impact of the fibroid on the endometrial cavity, the greater the effect on fertility. Hence, submucosal, intramural and subserosal fibroids have a decreasing impact on fertility in that order.

5.3 Submucosal Fibroids and Fertility

Studies have demonstrated that submucosal fibroids have the most significant adverse effect on fertility by decreasing implantation rate and increasing the risk of miscarriage in spontaneous pregnancies and assisted reproduction cycles [13–15]. A systematic review from 2001 looking into the effect of fibroids and infertility demonstrated lower pregnancy rates (RR 0.30; 95% confidence interval [CI]: 0.13–0.70) and implantation rates (RR 0.28; 95% CI: 0.10–0.72) in women with submucosal fibroids when compared to infertile women without fibroids [13].

A newer meta-analysis from 2009 investigated the effect of submucosal fibroids on fertility [16]. The results showed that women with submucosal fibroids had significant lower fertility, clinical pregnancy and ongoing pregnancies/birth rates, and higher miscarriage rates [16].

Several studies have demonstrated an increase in spontaneous conception, reduced miscarriage rate and improved IVF outcomes following the removal of submucosal fibroids [17, 18]. Casini et al. demonstrated a significantly higher spontaneous pregnancy rate at 12 months following myomectomy compared to patients without myomectomy (43.3% vs. 27.2%) [19]. A randomized matched control study of 215 women with submucosal fibroids showed increased fertility rates following hysteroscopic myomectomy of grade 0 and 1 fibroids, but not of grade 2 fibroids [20].

5.4 Intramural Fibroids and Fertility

Infertility and recurrent miscarriage have been associated with submucosal fibroids or intramural fibroids distorting the uterine cavity [16, 21–23].

The greatest inconsistency has been on the effect of intramural fibroids not distorting the uterine cavity. The first systematic review on fibroids and infertility did not show an effect of intramural fibroids on infertility [13]. An updated systematic review by the same author demonstrated a possible negative effect of intramural fibroids on reproductive outcomes [16]. Women with intramural fibroids had significantly lower clinical pregnancy rates, implantation rates, ongoing pregnancy/live birth rates and significantly higher miscarriage rates [16]. However, most of the studies had a poor evaluation of the uterine cavity [16].

A more recent systematic review has suggested that the presence of intramural fibroids without cavity distortion has a negative impact on IVF outcomes [21].

A significant decrease in clinical pregnancy (RR = 0.85, 95% CI: 0.77–0.94, p = 0.002) and live birth rates (RR = 0.79, 95% CI: 0.7–0.88, p < 0.0001) after IVF treatment has been found in women with intramural fibroids without uterine cavity involvement when compared to women without fibroids [21]. A significant negative effect of intramural fibroids for conception (OR = 0.8, 95% CI: 0.6–0.9) and delivery (OR = 0.7, 95 % CI: 0.5–0.8) was also reported in a different systematic review of fibroids in female reproduction [19].

The most recent systematic review and meta-analysis initially showed a negative impact of intramural fibroids on clinical pregnancy rates, but not on live birth or miscarriage rates [24]. However, there was no significant effect of intramural fibroids without cavity distortion on clinical pregnancy rate (OR = 0.74, 95% CI: 0.5–1.04), live birth rate (OR = 1.17, 95% CI: 0.62–2.22) or miscarriage rate (OR = 1.88, 95% CI: 0.61–4.2), when only the highest-quality studies were included [24]. This is in contrast to the two recent meta-analyses [16, 21], which can be explained by the way confounding factors such as age and involvement of the uterine cavity were analysed. In addition, a low number of high-quality studies and significant statistical heterogeneity between the included studies were identified [24]. The same review could not identify a significant effect on clinical pregnancy rates (OR = 1.88, 95% CI: 0.57–6.14) or miscarriage rates (OR = 0.89, 95% CI: 0.14–5.48) following myomectomy for intramural fibroids [24]. High-quality studies are desperately needed regarding the effect of intramural fibroids on reproductive outcomes.

Even if intramural fibroids reduce fertility, the question is whether removal of those fibroids would improve reproduction.

Given the risks of surgery, including bleeding, infection, damage to internal organs and postoperative adhesions, the decision for a myomectomy should not be taken lightly if there is uncertain benefit. According to a systematic review there is no significant difference in reproductive outcomes when the laparoscopic and abdominal approaches for myomectomy are compared [25]. Nevertheless, removal of intramural fibroids did not seem to significantly improve fertility outcome [16, 19].

It is advisable to manage women with intramural fibroids on an individual basis, as there is insufficient evidence about the effect of intramural fibroids on fertility. Age and other reasons for infertility as well as number, size, location and presence of other fibroids need to be taken into consideration. In addition, it is important to check for any involvement of the uterine cavity. Many clinicians consider removing larger intramural fibroids (>5 cm). Future high-quality research is needed on the treatment of intramural fibroids, with a description of size and number of fibroids as well as their proximity to the endometrium.

5.5 Subserosal Fibroids and Fertility

A meta-analysis from 2009 did not reveal an effect of subserosal fibroids on fertility, implantation rates and clinical pregnancy rates [16], and there is currently insufficient evidence that removal of a subserosal fibroid improves fertility in women who are otherwise asymptomatic [26]. However, surgery may be considered if the subserosal fibroid is large and causing symptoms or is distorting the pelvic anatomy, leading to difficult access to the ovaries for egg retrieval.

5.6 Conclusion

Uterine fibroids are commonly found in women of reproductive age. They can lead to reduced fertility and adverse pregnancy outcomes. Fertility outcomes are decreased in women with submucosal fibroids, and removal seems to be beneficial. Subserosal fibroids do not affect fertility outcomes, and removal does not show any benefit. Intramural fibroids appear to decrease fertility, but there is still some uncertainty and controversy regarding the management of intramural uterine fibroids. Intramural fibroids with a submucosal component reduce reproductive outcomes, and myomectomy may be considered to increase the pregnancy chances. Therefore, it is important to exclude any involvement of the uterine cavity. More high-quality studies are needed to determine the impact of intramural fibroids on fertility and the effect of myomectomy on reproductive outcomes. Therefore, counselling and individualized planning is recommended when dealing with subfertile women diagnosed with uterine fibroids.

References

1. Baird D, Dunson DB, Hill MC, Cousins D, Schectman JM. High cumulative incidence of uterine leiomyoma in black and white women: ultrasound evidence. *Am J Obstet Gynecol* 2003;**188**:100–7.

2. Bulun S. Uterine fibroids. *N Engl J Med* 2013;**369**:14.

3. Donnez J, Jadoul P. What are the implications of myomas on fertility? A need for a debate? *Hum Reprod* 2002;**17**:1424–30.

4. Hart R. Unexplained infertility, endometriosis and fibroids. *Br Med J* 2003;**327**(7417):721–4.

5. Segars JH, Parrott EC, Nagel JD, et al. Proceedings from the Third National Institutes of Health International Congress on Advances in Uterine Leiomyoma Research: comprehensive review, conference summary and future recommendations. *Hum Reprod Update* 2014;**20**(3):309–33.

6. Cramer SF, Patel A. The frequency of uterine leiomyomas. *Am J Clin Pathol* 1990;**94**(4):435–8.

7. Wallach EE, Vu KK. Myomata uteri and infertility. *Obstet Gynecol Clin North Am* 1995;**22**(4):791–9.

8. Catherino WH, Eltoukhi HM, Al-Hendy A. Racial and ethnic differences in the pathogenesis and clinical manifestations of uterine leiomyoma. *Semin Reprod Med* 2013;**31**(5):370–9.

9. Khaund A, Lumsden MA. Impact of fibroids on reproductive function. *Best Pract Res Clin Obstet Gynaecol* 2008;**22**(4):749–60.

10. Somigliana S, Vercellini P, Daguati R, et al. Fibroids and female reproduction: a critical analysis of the evidence. *Hum Reprod Update* 2007;**13**:465–76.

11. Sinclair DC, Mastroyannis A, Taylor HS. Leiomyoma simultaneously impair endometrial BMP-2-mediated decidualization and anticoagulant expression through secretion of TGF-β3. *J Clin Endocrinol Metab* 2011;**96**:412–21.

12. Galliano D, Bellver J, Días-Garcia C, Simón C, Pellicer A. ART and uterine pathology: how relevant is the maternal side for implantation? *Hum Reprod Update* 2015;**21**:13–38.

13. Pritts EA. Fibroids and infertility: a systematic review of the evidence. *Obstet Gynecol Surv* 2001;**56**(8):483–91.

14. Farhi J, Ashkenazi J, Feldberg D, et al. Effect of uterine leiomyomata on the results of in-vitro fertilization treatment. *Hum Reprod* 1995;**10**(10):2576–8.

15. Eldar-Geva T, Meagher S, Healy DL, et al. Effect of intramural, subserosal and submucosal uterine fibroids on the outcome of assisted reproductive technology treatment. *Fertil Steril* 1998;**70**(4):687–91.

16. Pritts EA, Parker WH, Olive DL. Fibroids and infertility: an updated systematic review of the evidence. *Fertil Steril* 2009;**91**:1215–23.

17. Bernard G, Darai E, Poncelet C, Benifla JL, Madelenat P. Fertility after hysteroscopic myomectomy: effect of intramural myomas associated. *Eur J Obstet Gynecol Reprod Biol* 2000;**88**(1):85–90.

18. Narayan R, Rajat, Goswamy K. Treatment of submucous fibroids, and outcome of assisted conception. *J Am Assoc Gynecol Laparosc* 1994;**1**(4 Pt 1):307–11.

19. Casini ML, Rossi F, Agostini R, Unfer V. Effects of the position of fibroids on fertility. *Gynecol Endocrinol* 2006;**22**(2):106–9.

20. Shokeir T, El-Shafei M, Yousef H, Allam AF, Sadek E. Submucous myomas and their implications in the pregnancy rates of patients with otherwise unexplained

primary infertility undergoing hysteroscopic myomectomy: a randomized matched control study. *Fertil Steril* 2010;**94** (2):724–9.

21. Sunkara SK, Khairy M, El-Toukhy T, Khalaf Y, Coomarasamy A. The effect of intramural fibroids without uterine cavity involvement on the outcome of IVF treatment: a systematic review and meta-analysis. *Human Reprod* 2010;**25**:418–29.

22. Yan LMD, Ding L, Li C, et al. Effect of fibroids not distorting the endometrial cavity on the outcome of in vitro fertilization treatment: a retrospective cohort study. *Fertil Steril* 2014;**101**:716–21.

23. Zepiridis LI, Grimbizis GF, Tarlatzis BC. Infertility and uterine fibroids. *Best Pract Res Clin Obstet Gynaecol* 2015;**S1521–6934**: 00235–7.

24. Metwally M, Farquhar CM, Li T-C. Is another meta-analysis on the effects of intramural fibroids on reproductive outcomes needed? *Reprod Biomed Online* 2011;**23** (1):2–14.

25. Metwally M, Cheong YC, Horne AW. Surgical treatment of fibroids for subfertility. *Cochrane Database Syst Rev* 2012;(11): CD003857.

26. Practice Committee of the American Society for Reproductive Medicine. Removal of myomas in asymptomatic patients to improve fertility and/ or reduce miscarriage rate: a guideline. *Fertil Steril* 2017;**108** (3):416–25.

Fibroids and Reproduction

Elizabeth A. Pritts

6

Fibroids have long been labelled by clinicians as a factor resulting in adverse reproductive outcomes, from conception to parturition. However, despite the widespread belief that fibroids are a detriment to reproduction, there have been surprisingly few high-quality studies addressing these issues and even fewer that have examined the value of intervention via treatment trials. This chapter will discuss the role of fibroids in hindering fertility, early pregnancy, and late pregnancy. In this, we will examine the existing data, the quality of that data, and attempt to draw conclusions consistent with the best available evidence to aid in the clinical approach to these tumours.

6.1 Issues with Existing Data

The primary problem with studying the disease 'uterine fibroids' is that leiomyomas are quite heterogeneous in their characteristics from patient to patient and even within the same patient. Fibroids vary in the number present per patient, the size, the location within the uterus, the location in relation to the uterine cavity, and histology/biochemistry. To further complicate the issue, the description of these factors is varied and inconsistent throughout the literature.

An additional problem confronting researchers is the large number of confounding variables when comparing women with fibroids to those without. Women with fibroids are often older, have an increased body mass index, are more likely of African descent, are more likely to suffer from diabetes pre-pregnancy as well as gestational diabetes, and more likely to have pre-pregnancy hypertension as well as hypertensive disorders during pregnancy. They are less likely to smoke cigarettes, but are more likely to consume alcohol.

6.2 Classification

Fibroids may be present just below the serosal surface of the uterus (subserosal), within the wall of the uterus (intramural), or extending into the uterine cavity (submucosal). The ability to differentiate a submucosal from an intramural location may be particularly critical, but is often exceedingly difficult due to the nature of available diagnostic tests. Unfortunately, non-uniformity of criteria for this classification adds considerable confusion to the literature. Furthermore, many published studies inadequately classify women with fibroids or omit this parameter altogether.

To classify a fibroid as submucosal, some authors require the fibroid to be within 4 mm of the endometrium, while some just subjectively determine that a tumour is 'abutting' or 'impinging upon' the endometrium. Others may rely upon operative report descriptions or specific tests used to determine if the cavity is invaded. For intramural fibroids, many authors rely upon measurements of 4 or 10 mm from the endometrium, while others simply determine the location subjectively. Some use 'depth of the fibroid into the myometrium' of 70–100% to classify a fibroid as a submucosal, but call the fibroids intramural in location if the depth is 30–70% into the myometrium. Even subserosal location definitions vary, with some authors using >50% outside the muscularis and others requiring 'most' of the fibroid outside the myometrium.

Recently, Munro and colleagues put forth a subclassification system to ensure uniformity for practitioners and authors when speaking about fibroids and their location (Figure 6.1). Unfortunately, many authors have ignored this system, further promoting heterogeneity within the literature.

6.3 Diagnostic Methodology

When an attempt is made to determine the type(s) of fibroids present in a patient, the most common pre-operative tests are the hysterosalpingogram (HSG) and transvaginal ultrasonography (TVUS). Both of

37

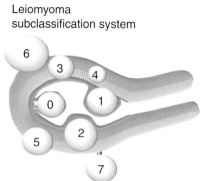

Leiomyoma subclassification system

S – Submucosal	0	Pedunculated intracavitary
	1	>50% intracavitary
	2	≤50% intracavitary
O – Other	3	Contacts endometrium; 0% intracavitary
	4	Intramural
	5	Subserosal ≥50% intramural
	6	Subserosal <50% intramural
	7	Subserosal pedunculated
	8	Other

Figure 6.1 (Reproduced with permission from Munro [1].)

these techniques have limited accuracy due to significant limitations.

HSGs may have sensitivities as low as 50% and positive predictive values as low as 28.6% for intrauterine lesions [2]. Furthermore, specificity may be as low as 20% [3]. Thus, if evaluation of the uterine cavity is limited to hysterosalpingography, imprecise fibroid localization is highly likely.

TVUS was once thought to be an accurate tool for diagnosis of submucosal fibroids, with initial studies showing sensitivity and specificity of 100% and 94%, respectively, with positive predictive values of 81% and negative predictive values of 100% when compared with hysteroscopy as the 'gold standard' [4]. However, current studies have failed to duplicate this high level of accuracy, with sensitivities as low as 69% and positive predictive values as low as 47% [5].

Sonohysterogram, hysteroscopy, and magnetic resonance imaging (MRI) are the most accurate techniques available to localize the fibroid outside of pathologic evaluation of the extirpated uterus. This is particularly true when differentiating between submucosal and intramural fibroids. In 1993, Fukuda found that when attempting to classify fibroids as intramural or submucosal, sonohysterogram misdiagnosed only 1 of 22 of these myomas [6]. In a second study, sonohysterography and hysteroscopy had sensitivity, specificity, and predictive values of 100% [7].

MRI, while expensive and time-consuming, is likely the most accurate of all. In a study comparing sonography, hysteroscopy, and MRI in 106 women scheduled for hysterectomy – with the gold standard being pathologic examination – MRI proved to perform the best, with 100% sensitivity and 91% specificity [8]. The value of MRI, however, may extend beyond mere classification of fibroids. The junctional zone of myometrium is ontogenetically, structurally, and hormonally different from the outer myometrium and MRI alone can successfully distinguish these histologic interfaces. This may prove to be of value as investigations become more precise in their research questions and hypotheses [9].

6.4 Fibroids and Infertility

Since 2001, when the first systematic review and meta-analysis was published addressing the issue of uterine fibroids and infertility, there have been nine additional systematic reviews/meta-analyses [10]. To date, there are 31 total studies with control groups: 10 prospective (with 2 randomized) and 21 retrospective. There are only seven treatment trials, and one of those was recently redacted [11].

6.4.1 What Effect Does Fibroid Location Have upon Fertility Status?

For submucosal fibroids, the data combined from only a few studies show a decrease in clinical pregnancy rate, but no differences in implantation or ongoing pregnancy/delivery rates. However, due to the limited amount of data the robustness of these findings is questionable [5] (Table 6.1).

The role of intramural myomas is of intense interest and has long been controversial. We examined the existing data in 2012 and it suggested that women have significantly lower rates of implantation and ongoing pregnancy/delivery rates in the presence of these myomas (Table 6.2).

Table 6.1 Effect on fertility of submucosal fibroids

Submucosal fibroids: effect on fertility				
Outcome	Number of studies	Relative risk	95% Confidence interval	Significance
Clinical pregnancy rate	5	0.560	1.315–0.997	p=0.049
Implantation rate	3	0.517	0.168–1.590	Non-significant
Ongoing/live birth rate	2	0.595	0.117–2.007	Non-significant

Table 6.2 Effect on fertility of intramural fibroids

Intramural fibroids: effect on fertility				
All studies: regardless of diagnostic modality				
Outcome	Number of studies	Relative risk	95% Confidence interval	Significance
Clinical pregnancy rate	18	0.911	0.821–1.010	Non-significant
Implantation rate	12	0.827	0.688–0.993	p<0.042
Ongoing/live birth rate	15	0.797	0.698–0.910	p<0.001

In an attempt to improve the quality of those meta-analytic data, our group performed subset analyses. When only those studies that used ultrasound and hysteroscopy in all subjects are included, the differences above disappear (Table 6.3).

Recently, an analysis was performed on data from a randomized controlled trial addressing intramural fibroids. The initial study included 900 couples, and different treatment regimens were evaluated for fertility outcomes. Of those couples, 11% were found to

Table 6.3 Effect on fertility of intramural fibroids: results from studies that used ultrasound and hysteroscopy in all subjects

Intramural fibroids: effect on fertility				
Studies using ultrasound and hysteroscopy in all subjects.				
Outcome	Number of studies	Relative risk	95% Confidence interval	Significance
Clinical pregnancy rate	6	0.878	0.722–1.068	Nonsignificant
Implantation rate	4	0.803	0.617–1.044	Nonsignificant
Ongoing/live birth rate	6	0.831	0.649–1.065	Nonsignificant

have intramural fibroids without intracavitary involvement. Once adjusted for confounders, there were no differences in conception, clinical pregnancy, pregnancy loss, or live birth rates in women with intramural fibroids compared to control subjects without fibroids [12].

Although it is possible that intramural fibroids without intracavitary involvement may affect fertility, the best evidence thus far does not support this theory.

For fibroids that are primarily subserosal in location, the studies consistently report no differences in clinical pregnancy rates, implantation rates, or ongoing/live birth rates. These data did include studies evaluating women undergoing assisted reproductive techniques as well as those attempting spontaneous conception [13] (Table 6.4).

6.4.2 Does Fibroid Size Affect Fertility?

An important clinical question is whether there is a particular size of fibroid that results in decreased fertility. Once that size is identified, the follow-up question would be whether or not surgical removal of the fibroid will enhance fertility.

To better understand the relationship between size and fertility, we attempted to perform a systematic review of the studies addressing this issue. Due to the

heterogeneity of studies, we were unable to perform a meta-analysis. Below is a summary of the studies addressing outcomes from comparing women that have smaller fibroids with those without fibroids. There appear to be no differences in clinical pregnancy rates, implantation rates, or ongoing pregnancy/delivery rates (Table 6.5) [14–20].

When addressing fibroids that are larger, the data are more conflicting. If all data are included, no matter the diagnostic criteria for classification, there is some variability in study findings (Table 6.6) [21–26].

However, if only those studies that utilize adequate methods of diagnosing the location (hysteroscopy and ultrasound, or sonohysterography) are examined, then the number is limited to three investigations. All are retrospective, and in one, the cohort of women suffering from larger fibroids is older than those with smaller fibroids (Table 6.7) [22, 24, 25].

If the studies are further limited to those that control for age, there are only two studies evaluable. There are no differences in either clinical pregnancy rates, implantation rates, or ongoing pregnancy rate. However, one study did note that a second in vitro fertilization cycle was necessary for those with larger fibroids to achieve the same success rate (Table 6.8) [22, 24].

Table 6.4 Effect on fertility of subserosal fibroids

Subserosal fibroids: effect on fertility

Outcome	# Studies	Relative risk	95% Confidence interval	Significance
Clinical pregnancy rate	7	0.918	0.718–1.172	0.492
Implantation rate	3	0.916	0.653–1.286	0.614
Ongoing/live birth rate	4	0.963	0.651–1.424	0.851

Table 6.5 The effect of fibroid size on fertility: studies comparing outcomes in women with small fibroids versus no fibroids

Fertility comparisons with size <5–6 cm

Study Location	Sizes	Findings
Bozdag] [14] Intramuscular	0.5–4.3 cm	No differences
Gianaroli [15] Intramuscular/submucosal	<1, 1–3 , ≥3 cm	No differences
Jun [16] All locations	<1.05, 1.06–1.5, 1.6–2.3, >2.3 cm	No differences
Manzo [17] No cavity distortion	<2, 2–5, ≥5 cm (1 pt)	No differences
Somigliana [18] No cavity encroachment	<2, 2–4, >4 cm (maximum 5 cm)	No differences
Surrey [19] Intramuscular	2 ± 0.2, 3.1 ± 0.5 cm	No differences
Wang [20] Intramuscular/submucosal	<3, 3–6, >6 cm (1 patient)	No differences

Thus, from the best available evidence, it is observed that fibroids that are less than 5–6 cm probably do not affect fertility. When looking at women with larger fibroids, there is more ambiguity as to whether or not they produce an adverse effect due to size alone.

6.4.3 Does the Number of Fibroids Affect Fertility?

A number of studies have addressed this issue, and the majority are quite consistent in demonstrating that there is no effect on fertility potential with

Table 6.6 The effect of fibroid size on fertility: studies of outcomes in women with larger fibroids (CPR, clinical pregnancy rate; DR, delivery rate; IR, implantation rate; ROC, receiver operating characteristic; SAB, spontaneous abortion)

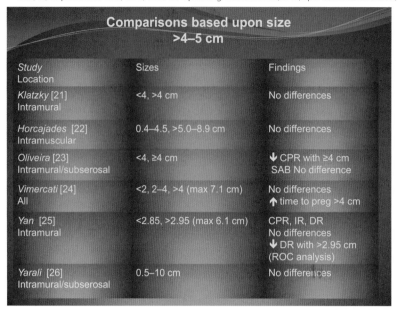

Comparisons based upon size >4–5 cm		
Study Location	Sizes	Findings
Klatzky [21] Intramural	<4, >4 cm	No differences
Horcajades [22] Intramuscular	0.4–4.5, >5.0–8.9 cm	No differences
Oliveira [23] Intramural/subserosal	<4, ≥4 cm	↓ CPR with ≥4 cm SAB No difference
Vimercati [24] All	<2, 2–4, >4 (max 7.1 cm)	No differences ↑ time to preg >4 cm
Yan [25] Intramural	<2.85, >2.95 (max 6.1 cm)	CPR, IR, DR No differences ↓ DR with >2.95 cm (ROC analysis)
Yarali [26] Intramural/subserosal	0.5–10 cm	No differences

Table 6.7 The effect of larger fibroids on fertility: studies using hysteroscopy and/or sonohysterography for diagnosis

Hysteroscopy or Sonohysterogram for diagnosis of location		
Study *Diagnosis	Sizes	Findings
Horcajades [22] *Diagnosis: Hysteroscopy or Sonohysterography	0.4–4.5,>5.0–8.9 cm	No differences
Vimercati [24] *Diagnosis: Ultrasonography and Hysteroscopy	<2, 2–4, >4 (maximum 7.1 cm)	No differences (increased time to pregnancy if fibroid >4 cm
Yan [25] *Diagnosis: Hysteroscopy	<2.85, >2.95 (maximum 6.1 cm)	Clinical pregnancy, implantation and ongoing pregnancy rates not different. decreased delivery rates if >2.95 cm

increasing numbers of fibroids, at least when the number of fibroids is easily countable (Table 6.9) [15, 17, 18, 21–27].

6.5 Fibroids and Early Pregnancy Loss

It has long been hypothesized that uterine fibroids can increase the risk of early pregnancy loss.

Mechanisms that have been postulated include anatomic distortion resulting in abnormal uteroplacental circulation, increased early uterine contractility, adverse mechanical effects, and biochemical impairment of developing pregnancies [28].

The data regarding miscarriages and fibroids have been questionable at best. Most studies are

Table 6.8 The effect of larger fibroids on fertility: studies of age-matched samples using hysteroscopy and/or sonohysterography for diagnosis (HSC, hysteroscopy; IVF, in vitro fertilization; US, ultrasound)

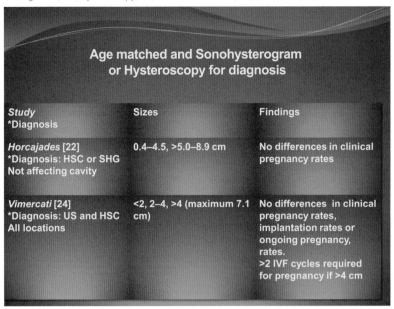

Age matched and Sonohysterogram or Hysteroscopy for diagnosis		
Study *Diagnosis	Sizes	Findings
Horcajades [22] *Diagnosis: HSC or SHG Not affecting cavity	0.4–4.5, >5.0–8.9 cm	No differences in clinical pregnancy rates
Vimercati [24] *Diagnosis: US and HSC All locations	<2, 2–4, >4 (maximum 7.1 cm)	No differences in clinical pregnancy rates, implantation rates or ongoing pregnancy, rates. >2 IVF cycles required for pregnancy if >4 cm

Table 6.9 Effect on fertility of number of fibroids

Comparisons based upon number		
Study	Numbers	Findings
Check [27]	1–7	No differences
Gianaroli [15]	≤3, >3	↑ Spontaneous abortion ↓ Implantation with >3 fibroids
Horcajadas [22]	1, 2, >3	No differences
Klatzky [21]	single, multiples	No differences
Manzo [17]	1, 2, 3, 4	No differences
Oliveira [23]	1–4	No differences
Somigliana [18]	1, ≥2	No differences
Vimercati [24]	1, 2, >2	No differences
Yan [25]	1, ≥2	No differences
Yarali [26]	1–8	No differences

retrospective, location is inconsistently and often suboptimally evaluated, and confounding factors such as age are rarely adjusted for.

We published a meta-analysis in 2009 that suggested an increased risk of spontaneous abortion in the presence of either submucosal or intramural fibroids. Three studies were subsequently published that, when added to the results of the meta-analysis, demonstrated a higher rate of spontaneous abortion for all types of fibroids [5].

More recently, however, Hartmann and colleagues conducted a prospective cohort study of 5,512 participants. All had uniform evaluation and outcome assessment. While an association appeared between

Table 6.10 Relationship between number of fibroids and rate of spontaneous abortion

Spontaneous abortion: number of fibroids

Hartmann [29]

#	Number of patients	Hazard ratio	95% CI
0	4,225	1.0	Referrant
1	344	0.84	0.62–1.15
2	141	0.79	0.53–1.23

Data from Hartmann et al. [29].

Table 6.11 Relationship between type of fibroid and rate of spontaneous abortion

Type of fibroids and SAB

Type of fibroid	Number of patients	Hazard ratio	95% Confidence interval
No fibroids	4225	1.0	Referrant
Subserosal	206	0.64	0.42–0.98
Submucosal	95	0.92	0.56–1.50
Intramural	216	1.05	0.75–1.47

fibroids and spontaneous abortion in the crude data, adjustment for confounding factors eliminated this association. Furthermore, fibroid location was not of predictive importance [29] (Table 6.10).

A recent high-quality meta-analysis found similar results [30]. Five studies comparing women with fibroids to the general population without fibroids found no difference in spontaneous abortion rate between groups. The researchers were careful to include only those studies that documented fibroids or no fibroids with ultrasound, and the study must not have been limited to special populations of

Table 6.12 Relationships between size and number of fibroids and rates of early pregnancy failure

Size and number and spontaneous abortion			
Benson [31]			
No fibroids versus all sizes	Comparison between sizes	No fibroid versus single fibroid	Single fibroid versus multiple fibroids
7.6% versus 14% p<0.05	<2 cm = 20.5% 2–4 cm = 8.6% >4 cm = 15.2% p = 0.24	7.6% versus 8%	8% versus 23.6% p<0.05

Data from Benson et al. [31].

women. Confounders were adjusted for in only one study, so in the remaining four studies they approximated adjusted point estimates based upon the single study that did adjust (Table 6.11).

Size of myomas and number of fibroids have also been evaluated as possible contributors to early pregnancy failure. In the two studies examining size, no effect was seen between small versus large fibroids [29, 31] (Table 6.12). Three studies have evaluated fibroid number. None showed an increased risk of miscarriage in the presence of one or two fibroids, but two studies suggested a higher pregnancy failure rate if more than two fibroids are present. However, the best study [29], which adjusted for confounders, failed to find any difference in spontaneous abortion rates even with more than two fibroids.

Thus, despite the suggestion from early studies that fibroids are associated with an increase in spontaneous abortion, current best available evidence would suggest that this is not the case, regardless of location, size, and number.

6.6 Late Pregnancy Complications

Although the majority of women with fibroids have normal pregnancies, a large number of complications of late pregnancy have been linked to their presence [32]. Many investigators have attempted to determine which complications are more common with fibroid uteri, and if so how much is the risk increased. In examining these studies, however, the evidence evaluating such complications is of varying quality and reliability. Of the 22 studies found by the authors, only 4 are prospective in design. Eighteen used control groups, but only five made use of controls matched for one or more known confounders. Fifteen studies collected data on confounders, and 12 attempted to adjust for these via regression analysis.

Data on fibroids were also widely variable. Fifteen studies attempted to categorize fibroids by size, 13 by location, 11 by number, and only 4 calculated total fibroid volume.

6.6.1 Excessive Blood Loss at Delivery

Two retrospective studies have examined the issue of blood loss at delivery, and both showed greater blood loss at delivery in the presence of fibroids [33, 34]. Both used age-matched controls and adjusted for confounders via regression analysis. In both studies, the excessive blood loss was only seen in women with fibroids greater than 5 cm in diameter. In these women with large fibroids, one study found an increased rate of transfusion [34] and also noted a correlation between transfusion rate and total fibroid volume.

6.6.2 Caesarean Section Rate

Fifteen studies have examined the rate of caesarean section in the presence and absence of fibroids, with 13 of the 15 showing an increased rate. Of the 11 studies that adjusted for confounders via regression analysis, all 11 demonstrated an increased rate [33, 35–44]. Additionally, a meta-analysis recently examined this issue, including 10 of these studies. The authors found an increased risk with an odds ratio of 2.60 (95% CI: 2.02–3.18).

Six studies have examined the effect of fibroid size on caesarean section rate, with three showing no effect [35, 37, 39] and three showing that size does matter [33, 38, 44]. Four studies determined the relationship between fibroid number and c-section rate, with two showing an increased rate [35, 43] and two not showing a difference [37, 41]. Total fibroid volume combines both of these variables, and the two studies that calculated the correlation between volume and rate of caesarean section both found a mildly increasing rate with volume increase [38, 42]. Two studies demonstrated no rate change with fibroid location [42, 43], while one claimed a higher c-section rate with fibroids in the lower uterine segment [37].

In summary, it appears that women with fibroids in pregnancy are indeed at increased risk for having a caesarean section, even when adjusting for the many confounding factors that affect this decision. However, it is not clear which women with fibroids are at heightened risk based on the number and characteristics of their tumours.

6.6.3 Malpresentations

Seven studies examined whether the presence of fibroids leads to a higher rate of fetal malpresentation, and five concluded that this was indeed the case. Of the five studies utilizing multivariate regression for correction of confounding variables, all showed an increased risk of malpresentation at delivery [39–41, 43, 44]. Furthermore, a recent meta-analysis showed a significant association between fibroids and malpresentation at term, with an odds ratio of 2.65 (95% CI: 1.0–3.70) [45].

6.6.4 Dysfunctional Labour

It has been theorized that uterine fibroids might cause abnormal labour patterns due to disruption of normal uterine contractility patterns. One population-based study from Israel, with prospective data collection but a retrospective research direction, has examined this issue. The authors found that there was a significant increase in the rate of failing to progress during the first stage of labour in women with fibroids but not in the second stage [40]. Unfortunately, the data were not analysed to correct for confounders. A second study found no difference in length of either first or second stage, but this investigation was limited to women who delivered vaginally [39]. Finally, Coronado and colleagues examined the rate of dysfunctional labour with adjustments for multiple confounders and revealed an increased odds ratio of 1.85 (95% CI: 1.65–2.18) [36]. Thus, the idea of fibroids leading to abnormal labour is plausible, and limited data seem to bolster this hypothesis.

6.6.5 Postpartum Haemorrhage

Five studies have examined aspects of the relationship between uterine fibroids and postpartum haemorrhage, all retrospective in research direction. Two found postpartum haemorrhage to be more common in women with fibroids [39, 43], both utilizing large population-based databases and regression analysis to correct for confounding variables. A third study found no difference, but did find an increase in transfusion rate when postpartum haemorrhage occurred [40]. Size has been claimed to play a role, with one investigation showing a higher rate of postpartum haemorrhage with larger fibroids [43] and a second showing more frequent transfusions when large fibroids (>5 cm) were present [34]. Finally, location may also play a role, with higher rates of haemorrhage seen when fibroids are intramural [43] or low in the uterus or cervix [37], as opposed to other locations. Thus, fibroids seem to enhance the likelihood of severe postpartum haemorrhage, and this is particularly true if the fibroid(s) is large, intramural, or low-lying.

6.6.6 Hysterectomy

Two retrospective studies have examined the rate of caesarean hysterectomy in women with fibroids, one finding an 18-fold increase in the rate (5.3% vs. 0.3% in controls) [46] and the other a 75-fold increase (2.9% vs. 0.04%) [47]. This does appear to be a real complication and worthy of further investigation to help delineate more specific risk factors.

6.6.7 Retained Placenta

Three retrospective analyses have addressed the issue of retained placenta rate in the presence of fibroids. Two studies found no relationship [34, 42]. The third study [40] found a significant increase in retained placenta rate (1.2% vs. 0.5% in controls), but this disappeared when adjusted for confounders using multivariate analysis. There is no evidence that fibroids in pregnancy increase the chances of retained placenta after delivery.

6.6.8 Chorioamnionitis and Endomyometritis

Only one research group has examined the rate of chorioamnionitis in pregnancies with and without fibroids [39]. In this 10-year retrospective evaluation, there was no difference in the chorioamnionitis rate between groups. The same team also examined the rate of endomyometritis [39]. There was a non-significant trend towards more infection in the fibroid patients compared to controls (5.5% vs. 3.6%). However, even this trend disappeared when the rates were adjusted for mode of delivery.

6.6.9 Intrauterine Growth Restriction and Small for Gestational Age Newborns

Seven studies have investigated intrauterine growth restriction (IUGR) in women with fibroids. Six of these found no difference in the risk between women with fibroids and controls [33, 34, 41, 42, 46, 47], while one study that did show a difference (6.8% with fibroids vs. 1.9% for controls) made no adjustment for confounders [40]. Thus, there is little evidence that fibroid uteri predispose to IUGR. Seven studies have examined birth weight: five show no difference due to the presence of fibroids [34–36, 46, 48] while the two demonstrating a difference found the decrease to be on average only 14–177g [49, 50]. It has been suggested by data from Knight et al. that large, retroplacental fibroids are more likely to result

in poor fetal growth [50], but this issue has not been thoroughly examined.

6.6.10 Preterm Labour

Three studies have attempted to determine the relationship between preterm labour (PTL) and the presence of fibroids. All three are of relatively poor quality in that none adjusted for potential confounders. One study found no difference between women with fibroids and those without [33], one found a substantial increase in PTL in the presence of fibroids (16.3% vs. 9.7% in controls) [45], and the third uncovered an increase only when fibroids were larger than 3 cm [46]. It remains unclear whether or not there is an association between PTL and fibroid uteri.

6.6.11 Preterm Delivery

Twelve studies have addressed this issue. Ten have investigated whether preterm delivery (PTD) is more common in women with fibroids, with six showing an increased risk [34, 35, 39, 41, 49, 51] and four showing no difference between women with fibroids and those without [42–44, 48]. However, five of the six that adjusted the risk ratio for known confounders found an increase, lending greater credence to the theory that fibroids do influence PTD [35, 39, 41, 43, 49, 51]. If there is an increased risk, it is also unclear whether or not the fibroid number changes that risk, with one study saying the risk is higher with multiple myomas [37] and one claiming no difference [39]. Finally, a single study suggests location (anterior vs. posterior) does not matter [48]. In summary, it remains unclear whether or not fibroids increase PTD risk, but the best available evidence would suggest that they do.

6.6.12 Placenta Praevia

Eight studies have investigated the occurrence rate of placenta praevia in the presence of fibroids, with six being cohort studies and two being matched case–control studies. Of these, four show no difference in the rate of placenta praevia in fibroid uteri vs. control uteri [34, 35, 42, 43], while four studies show an increased occurrence rate [39–41, 44]. Four of the investigations adjust for confounders, with three claiming an increased risk of praevia [39, 41, 44] and the fourth showing a trend (adjusted OR = 1.1, 95% CI: 1.0–1.3) [43].

A recent meta-analysis has also investigated this relationship [52]. The authors found no correlation between fibroids and placenta praevia in the studies that used crude analysis, while including only the studies with odds ratios adjusted for confounders led to an increase in placenta praevia when fibroids are present (OR = 2.21, CI: 1.48–2.94). They also found that when only large fibroids of 5 cm or more are considered, the association is still present (OR = 3.53, 95% CI: 1.02–6.05).

In summary, the data regarding the predilection of placenta praevia occurring when fibroids are present is varied, but the best evidence would suggest that a relationship does indeed exist, with the possibility that larger fibroids contribute more to the formation of this pathology.

6.6.13 Placental Abruption

Twelve studies have evaluated the issue of placental abruption and its relationship to fibroids in the pregnant uterus. Of these, five studies have shown a significant increase in the incidence of abruption (odds ratios 2.1–3.7) [36, 40, 41, 46, 47], while seven studies failed to show any difference between fibroid uteri and controls [33–35, 39, 42–44]. Of interest is the fact that three of the negative studies used matched controls and had little power to detect small differences. Additionally, a meta-analysis recently investigated this relationship, including nine of these studies [53]. Among all the studies included, there was a significant increase in the rate of abruption (OR = 2.63, 95% CI: 1.38–3.88). When including only the studies with adjustments for confounders, the significance in the difference was maintained (OR = 2.29, 95% CI: 1.62–2.96).

If abruption is more common in fibroid uteri, it is of value to understand which fibroid characteristics are responsible for this adverse occurrence. Three studies examined fibroid number and found no effect [35, 39, 43]. Two studies have investigated fibroid size and risk of abruption, with one showing no effect [43] and the other noting that myomas greater than 200 cm^3 volume increased the rate of abruption [47]. Myoma location within the uterus has been culled out twice, with one study showing no effect by location [43] and another claiming that submucosal myomas significantly increase the risk [47].

Finally, two studies specifically examined the effect of fibroids when located retroplacentally [46, 47], with both finding this location to drastically elevate the risk of abruption. In fact, Rice and colleagues found abruption occurred in 8 of 14 women with retroplacental fibroids, while it occurred in only 2 of 79 women with fibroids in other locations [46]. This specificity of effect may be responsible for variation in study results, as the relationship between fibroid and placenta is not identified in most reports.

In summary, there is a likely relationship between fibroids in the pregnant uterus and the chance of abruption, but it may be limited to fibroids near to or superimposed upon the placental implantation site.

6.6.14 Premature Rupture of Membranes

Seven studies have investigated whether or not fibroids influence the rate of premature rupture of membranes (PROM). Five of the seven showed no difference in risk, with four of the five using regression analysis to correct for confounding variables [33, 39, 43, 44, 47]. Of the two studies that did find a difference, one failed to correct for confounders [40] and the other showed a small increase in the risk (adjusted OR = 1.79, 95% CI: 1.2–2.68) [36]. Similarly, when fibroid characteristics were analysed, there was no increased risk of PROM with increasing fibroid size [39, 43], number [39, 43], or location [43]. Thus, it is highly unlikely that fibroids play a role in promoting PROM in the pregnant uterus.

6.6.15 Preterm Premature Rupture of Membranes

Preterm premature rupture of membranes (PPROM) and its association with uterine fibroids has been evaluated in six studies. Three found no difference in the risk compared to normal uteri [33, 42, 51], but two of the three found absolute differences that did not reach statistical significance, possibly due to inadequately powered comparisons [33, 51]. In fact, one 'negative' study showed the rate of PPROM to be twice as high in women with large fibroids (8.89%) compared to women with only small fibroids (4.02%) or no fibroids (4.3%) [33]. Alternatively, three studies found the risk of PPROM to be elevated when fibroids are present [34, 35, 41], with two using matched controls and the other being a population-based cohort study. While the overall risk was not large (adjusted OR = 1.3, 95% CI: 1.0–1.7) [41], all three found larger fibroids to increase the risk of PPROM when compared to small fibroids or no myomas. It appears that this question remains open and deserves future high-quality investigation.

6.7 Treatment of Fibroids for Reproductive Enhancement

6.7.1 Myomectomy

While it is not clear that fibroids are in fact detrimental to fertility and maintenance of early pregnancy, myomectomies are commonly carried out as a means of enhancing fertility potential. Nearly a decade ago, we evaluated the evidence to support such interventions [13].

Submucosal myomas are the fibroids generally believed to be the most damaging to fertility and early pregnancy. However, despite widespread use of myomectomy to remove these tumours in an attempt to enhance fertility, there are few data to evaluate the efficacy. In women who have undergone myomectomy, there is an increased clinical pregnancy rate when compared to women with submucosal myomas in situ (Table 6.13). Furthermore, when compared to other infertile women without fibroids, women with submucosal myomas removed via myomectomy have

similar pregnancy rates, suggesting that once the fibroids are removed they respond to infertility treatments like all other women (Table 6.14). Despite the poor and limited quality of data, it appears as if there is likely to be benefit from removal of submucosal myomas in fertility promotion.

The most controversial area of fibroid management for fertility enhancement is the role of myomectomy for intramural myomas. In our meta-analysis, we found a paucity of studies, and those that existed failed to show any improvement in fertility or miscarriage rate following myomectomy [13] (Table 6.15).

Subserosal fibroids have not been implicated in fertility reduction, and there are no studies and thus no evidence that subserosal myomectomy is of reproductive benefit.

Other characteristics aside from location have been thought to influence the need for myomectomy. Many clinicians believe that larger fibroids may decrease fertility, and the appropriate follow-up question to ask would be if myomectomy can reverse this effect. Two studies have addressed this issue. Bulletti and his colleagues first investigated this subject in a study published in 1999. They included three groups of women: (1) those with one or more fibroids, 4–6 cm, (2) those with three or more fibroids >6 cm, and (3) a control group with either unexplained infertility or recurrent abortion. The location and size of fibroids

Table 6.13 Relationship between myomectomy of submucosal fibroids and pregnancy outcome: comparison with fibroids in situ

Submucosal fibroids: effect of myomectomy

Controls: fibroids in situ (no myomectomy)

Outcome	# Studies	RR	95% CI	Significance
Clinical pregnancy rate	2	2.034	1.081–3.826	p = 0.028
Ongoing/live birth rate	1	2.654	0.920–7.658	NS
Spontaneous abortion rate	1	0.771	0.359–1.658	NS

Table 6.14 Relationship between myomectomy of submucosal fibroids and pregnancy outcome: comparison with no fibroids

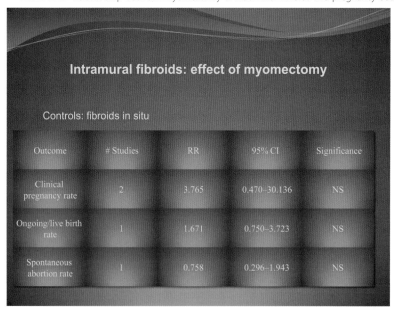

Submucosal fibroids: effect of myomectomy

Controls: infertile women with no fibroids

Outcome	# Studies	RR	95% CI	Significance
Clinical pregnancy rate	2	1.545	0.998–2.391	NS
Implantation rate	2	1.116	0.906–1.373	NS
Ongoing/live birth rate	3	1.128	0.959–1.326	NS
Spontaneous abortion rate	2	1.241	0.475–3.242	NS

Table 6.15 Relationship between myomectomy of intramural fibroids and pregnancy outcome: comparison with fibroids in situ

Intramural fibroids: effect of myomectomy

Controls: fibroids in situ

Outcome	# Studies	RR	95% CI	Significance
Clinical pregnancy rate	2	3.765	0.470–30.136	NS
Ongoing/live birth rate	1	1.671	0.750–3.723	NS
Spontaneous abortion rate	1	0.758	0.296–1.943	NS

was diagnosed only by ultrasonography. The patients had surgery depending upon 'consultation with an outside evaluator'. There was no size comparison, no age comparison, and no inclusion of women with smaller fibroids. There was no control for number of fibroids or for location. The authors found higher clinical pregnancy rates and delivery rates in women undergoing the surgery, compared with women with in situ fibroids [54].

In 2004, Bulletti et al. published a second report, looking prospectively at women who had from one to five fibroids, at least one >5 cm, that were either intramural or subserosal in location. Diagnostic modalities included ultrasound and/or hysterosalpingogram and/or hysteroscopy. Ages were not reported, women with smaller fibroids were not included, and the patients themselves made the choice of surgery or not. Again, women undergoing myomectomy were found to have an increased clinical pregnancy and delivery rate following treatment [55].

These studies are difficult to utilize as justification for surgical intervention in infertile women with large fibroids. Location of the fibroid was not provided, and the allocation to surgery or no surgery is not randomized but based on clinical opinion and patient choice. Furthermore, countless confounding factors that might influence fertility are not included, much less adjusted for. In summary, it is unclear whether or not large fibroids, simply due to size, reduce fertility. However, there is no good evidence that removing these large fibroids will enhance fertility. In fact, there is a distinct possibility that such surgery might prove detrimental to fertility potential.

The effect of myomectomy in improving late pregnancy outcomes has barely been examined. A single study looked retrospectively at women who underwent myomectomy prior to pregnancy versus those that did not [56]. The study showed that delivery outcomes after myomectomy were worse, with an increase in PTD, caesarean section, and blood loss compared with women that had fibroids >5 cm left in situ. The patients had similar ages, gravity, parity, twin, and placenta praevia rates. There were no differences in abruption, birth weight, neonatal morbidity, or postpartum infection. Thus, to date there is no evidence that myomectomy will improve any of the late obstetrical problems that are increased by fibroids.

6.7.2 Uterine Artery Embolization

Uterine artery embolization (UAE) is a procedure performed by interventional radiologists who occlude the vascular supply to the uterus and thus any fibroids present, resulting in decrease in size and metabolic activity of the tumours. The procedure has been well established for treatment of other fibroid symptoms, but until recently, there was limited information regarding subsequent reproduction in such patients. There are no studies utilizing this intervention to improve fertility. However, there are 17 total studies addressing pregnancy outcomes, including almost 1,000 patients. There is a single randomized controlled trial, 2 cohort studies, and 14 case series [57].

In the randomized trial, 121 women were randomized to either uterine artery embolization or myomectomy. They had similar baseline characteristics including age, size of fibroids, and follicle-stimulating hormone (FSH) values. The fibroids had to be intramural and measure at least 4 cm average diameter. The pregnancy rates were similar at 50% and 78%, respectively, but the spontaneous abortion rates were significantly higher after UAE at 60%, compared with only 20% after myomectomy ($p < 0.05$).

When looking at the two prospective cohort studies, pregnancy rates were 51% and 69% for women after UAE, and 47% and 67% in the comparative groups that underwent laparoscopic uterine artery occlusion (LUAO) (non-significant). However, miscarriage rates were 56% and 45% after UAE and 11% and 38% after LUAO ($p < 0.001$).

Of the 14 case series, 8 were prospective and 6 were retrospective without control groups. Women underwent UAE for symptomatic uterine fibroids and the studies were not designed to evaluate pregnancy or miscarriage rates. Pregnancy rates ranged from 14% to 61%, and miscarriage rates ranged from 2% to 100%. The median pregnancy rate after UAE was 29% ($I^2 = 89.7\%$) and the median miscarriage rate was 25% ($I^2 = 54.4\%$) [57].

There are also reports of uterine ischaemia leading to endometrial atrophy, intracavitary protrusion of fibroids, fistulae between the fibroid and the endometrial cavity, and adhesive disease [58]. Based upon these data, at this time, most clinicians recommend against UAE for women interested in future family building.

Table 6.16 Pregnancy outcomes after high-intensity focused ultrasound or thermal ablation (C/S, caesarean section; HIFU, high-intensity focused ultrasound; SAB, spontaneous abortion; TAB, therapeutic abortion; VD, vaginal delivery)

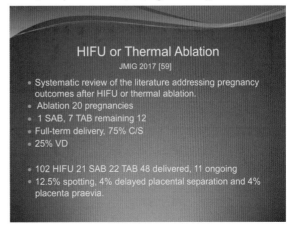

6.7.3 High-Intensity Focused Ultrasound and Thermal Ablation

High-intensity focused ultrasound (HIFU) is a new technique designed to destroy uterine fibroid tissue in situ. To date, there are approximately 102 pregnancies reported after HIFU treatment prior to pregnancy. When compared either with women with untreated fibroids or with the normal population, it appears that outcomes do not differ significantly [59] (Table 6.16).

Thus, while both HIFU and thermal ablation are of value in treating symptomatic fibroids, there is no evidence that either improves fertility or pregnancy outcome.

References

1. Munro MG, *Abnormal Uterine Bleeding*. Cambridge, UK: Cambridge University Press, 2010.

2. Soares S, dos Reis MMB, Camargos A. Diagnostic accuracy of sonohysterogram, transvaginal sonography, and hysterosalpingography inpatients with uterine cavity diseases. *Fertil Steril* 2000;73:406–11.

3. Keltz MD, Olive DL, Kim AH, Arici A. Sonohysterogram for screening in recurrent pregnancy loss. *Fertil Steril* 1997;67:670–4.

4. Fedele L, Bianchi S, Dorta M, et al. Transvaginal ultrasonography versus hysteroscopy in the diagnosis of uterine submucous myomas. *Obstet Gynecol* 1991;77:745–8.

5. Pritts EA, Olive DL. When should uterine fibroids be treated. *Curr Obstet Gynecol Rep* 2012;1:71–80.

6. Fukuda M, Shimizu T, Fukuda K, et al. Transvaginal hysterosonography for differential diagnosis between submucosal and intramural myoma. *Gynecol Obstet Invest* 1993;35:236–9.

7. Cicinelli E, Romano F, Anastasio PS, et al. Transabdominal sonohysterography, transvaginal sonography, and hysteroscopy in the evaluation of submucosal myomas. *Obstet Gynecol* 1995;85:42–7.

8. Dueholm M, Lundorf E, Hansen ES, et al. Evaluation of the uterine cavity with magnetic resonance imaging, transvaginal sonography, hysterosonographic examination and diagnostic hysteroscscopy. *Fertil Steril* 2001;76:350–7.

9. Johnson G, MacLehose RF, Baird DD, et al. Uterine leiomyomata and fecundability in the Right From the Start study. *Hum Reprod* 2012;27:2991–7.

10. Pritts EA. Fibroids and infertility: a systematic review of the evidence. *Obstet Gynecol Surv* 2001;58:483–91.

11. Shokeir T, El-Shafei M, Yousef H, et al. Submucous myomas and their implications in the pregnancy rates of patients with otherwise unexplained primary infertility undergoing hysteroscopic myomectomy: a randomized matched control study. *Fertil Steril* 2010;94 (2):724–9.

12. Styer AK, Jin S, Liu D, et al. Association of uterine fibroids and pregnancy outcomes after ovarian stimulation-intrauterine insemination for unexplained infertility. *Fertil Steril* 2017;107 (3):756–62.

13. Pritts EA, Olive DL, Parker WH. Fibroids and infertility: an updated systematic review of the evidence. *Fertil Steril* 2009;91 (4):1215–23.

14. Bozdag G, Esinler I, Boynukalin K, et al. Single intramural leiomyoma with normal hysteroscopic findings does not affect ICSI-embryo transfer outcome. *RBM Online* 2009;19 (2):276–80.

15. Gianaroli L. Effect of inner myometrium fibroid on reproductive outcome after IVF. *Reprod Biomed Online* 2005;10:633–40.

16. Jun SH, Ginsburg ES, Racowsky C, et al. Uterine leiomyomas and their effect on in vitro fertilization outcome: a retrospective study. *J Assist Reprod Genet* 2001;18 (3):139–43.

17. Manzo AB, Delgadillo JCB, Rueda SO, et al. Efecto de los miomas intramurales y subserosos en los ciclos de fertilizacion in vitro y sus resultados perinatales. *Ginecol Obstet Mex* 2006;74:55–65.

18. Somigliana E, De Benedictis S, Vercellini P, et al. Fibroids not encroaching the endometrial cavity and IVF success rate: a prospective study. *Hum Reprod* 2011;26(4):834–9.

19. Surrey ES, Lietz AK, Schoolcraft WB. Impact of intramural leiomyomata in patients with a normal endometrial cavity on in vitro fertilization-embryo transfer cycle outcome. *Fertil Steril* 2001;75:405–10.

20. Wang W, Check JH. Effect of corporal fibroids on outcome following embryo transfer in donor-oocyte recipients. *Clin Exp Obstet Gynecol* 2004;31:263–4.

21. Klatzky PC, Lane DE, Ryan IP, et al. The effect of fibroids without cavity involvement on ART outcomes independent of ovarian age. *Hum Reprod* 2007;22:521–6.

22. Horcajadas JA, Goyri E, Higon MA, et al. Endometrial receptivity and implantation are not affected by the presence of uterine intramural leiomyomas: a clinical and functional genomics analysis.

J Clin Endocrinol Metab
2008;**93**:3490–8.

23. Oliveira FG, Abdelmassih VG, Diamond MP, et al. Impact of subserosal and intramural uterine fibroids that do not distort the endometrial cavity on the outcome of in vitro fertilization-intracytoplasmic sperm injection. *Fertil Steril* 2004;**81**:582–7.

24. Vimercati, A, Scioscia M, Lorusso F, et al. Do uterine fibroids affect IVF outcomes? *RMB Online* 2007;**15**(6):686–91.

25. Yan L, Ding L, Li C, et al. Effect of fibroids not distorting the endometrial cavity on the outcomes if in vitro fertilization treatment: a retrospective cohort study. *Fertil Steril* 2014;**101** (3):716–21.

26. Yarali H, Bukulmez O. The effect of intramural and subserous uterine fibroids on implantation and clinical pregnancy rates in patients having intracytoplasmic sperm injection. *Arch Gynecol Obstet* 2002;**266**:30–3.

27. Check JH, Choe JK, Lee G, et al. The effect on IVF outcomes of small intramural fibroids not compressing the uterine cavity as determined by a prospective matched control study. *Hum Reprod* 2002;**17**:1244–8.

28. Ezzedine D, Norwitz ER. Are women with uterine fibroids at increased risk for adverse pregnancy outcome? *Clin Obstet Gynecol* 2016;**59**(1):119–27.

29. Hartmann KE, Velez EDR, Savitz DA, et al. Prospective cohort study of uterine fibroids and miscarriage risk. *Am J Epidemiol* 2017 Nov 15;**186**(10):1140–8.

30. Sundermann AC, Velez Edwards, DR, Bray MJ, et al. Leiomyomas in pregnancy and spontaneous abortion. *Obstet Gynecol* 2017;**130** (5):1065–72.

31. Benson CB, Chow JS, Chang-Lee W, et al. Outcome of pregnancies in women with uterine leiomyomas identified by sonography in the first trimester. *J Clin Ultrasound* 2001;**29**:261–4.

32. Segars JH, Parrott EC, Nagel JD, et al. Proceedings from the Third National Institutes of Health International Congress on Advances in Uterine Leiomyoma Research: comprehensive review, conference summary and future recommendations. *Hum Reprod Update* 2014;**20**:309.

33. Martin J, Ulrich NC, Duplantis S, et al. Obstetrical outcomes of ultrasound identified uterine fibroids in pregnancy. *Am J Perinatol* 2016;**33**:1218–22.

34. Shavell VI, Thakur M, Sawant A, et al. Adverse obstetric outcomes associated with sonographically identified large uterine fibroids. *Fertil Steril* 2012;**97**:107–10.

35. Ciavattini A, Clemente N, Delli Carpini G, et al. Number and size of uterine fibroids and obstetric outcomes. *J Matern Fetal Neonatal Med* 2015;**28**(4): 484–8.

36. Coronado GD, Marshall LM, Schwartz SM. Complications in pregnancy, labour and delivery with uterine leiomyomas: a population-based study. *Obstet Gynecol* 2000;**95**:764–9.

37. Lam SJ, Best S, Kumar S. The impact of fibroid characteristics on pregnancy outcome. *Am J Obstet Gynecol* 2014;**211**:395. e1–5.

38. Michels KA, Edwards DRV, Baird DD, et al. Uterine leiomyomata and cesarean birth risk: a prospective cohort with standardized imaging. *Ann Epidem* 2014;**24**:122–6.

39. Qidwai GI, Caughey AB, Jacoby AF. Obstetric outcomes in women with sonographicallly identified uterine leiomyomata. *Obstet Gynecol* 2006;**107**(2):376–82.

40. Sheiner E, Bashiri A, Levy A, et al. Obstetric characteristics and perinatal outcome of pregnancies with uterine leiomyomas. *J Reprod Med* 2004;**49**:182–6.

41. Stout MK, Odibo AO, Graseck AS. Leiomyomas at routine second-trimester ultrasound examination and adverse obstetric outcomes. *Obstet Gynecol* 2010;**116**:1056–63.

42. Vergani P, Ghidini A, Strobelt N, et al. Do uterine leiomyomas influence pregnancy outcome? *Am J Perinatol* 1994;**11**(5):356–8.

43. Zhao R, Wang X, Zou L, et al. Adverse obstetric outcomes in pregnant women with uterine fibroids in China: a multicenter survey involving 112,403 deliveries. *PLoS ONE* 2017;**12**(11): e0187821.

44. Vergani P, Locatelli A, Ghidini A, et al. Later uterine leiomyomata and risk of cesarean delivery. *Obstet Gynecol* 2007;**109** (2):410–14.

45. Jenabi E, Khazaei S. The effect of uterine leiomyoma on the risk of malpresentation and cesarean: a meta-analysis. *J Matern Fetal Neonatal Med* 2018;**31**(1):87–92.

46. Rice JP, Kay HH, Mahony BS. The clinical significance of uterine leiomyomas in pregnancy. *Am J Obstet Gynecol* 1989;**160**:1212–16.

47. Exacoustos C, Rosati P. Ultrasound diagnosis of uterine myomas and complications in pregnancy. *Obstet Gynecol* 1993;**82**:97–101.

48. Deveer M, Deveer R, Engin-Ustun Y, et al. Comparison of pregnancy outcomes in different localizations of uterine fibroids. *Clin Exp Obstet Gynecol* 2012;**39**(4): 516–18.

49. Chen Y, Lin H, Chen S, et al. Increased risk of preterm births among women with uterine leiomyoma: a nationwide population-based study. *Hum Reprod* 2009;**24**(12):3049–56.

50. Knight JC, Elliot JO, Amburgey OL. Effect of maternal retroplacental leiomyomas on fetal growth. *J Obstet Gynaecol Can* 2016;**38**(12):1100–4.

53

51. Lai J, Caughey AB, Qidwai GI, et al. Neonatal outcomes in women with sonographically identified uterine leiomyomata. *J Matern Fetal Neonatal Med* 2012;**25**(6):710–13.

52. Jenabi E, Fereidooni B. The uterine leiomyoma and placenta previa: a meta-analysis. *J Matern Fetal Neonatal Med* 2017;doi: 10.1080/ 14767058.2017.1400003.

53. Klatzky PC, Tran ND, Caughey AB, et al. Fibroids and reproductive outcomes: a systematic literature review from conception to delivery. *Am J Obstet Gynecol* 2008;**198**(4):357–66.

54. Bulletti C, De Ziegler D, Polli V, et al. The role of leiomyomas in infertility. *J Am Assoc Gynecol Laparosc* 1999;**6**:441–5.

55. Bulletti C, De Ziegler D, Sett PL, et al. Myomas, pregnancy outcomes, and invitro fertilization. *Ann N Y Acad Sci* 2004;**1034**:84–92.

56. Kinugasa-Taniguchi Y, Ueda Y, Hara-Ohyagi C, et al. Impaired delivery outcomes in pregnancies following myomectomy compared to myoma complicated pregnancies. *J Reprod Med* 2011;**56**(3–4): 142–8.

57. Karlsen K, Hrobjartsson A, Korsholm M, et al. Fertility after uterine artery embolization of fibroids: a systematic review. *Arch Gynecol Obstet* 2018;**297**:13–25.

58. Mara M, Fucikova Z, Kuzel D, et al. Hysteroscopy after uterine fibroid embolization in women of fertile age. *J Obstet Gynaecol Res* 2007;**33**(3):316–24.

59. Keltz J, Levie M, Chudnoff S. Pregnancy outcomes after direct myoma thermal ablation: review of the literature. *J Minim Invasive Gynecol* 2017;**24**(4):538–45.

Chapter 7

Open Myomectomy

Tin-Chiu Li and Jacqueline P. W. Chung

7.1 Introduction

Uterine fibroids or leiomyomas are the most common benign gynaecological tumours; up to 25–30% of women may be diagnosed with fibroids during their lifetime [1]. Women with uterine fibroids may be asymptomatic, or they may present with menstrual symptoms such as menorrhagia and dysmenorrhoea, pressure symptoms, infertility, recurrent miscarriage or complications during pregnancy like red degeneration.

The management of uterine fibroids depends on the presenting symptom, number, size and location of the fibroid within the uterus and the patient's fertility wish. The risk of malignancy is extremely rare in slow-growing fibroids. However, in suspiciously fast-growing fibroids, the risk of malignancy can be up to 0.27% [2].

Small asymptomatic fibroids are usually managed expectantly. However, for those with large symptomatic fibroids, surgery may be required. In those who have completed childbearing, hysterectomy may be appropriate, but for women who still wish to conceive in the future, myomectomy could be considered. Myomectomy can be performed via hysteroscopy, laparoscopy or laparotomy (open myomectomy); the choice being primarily dependent on the location of the fibroids, as well as on the size, number, available expertise and facilities.

7.2 Open Myomectomy

7.2.1 Why Laparotomy?

Up till now, increasing number of intramural and subserosal fibroids are being removed laparoscopically, for several reasons [3]. It is minimally invasive with reduced need for postoperative analgesia and hospital stay. It is often quoted that recovery following laparoscopic myomectomy is speedier than open myomectomy. Whilst this is still true, the difference is becoming less significant as women after open myomectomy in many modern units are being mobilized earlier, allowed to eat early and discharged home after 24–48 hours. In recent years, it appears that open myomectomy is regaining favour in women who wish to conceive again, as the risk of scar rupture during pregnancy following laparoscopic myomectomy is perceived to be higher than that after open myomectomy.

In addition, open myomectomy remains necessary in several situations, such as a huge subserosal or intramural fibroids, multiple fibroids or when entry into the uterine cavity is expected [4]. Open myomectomy is also preferred in cases with vascular fibroids or fibroids with suspected sarcomatous change, and in women who would not wish to consider blood transfusion (Jehovah's witness).

7.3 Preoperative Counselling and Preoperative Preparation

Whilst many aspects of preoperative counselling and preparation apply to both laparoscopic and open myomectomy, given that the size of the fibroid or number of fibroids are often larger in the case of open myomectomy, detailed counselling on the possible (immediate and delayed) complications of myomectomy and preoperative preparations to minimize the various complications are particularly important.

7.3.1 Preoperative Counselling

Women considering myomectomy should be fully counselled regarding the various possible risks, including anaesthetic complications, infection, visceral injury, bleeding, blood transfusion, hysterectomy (~1%), recurrence and adhesion formation.

7.3.2 Preoperative Preparation

Women undergoing myomectomy should have their baseline haemoglobin level checked. Anaemia if present should be treated before the planned surgery as it is known to increase surgical morbidities. The anaemia can be corrected with oral iron supplements or blood transfusion depending on urgency. The use of hormone treatment to suppress menstruation for a few months prior to surgery may be considered if there is significant menorrhagia. Cross-matching of blood should be performed if excessive blood loss is anticipated. Bowel preparation is not routinely necessary but may be considered in those with high risk of intra-abdominal adhesions. Prophylactic measures against thromboembolism such as elastic stockings or subcutaneous heparin should be undertaken.

7.3.3 GnRH Analogues

Prior to surgery, a GnRH agonist can be used to induce amenorrhea, which can improve preoperative haemoglobin as well as reduce intraoperative blood loss [5]. Moreover, it can shrink the fibroid and uterine size and may, in some cases, enable a pfannenstiel incision to be made instead of a midline incision.

Yet many surgeons do not advocate the routine use of GnRH analogues, for many reasons. Firstly, it makes the surgical planes less distinct and thus more difficult for surgeons to enucleate the fibroids during the operation. This may then increase the difficulty of the operation and prolong the operative time [4]. Secondly, some surgeons believe that it causes small fibroids to shrink (temporarily) and so become more difficult to be detected during the operation, which may therefore increase the recurrence rate. In addition, GnRH agonist therapy is associated with unwanted side effects and increases the overall cost of the treatment.

7.3.4 Ulipristal Acetate (UPA)

Ulipristal acetate (UPA) is a selective progesterone receptor modulator (SPRM) and has been recently introduced in the treatment of uterine fibroids [6]. It has been shown to be effective in reducing menorrhagia and fibroid size and may be an alternative to preoperative GnRH agonist therapy. There is increasing use of UPA for uterine shrinkage before surgery nowadays [6, 7]. However, it is unclear if it makes the enucleation of the fibroid more difficult, as in the case of GnRH agonist therapy.

7.3.5 Preoperative Fibroid Mapping

It is useful to ascertain the number and location of fibroids before the operation. This can usually be performed with a careful ultrasound examination. A 3D saline infusion sonography may from time to time provide additional information. In more complex cases, magnetic resonance imaging may be needed [8]. Fibroid mapping before the operation allows better surgical planning, including a decision regarding the choice of laparoscopic or open myomectomy, whether special equipment is required and the likely operation time.

7.4 Operation Techniques

7.4.1 Microsurgical Principles

It is important to follow microsurgical techniques during open myomectomy. Minimal handling of tissue with meticulous haemostasis throughout the operation is crucial. Atraumatic instruments should be used when handling tissue. Moreover, the operative field should be kept moist with continuous irrigation [4].

7.4.2 Abdominal Incision

A suprapubic transverse pfannenstiel incision is sufficient in most of the cases. It is not only aesthetically acceptable to the patient but is also shown to be associated with less postoperative pain and quicker postoperative recovery. Even when the size of the fibroid uterus means that it is well above the umbilicus, it is often possible to shrink it down to the level of the umbilicus with GnRH analogues [9], so that a suprapubic transverse pfannenstiel skin incision is sufficient. A midline incision is required only in cases where the uterine size remains huge despite GnRH down-regulation, and when difficulty with access such as those with obesity or dense adhesion is encountered. When there is already an existing midline incision scar, it is still preferable to perform the laparotomy via a new pfannenstiel incision.

7.4.3 Reducing Blood Loss

Reducing blood loss is the most important aspect of myomectomy surgery. The risk of hysterectomy has been quoted to be 1–2%, and up to 20–30% of patients may require blood transfusion during the operation [10]. Many techniques for reducing blood loss are applicable to both laparoscopic and open surgery, while some methods are specific for open myomectomy.

7.4.3.1 Methods Specific to Open Myomectomy

Rubber Tourniquets

Tourniquets have been used to reduce the blood flow from the main feeding vessels. When a single tourniquet is used, the tourniquet is applied around the cervix to occlude both uterine arteries. When triple tourniquets are used, the ovarian vessels are occluded lateral to the ovaries [11]. The broad ligament is opened anteriorly with the bladder reflected. After the surgeon creates a small opening in the avascular leaf of the broad ligament on either side of the uterine isthmus superior to the uterine vessels, a rubber tourniquet can be threaded through the holes and tied anterior around the cervix at the level of the internal os to compress the uterine arteries. In addition, two further tubings can be threaded through the defect over the broad ligament and looped around the infundibulopelvic ligament lateral to the fallopian tube and ovaries to compress the ovarian vessels.

A recent randomized controlled trial (RCT) by Al et al. [12] involving 48 patients found no significant difference in the outcome of blood loss between triple and single uterine tourniquets (322 ± 223 vs. 426 ± 355 mL, p = 0.230) at open myomectomy. In another RCT, triple tourniquets have been shown to be effective in reducing bleeding and transfusion rates and appear to have no obvious adverse effect on uterine perfusion or ovarian function when compared to controls [13]. Some surgeons have used the Foley catheter as a tourniquet as it is easily available in theatres [14].

Bonney's Myomectomy Clamp

Victor Bonney was the pioneer for open myomectomy, and modern myomectomy technique has changed very little since he described his technique in 1946. He developed a technique to reduce the blood supply to the uterus and fibroid by using a paracervical mechanical clamp also known as the Bonney myomectomy clamp [15]. This clamp is placed at the level of the cervix to temporarily compress the uterine arteries during the operation. It can be used in conjunction with rubber tourniquets to occlude the ovarian vessels. The ureters should be traced before applying the clamps. The clamps can be released every 15 minutes to reduce the chance of irreversible ischaemic damage.

Haemostatic Suture

A further advantage of open myomectomy over that of laparoscopic myomectomy is that haemostatic suture can be applied promptly in case of brisk bleeding from a major feeding vessel. Active bleeding can be controlled immediately with manual compression or the application of a clamp, followed by the application of an haemostatic suture. There is little doubt that effective haemostasis can be achieved more quickly during open myomectomy compared with laparoscopic myomectomy.

Uterine Artery Ligation

Uterine artery ligation involves the suturing of both uterine arteries. Its efficacy remains controversial. Sampaz et al. [16] showed that intraoperative blood loss was lower with bilateral ligation of the ascending branches of the uterine artery when compared to tourniquet methods during myomectomy. They found that the effect of ligation on haemorrhage continues in the postoperative period. Moreover, Helel et al. [17] performed an RCT to compare the effectiveness of preliminary uterine artery ligation versus pericervical mechanical tourniquet in reducing haemorrhage during myomectomy. Their study included a total of 103 patients undergoing myomectomy. The operative blood loss was found to be significantly less with uterine artery ligation than with tourniquet (434 vs. 823 mL, p < 0.001). The mean operation time (51 vs. 76 minutes, p < 0.001) and postoperative hospital stay (4.1 vs. 5.1 days, p < 0.001) were also significantly shorter than in the tourniquet group. Their study concluded that uterine artery ligation was more effective than pericervical tourniquet in reducing blood loss during abdominal myomectomy.

However, there are concerns that uterine artery ligation may adversely affect wound healing, compromise ovarian blood supply, cause intrauterine adhesions and affect endometrial function. Further studies are required to assess if these concerns are justified.

7.4.3.2 Methods Feasible for Both Laparoscopic and Open Myomectomy

Vasopressin Injection

Vasopressin is a potent vasoconstrictor. Vasopressin may be injected into the broad ligament close to the insertion of ovarian and round ligaments and also superficially into the capsule of fibroids before incision (Figure 7.1). In an RCT performed by Frederick et al. [18], vasopressin was effective in preventing blood loss and reducing the need for blood transfusion during myomectomy. Another RCT involving 52 patients [19] compared the efficacy of perivascular vasopressin and tourniquet in minimizing bleeding during myomectomy. Vasopressin resulted in less blood loss (mean 287.3 mL vs. 512.7 mL for tourniquet, p = 0.036). Six out of 26 patients in the tourniquet group lost more than 1,000 mL of blood, whereas all of the vasopressin subjects lost less than this amount (p = 0.023). Their study concluded that vasopressin prevented blood loss better than tourniquet use during myomectomy.

However, vasopressin may rarely cause severe hypotension, bradycardia and even death [20], especially when it is inadvertently injected intravascularly. It is wise to aspirate before injection of vasopressin to avoid direct injection of vasopressin into a blood vessel. It is contraindicated in patients with vascular and renal diseases. The usual dose is 6 IU, at a dilution of 1 IU/mL normal saline.

GnRH Agonists (Preoperative)

GnRH agonists may be used to prevent blood loss during myomectomy. An earlier meta-analysis of 26 RCTs on the use of GnRH agonist before surgery for fibroids (either hysterectomy or myomectomy) has shown a beneficial impact on blood loss as well as pre- and postoperative haemoglobin and haematocrit level [9].

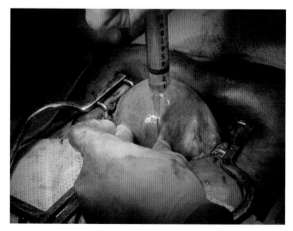

Figure 7.1 Injection of diluted vasopressin into the myometrium surrounding the fibroid before myomectomy.

Uterotonic Agents

Uterotonic agents are often used as first-line treatment during postpartum haemorrhage. Oxytocin is the most commonly used uterotonic agent, and oxytocin receptors have recently been demonstrated in fibroid uterus. Atashkhoei et al. [21] performed a double-blinded randomized controlled trial and found oxytocin safe and effective in decreasing blood loss during abdominal myomectomy. They randomized 40 women undergoing open myomectomy to the study group (with 30 IU in 500 mL normal saline given during myomectomy) and 40 women to the placebo group (pure normal saline given). The estimated intraoperative blood loss in the study group (189.5 mL) was significantly lower than in the placebo group (692.25 mL), p < 0.0001. They also found the need for blood transfusion was significantly lower in the study group. Blood transfusions were required for 3 (7.5%) women in the study group and 10 (25%) women in the placebo group.

Intravenous Tranexamic Acid

Intravenous tranexamic acid is an anti-fibrolytic agent commonly used to treat menorrhagia. In recent years, it has also been used to reduce blood loss during caesarean section. Wang et al. [22] have recently performed a meta-analysis of randomized controlled trials in assessing the efficiency and safety of tranexamic acid for reducing blood loss during open myomectomy. A total of four RCTs involving 328 patients were analysed. They found significant differences in terms of total blood loss, postoperative haemoglobin level, transfusion requirements and duration of surgery in those with tranexamic acid use when compared to those without. However, further high-quality RCTs are necessary to confirm the clinical benefit.

Uterine Artery Embolization

Preoperative uterine artery embolization (UAE) has been employed not only to shrink large fibroids but also to reduce blood loss during myomectomy. A retrospective study [23] showed a mean reduction of 77% in uterine volume and 46% in fibroid diameter among 20 patients who underwent open myomectomy after UAE. Whilst the results appeared encouraging, there are concerns regarding wound healing, ovarian blood supply and endometrial function, as in the case of uterine artery ligation.

Cell Saver

The use of autologous blood cell salvage has been suggested in women undergoing abdominal myomectomy. This can not only recycle the blood lost during the operation but also avoid the risks related to allogenic blood transfusion, including immunological reactions. Yamada et al. [24] found it useful in patients with heavy blood loss during open myomectomy. However, in a study involving 425 patients undergoing open myomectomy, Son et al. [25] suggested that routine use of cell salvage was not warranted. Cell salvage is not readily available in every unit and the set-up requires special expertise. It should be used in women who would not wish to consider blood transfusion (Jehovah's witnesses).

Gelatine Fibrin Matrix

FloSeal$^®$ (FloSeal Matrix; Baxter Healthcare Corp., Fremont, CA) is a gelatin fibrin matrix with both a bovine-derived gelatin matrix component and a human-derived thrombin component [26]. It is biocompatible and is completely reabsorbed within 6–8 weeks, which is consistent with normal wound healing. It has been widely employed in various specialties for haemostasis [27]. We have also been using it for haemostasis after laparoscopic ovarian stripping for ovarian endometriomas. After application to the bleeding sites, the special particles of the FloSeal$^®$ Matrix will swell approximately 10–20% upon contact with blood and provide an additional compression effect. It can achieve haemostasis within 2 minutes at the site of action. It works well in both wet and active bleeding sites but must not be injected directly into vessels due to the risk of thromboembolism. Raga's team have applied FloSeal$^®$ to the site of the uterine bleeding during myomectomy [28]. They found the use of FloSeal reduced haemorrhage during myomectomy. FloSeal$^®$ is particularly useful in situations when there is persistent oozing from serosal wound edge or suture holes, or when the bleeding occurs at locations difficult for suturing or diathermy, e.g. near the ureters following removal of a broad ligament fibroid.

7.4.4 Uterine Incision

7.4.4.1 How?

A serosal incision over the main bulk of the fibroid should be made. Incision with a scalpel is preferred to the use of diathermy to reduce the risk of subsequent scar rupture resulting from excessive diathermy. The incision is then extended towards the myometrium until the capsule of the fibroid is reached. The fibroid is then enucleated as described below.

7.4.4.2 Single versus Multiple Incision

If several fibroids are situated in close proximity, it may be possible to make a single incision to remove the multiple fibroids. Whilst it is desirable to reduce the number of incisions, this should not be done without due regard to other surgical factors. An anterior fibroid should be removed via an anterior incision and a posterior fibroid should be removed via a posterior wall incision to avoid unnecessary entry into the uterine cavity, which would increase the risk of subsequent scar rupture. The incision should be made over the maximal bulge of the fibroid. With open myomectomy, there is more flexibility in choosing a vertical, transverse or horizontal incision, to avoid getting too close to the cornual region (insertion of the fallopian tube), uterine vessels and bladder. In contrast, with laparoscopic myomectomy the choice of the incision is often influenced by how the surgeon is used to suturing in a particular position. Some surgeons prefer a transverse incision to avoid cutting through arcuate vessels, as this may reduce blood loss and allow better myometrial healing. In the case of a fundal fibroid, anterior incisions are preferred as posterior incisions are associated with an increased risk of adhesion formation. In the past, some surgeons would insist on making a single anterior incision regardless of the number of fibroids present, on the basis that adhesion formation after myomectomy is more common after a posterior wall incision; however, this is no longer regarded as necessary.

7.4.5 Enucleation

Once incision has been made, the fibroid capsule or the fibroid myometrial plane should be identified. Enucleation of the fibroid may be facilitated by applying traction to the fibroid using a myoma screw, separation of the fibroid from the capsule with a MacDonald dissector and the application of a twisting force towards the end of the enucleation process. During enucleation, bleeding from the feeding vessels can be controlled with diathermy or sutures. Excessive diathermy should be avoided as it may lead to poor healing of the myometrium and an increased risk of future uterine rupture. After enucleation, the uterine cavity should be checked for integrity. It is not always necessary to enucleate all fibroids; multiple small intramural fibroids that do not distort the uterine cavity may sometimes be left behind. In case the fibroid myometrial plane is difficult to distinguish, one should be beware of the possibility of adenomyosis and decide if the procedure should continue [29].

7.4.6 Closure

Once the fibroids are removed, it is important to carefully close the uterine defect and to ensure that any dead space is obliterated from the bottom up, using sutures to achieve good apposition and effective haemostasis. Careful reconstruction of the uterine wall is essential as it reduces the risk of scar dehiscence during a subsequent pregnancy. The uterine defect should be closed in two to three layers depending on the depth of myometrium. In closing a large defect, interrupted sutures may be considered for the deep, innermost layers. Several interrupted sutures may be placed along the entire length of the defect in the uterine wall; they are held separately by artery forceps but not tied until after all the sutures have been placed (Figures 7.2 and 7.3). The assistant is then asked to use fingers to bring the opposing edges of the uterine wall together to reduce tension on the sutures when the knots are tightly tied, one after the other (Figure 7.4). In this way, it will not

only ensure optimal closure of any dead space but also reduce the chances of the sutures cutting through the myometrium when they are tightened and tied (Figure 7.5).

In placing deep sutures, especially when the cavity has been entered, particular care must be exercised to avoid passing sutures through the endometrial cavity leading to its obliteration (Figure 7.6). When it happens, postoperative amenorrhea will inevitably follow.

In cases where the uterine defect is particularly large, redundant myometrium may be excised. Bonney described a 'hood' method of closure of the

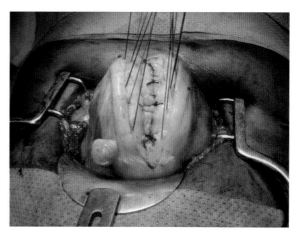

Figure 7.3 The second layer of closure: interrupted stitches are held with artery forceps.

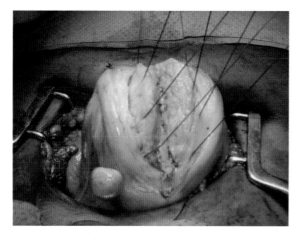

Figure 7.2 The placement of interrupted stitches in the first deep layer of the myometrium; the sutures are held by artery forceps till all the sutures have been placed, before they are tied one after the other.

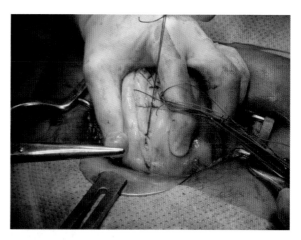

Figure 7.4 An assistant brings the uterine walls together for better tissue approximation and to reduce the tension when the interrupted sutures are tied.

uterine cavity defect after enucleation of a very large single posterior tumour [15]. This is performed by suturing the redundant flap of serosa to cover the myometrium over the fundus and the anterior wall to avoid adhesion formation.

A few additional penultimate horizontal subcuticular stitches may be applied to help regain a globular shape after reconstruction. The serosa is usually closed using a 'baseball' technique in which the edges are approximated closely with the serosa edge folded inwards to avoid exposure of the underlying myometrium. A fine non-absorbable or delayed absorption suture like 3-0 PDS is recommended for closure of the serosal layer.

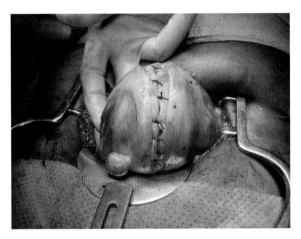

Figure 7.5 The uterus after two layers of myometrial closure using interrupted sutures.

7.4.7 Adhesion Prevention

Postoperative adhesion is a well-recognized complication of myomectomy, whether via laparoscopy or laparotomy. Meticulous haemostasis and gentle handling of the tissue should reduce the risk of adhesion formation. Continuous irrigation should be used instead of gauzes to clear the operative field and to keep the serosal layer moist and avoid desiccation, which predisposes to adhesion formation. Several mechanical adhesion barriers including Interceed, Hyalobarrier gel or Seprafilm have been used [4, 29], but so far none has been shown to be superior to any other.

Specifically, following open myomectomy, a free omental graft may be placed over the uterine incision after repair [4], anchored with fine 4-0 non-absorbable sutures or delayed absorbable sutures (Figures 7.7–7.9).

7.5 Postoperative Care

The vital signs of the patient should be monitored closely after the operation. A drop in haemoglobin or blood pressure or increase in pulse rate should alert to the possibility of postoperative haemorrhage. Excessive postoperative pelvic pain may signal the formation of haematoma in the uterus.

Contraception is advised for at least 3–6 months to allow time for the myometrium to heal. In case the uterine cavity has been entered, to reduce the risk of scar rupture, the patient should be advised to have elective caesarean section should pregnancy occur.

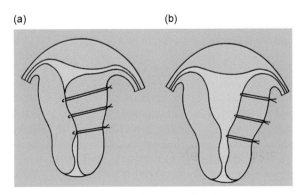

Figure 7.6 (a) Inadvertent obliteration of endometrial cavity by deep sutures. (b) Careful placement of deep sutures to avoid obliteration of uterine cavity.

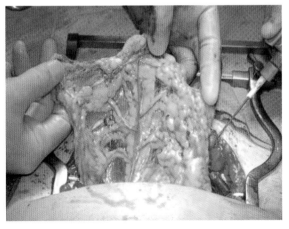

Figure 7.7 A piece of omentum is pulled down after myomectomy, ready to be excised for use as a free graft.

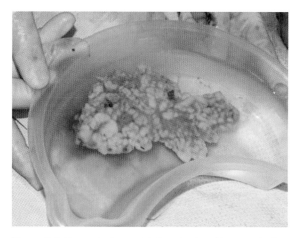

Figure 7.8 The excised omental tissue is placed in normal saline solution before being used as a graft to cover the uterine incision.

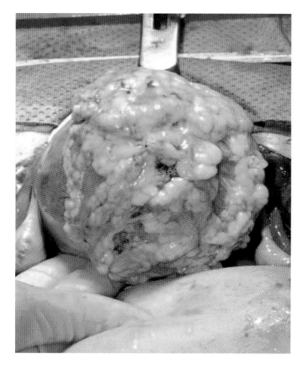

Figure 7.9 The omental graft covering the uterine incision has now been anchored with the use of several fine sutures.

7.6 Delayed Complications

7.6.1 Scar Rupture

After myomectomy, the risk of uterine rupture in a subsequent pregnancy is reported in the literature to be around 1% [30]. In general, the risk is higher if the uterine cavity has been entered during myomectomy; women in this situation should be advised to have elective caesarean section. It is difficult to compare the risk of scar rupture following laparoscopic and open myomectomy. There has never been any well-conducted, matched cohort study to address this question. Observational studies are likely to be biased because of patient selection, as fibroids in the laparoscopic group are more likely to be smaller and fewer than those in the open myomectomy group. Whilst evidence is lacking, it is likely that, if other things are equal, open myomectomy facilitates the placement of layered sutures to secure effective haemostasis and precise apposition of the myometrial and serosal layers, leading to better wound healing and therefore a reduced risk of scar rupture during subsequent pregnancy. An increasing number of reproductive specialists do now lower the threshold for open myomectomy (instead of laparoscopic myomectomy) in women who wish to conceive afterwards.

7.6.2 Recurrence

Women undergoing myomectomy must be fully counselled about the risk of recurrence. The risk of recurrence after myomectomy was found to be related to the number of uterine fibroids removed and uterine size during the operation. Solitary myomectomy and smaller intraoperative uterine size are associated with lower rates of fibroid recurrence. The 5-year cumulative rate for fibroid recurrence was 74% when multiple fibroids were removed and only 11% when a solitary fibroid was removed (p = 0.011) [31]. For all these reasons, it is not possible to compare the recurrence rates of fibroids following laparoscopic and open myomectomy, given the bias in selecting different types of fibroid for these two approaches.

7.7 Conclusion

Despite recent advances in laparoscopic myomectomy, open myomectomy continues to play an important role in women with large, multiple fibroids, or when entry to the uterine cavity is anticipated. The proper use of microsurgical techniques to minimize tissue injury and achieve effective haemostasis and accurate anatomical reconstruction – leading to better wound healing and reduced adhesion formation – will produce improved results and reduced complications.

References

1. Marshall LM, Spiegelman D, Barbieri RL, et al. Variation in the incidence of uterine leiomyoma among premenopausal women by age and race. *Obstet Gynecol* 1997;**90**:967–73.

2. Parker WH, Fu YS, Berek JS. Uterine sarcoma in patients operated on for presumed leiomyoma and rapidly growing leiomyoma. *Obstet Gynecol* 1994;**83**:414–18.

3. Bhave Chittawar P, Franik S, Pouwer AW, Farquhar C. Minimally invasive surgical techniques versus open myomectomy for uterine fibroids. *Cochrane Database Syst Rev* 2014;(10):CD004638.

4. McIlveen M, Li T-C. Myomectomy: a review of surgical technique. *Hum Fertil* 2005;**8**(1):27–33.

5. Conforti A, Mollo A, Alviggi C, et al. Techniques to reduce blood loss during open myomectomy: a qualitative review of literature. *Eur J Obstet Gynecol Reprod Biol* 2015;**192**:90–5.

6. Donnez J, Tatarchuk TF, Bouchard P, et al; PEARL I Study Group, Collaborators (57). Ulipristal acetate versus placebo for fibroid treatment before surgery. *N Engl J Med* 2012;**366**:409–20.

7. Trefoux Bourdet A, Luton D, Koskas M. Clinical utility of ulipristal acetate for the treatment of uterine fibroids: current evidence. *Int J Womens Health* 2015;**7**:321–30.

8. Saridogan E. Surgical treatment of fibroids in heavy menstrual bleeding. *Womens Health (Lond)* 2016;**12**:53–62.

9. Lethaby A, Vollenhoven B, Sowter M. Efficacy of pre-operative gonadotrophin hormone releasing analogues for women with uterine fibroids undergoing hysterectomy or myomectomy: a systematic review. *BJOG* 2002;**109**:1097–108.

10. Mukhopadhaya N, De Silva C, Manyonda IT. Conventional myomectomy. *Best Pract Res Clin Obstet Gynaecol* 2008;**22**:677–705.

11. Bieren R, McKelway W. The use of a tourniquet in uterine surgery. *Am J Obstet Gynecol* 1956;**71**:433–5.

12. Al RA, Yapca OE, Gumusburun N. A randomized trial comparing triple versus single uterine tourniquet in open myomectomy. *Gynecol Obstet Invest* 2017 [Epub ahead of print].

13. Taylor A, Sharma M, Tsirkas P, et al. Reducing blood loss at open myomectomy using triple tourniquets: a randomised controlled trial. *BJOG* 2005;**112**:340–5.

14. Alptekin H, Efe D. Effectiveness of pericervical tourniquet by Foley catheter reducing blood loss at abdominal myomectomy. *Clin Exp Obstet Gynecol* 2014;**41**:440–4.

15. Bonney V. The technique and results of myomectomy. *Lancet* 1931;**220**:171.

16. Sapmaz E, Celik H. Comparison of the effects of the ligation of ascending branches of bilateral arteria uterina with tourniquet method on the intra-operative and post-operative hemorrhage in abdominal myomectomy cases. *Eur J Obstet Gynecol Reprod Biol* 2003;**111**:74–7.

17. Helal AS, Abdel-Hady el-S, Refaie E, et al. Preliminary uterine artery ligation versus pericervical mechanical tourniquet in reducing hemorrhage during abdominal myomectomy. *Int J Gynaecol Obstet* 2010;**108**:233–5.

18. Frederick J, Fletcher H, Simeon D, Mullings A, Hardie M. Intramyometrial vasopressin as a haemostatic agent during myomectomy. *Br J Obstet Gynaecol* 1994;**101**:435–7.

19. Fletcher H, Frederick J, Hardie M, Simeon D. A randomized comparison of vasopressin and tourniquet as hemostatic agents during myomectomy. *Obstet Gynecol* 1996;**87**:1014–18.

20. Kitamura T, Saito Y, Yamada Y. Severe hypotension as a complication of intramyometrial injection of vasopressin: a case report. *Masui* 2008;**57**:1517–20.

21. Atashkhoei S, Fakhari S, Pourfathi H, et al. Effect of oxytocin infusion on reducing the blood loss during abdominal myomectomy: a double-blind randomised controlled trial. *BJOG* 2017;**124**:292–8.

22. Wang D, Wang L, Wang Y, Lin X. The efficiency and safety of tranexamic acid for reducing blood loss in open myomectomy: a meta-analysis of randomized controlled trials. *Medicine (Baltimore)* 2017;**96**:e7072.

23. McLucas B, Voorhees WD 3rd. The effectiveness of combined abdominal myomectomy and uterine artery embolization. *Int J Gynaecol Obstet* 2015;**130**:241–3.

24. Yamada T, Yamashita Y, Terai Y, Ueki M. Intraoperative blood salvage in abdominal uterine myomectomy. *Int J Gynaecol Obstet* 1997;**56**:141–5.

25. Son M, Evanko JC, Mongero LB, et al. Utility of cell salvage in women undergoing abdominal myomectomy. *Am J Obstet Gynecol* 2014;**211**:28.e1–8.

26. Baxter Healthcare Corporation. FLOSEAL© hemostatic matrix instructions for use. Hayward, CA: Baxter Healthcare Corporation.

27. Moriarty KT, Premila S, Bulmer PJ. Use of FloSeal© haemostatic gel in massive obstetric

haemorrhage: a case report. *BJOG* 2008;**115**:793–5.

28. Raga F, Sanz-Cortes M, Bonilla F, Casañ EM, Bonilla-Musoles F. Reducing blood loss at myomectomy with use of a gelatin-thrombin matrix hemostatic sealant. *Fertil Steril* 2009;**92**:356–60.

29. Jeffreys A, Akande V. Abdominal myomectomy. In: Metwally M, Li T-C, editors, *Reproductive Surgery in Assisted Conception.* London: Springer-Verlag; 2015.

30. Gambacorti-Passerini Z, Gimovsky AC, Locatelli A, Berghella V. Trial of labor after myomectomy and uterine rupture: a systematic review. *Acta Obstet Gynecol Scand* 2016;**95**:724–34.

31. Hanafi M. Predictors of leiomyoma recurrence after myomectomy. *Obstet Gynecol* 2005;**105**:877–81.

Laparoscopic and Robotic Myomectomy
Practical Tips

Ahmed M. El-Minawi

Uterine fibroids remain the most common cause of hysterectomy. Myomectomy is performed far less than hysterectomy despite what Victor Bonney stated in 1931: 'Since cure without deformity or loss of function must ever be surgery's highest ideal, the general proposition that myomectomy is a greater surgical achievement is incontestable'. In women seeking uterine conservation and improvement in reproductive outcomes, myomectomy remains the mainstay treatment of symptomatic leiomyomas. But other reasons exist: in a survey of 299 gynaecologists in the United Kingdom in 2017, 54% of respondents said that they would offer a myomectomy to a woman whose family is complete, but who wishes to retain her uterus because she feels a more 'complete woman' [1]. In this era where more women are delaying pregnancy till later in life, when fibroids are more symptomatic, it is imperative that surgeons embrace myomectomy and its newer techniques and alternatives.

8.1 Current State of Endoscopic Myomectomy

Minimally invasive surgery has one goal: getting patients back on their feet as quickly as possible with as little morbidity as possible. Modern instrumentation has made that possible in many surgical situations.

In the case of myomectomy, traditionally a very bloody procedure, newer instrument designs over the past century have changed the way gynaecologists deal with the condition.

In the twenty-first century, minimally invasive myomectomy is the gold standard in fertility-sparing surgery for intramural, subserosal and broad ligamentary myomas [2]. Laparoscopic myomectomy, since its introduction by Semm [3], remains underutilized due to its objective technical difficulty. Robotic assistance, since its first reported use by Advincula et al. [4], has facilitated wider adoption of

endoscopic myomectomy by newer generations. Despite major advances in the 1980s and 1990s, studies have shown that a disproportionately small number of surgeons do a small percentage of complicated surgeries by laparoscopy [5]. As regards submucosal fibroids, hysteroscopy is the gold standard for submucosal myomas, and the removal even of large (>4 cm) myomas is feasible this way [6].

Using traditional laparoscopic instruments, surgeons have to carry out every movement through a fulcrum action, moving their hand opposite to the instrument motion. Laparoscopic surgeons are at an ergonomic disadvantage, often forced to lean or bend uncomfortably while their arms are often held in excessive excursion/abduction in order to handle the long laparoscopic instruments. Cuschieri described a 'surgical fatigue syndrome' that occurs after lengthy laparoscopic surgery [7]. The lack of three-dimensional vision, the fulcrum effect of instruments and limited degrees of freedom of movement encountered with laparoscopic surgery all affect the efficiency of the surgeon. New instruments such as the FlexDex needle driver (FlexDex Inc., Brighton, MI) attempt to address some of these issues. It has a three-axis gimbal that attaches to a surgeon's wrist and leverages a series of mechanical components to translate the movement of the surgeon's hand to the tip of the instrument. The unique design of the instrument decouples these multiple degrees of freedom in a totally mechanical manner, something previously considered impossible without the use of computer control. FlexDex provides laparoscopic tactile feedback and robotic-like dexterity with six degrees of freedom (Figure 8.1)

Surgical robots, by contrast, are built ergonomically and the surgeon's hand movements are mirrored in the movements of the instrument. On a global level, laparoscopy will remain more popular than robotics in the foreseeable future, access to robots and costs being major deciding factors. Currently only two robotic platforms are readily available for

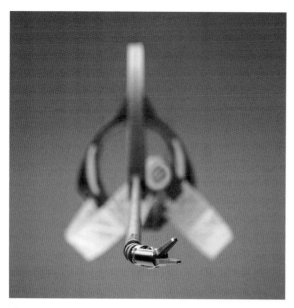

Figure 8.1 The FlexDex needle-holder offers robot-like dexterity for laparoscopists.

gynaecologic use, the da Vinci Surgical System (Intuitive Surgical Inc., Sunnyvale, CA) since 2000 and the recently FDA-approved Senhance (TransEnterix, Research Triangle Park, NC) that is just now coming onto market in 2018/2019. Both are approved for myomectomy and other gynaecologic procedures (Figures 8.2 and 8.3). The da Vinci has over 4,000 units installed worldwide and a base of over 18,000 trained surgeons. Intuitive Surgical is currently developing a single-port robot to be used for gynaecology and urology which allows for a reduced incision count versus the current 4-port techniques used. With the many thousands of robotic platforms currently installed, robotic surgery is here to stay, so it is inevitable that both young and experienced surgeons get to train in its usage [8].

Both robotic platforms utilize a console/patient-cart system with the surgeon seated at a console providing joy-stick-like controls to remotely regulate the robotic arms and instruments. But they differ in

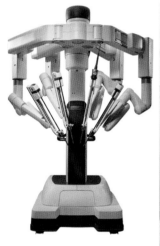
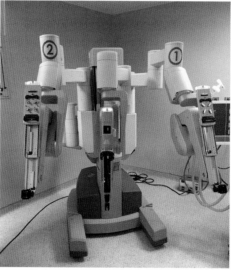

Figure 8.2 The da Vinci robotic platform.

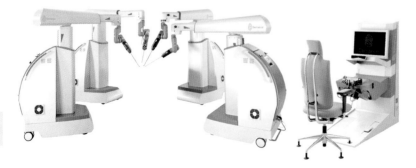

Figure 8.3 The Senhance robotic platform is the newest FDA-approved platform.

ergonomics. The older da Vinci has a periscope-like console at which the surgeon bends forward and views the 3D image through a binocular interface while controlling camera motion and instruments via joysticks and foot pedals. Since there is no direct or mechanical connection between the system's input and output, the surgeon receives no haptic feedback to gauge the forces exerted by the tool end effector. A single patient cart carries the articulated robotic arms and, with the new Xi system, any arm can hold the camera. The multiple actuators on the robotic arms translate the surgeon's input motions to the end-effector instrument inside the patient's body. Special trocars are needed.

The much newer Senhance robot platform is quite different. Each articulated robotic arm has a separate mobile cart. The trocars are regular laparoscopic trocars allowing instant removal of the robotic arms if urgently needed. The surgeon sits in front of an open console with a 3D monitor and his or her eye motion is tracked, allowing the camera to move to where the surgeon looks. Eye motion control also allows instrument assignment to the robotic arm desired and/or to the left or right steering handle. Together with a normal seating position, these features decrease eye and neck strain compared to sitting for long periods at a da Vinci console. The instrument joystick controls offer haptic feedback. No randomized comparative trials have yet been done to see the real value of these innovative ideas relative to the da Vinci experience. Alletti et al. [9] recently published a series of robotic-assisted total hysterectomies in obese women using the Senhance platform. Indication for total hysterectomy was early-stage (FIGO Stage IA) endometrial cancer in 100% of patients. The median operative time was 110 minutes (70–200). Median docking time was 10.5 minutes (5–25). The median estimated blood loss was 100 mL (50–200). No conversions to laparotomy were recorded. No intra- and 30-day postoperative complications were registered.

A recent meta-analysis of 20 studies involving 2,852 patients undergoing laparoscopic myomectomy (LM), robotic-assisted laparoscopic myomectomy (RALM) and abdominal myomectomy (AM) showed the numbers of complications (odds ratio [OR] 0.52, p = 0.009), estimated blood loss (EBL) (weighted mean difference [WMD] −33.03, p = 0.02), conversions (OR 0.34, p = 0.03) and postoperative bleeding (OR 0.18, p = 0.03) in RALM cases were significantly lower than in LM cases. Compared with LM and AM, RALM is associated with significantly fewer complications, significantly lower EBL, significantly fewer conversions than both LM and AM, and significantly less bleeding than LM [10]. These updated findings are in line with an older Cochrane review involving 808 women that reported laparoscopic myomectomy is a procedure associated with less subjectively reported postoperative pain, lower postoperative fever and shorter hospital stay compared with all types of open myomectomy [11].

Robotic assistance is very useful for inexperienced laparoscopists performing complex tasks such as knot tying, and they experience an early and persistent enabling effect. In case of experts, robotics is most useful for improving economy of motion, which may have implications for highly complex procedures in limited workspaces [12]. Such issues are of course moot for surgeons in developing countries where laparoscopy remains king due to cost issues. But even in Egypt, where we only have one robotic system, the improvement of visualization, better handling of tissues and better suturing was found to be particularly helpful in radical surgery [13]. Falcone notes that currently no evidence exists to support the routine use of robotic assistance at the time of laparoscopic myomectomy [14].

Minimally invasive procedures such as uterine artery embolization (UAE), non-invasive magnetic-resonance-guided high-frequency focused ultrasound surgery (MRgFUS) (Figure 8.4) and cryomyolysis are increasingly used to treat symptomatic fibroids. All these modern techniques offer alternatives to surgery. Whether these will prove to be the future remains to be seen. But I personally believe that many gynaecologists are steering their patients to these treatments due to the lack of minimally invasive surgical skills. Case in point, young doctors think of robotic surgery as 'easier' than laparoscopy because the learning curve for robotic suturing and skills is far shorter than for laparoscopy [5].

8.2 Planning the Procedure

A wise choice of surgical tools and materials by the surgeon performing an endoscopic myomectomy, whether laparoscopic or robot-assisted, will greatly facilitate his or her job. The following steps must be addressed in all cases:

1. Port placement and cameras
2. Haemostasis
3. Incision placement
4. Enucleation of the uterus/myoma(s)
5. Suturing of the myoma bed and closure of uterus
6. Tissue extraction.

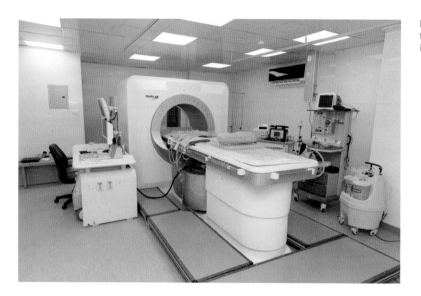

Figure 8.4 MRgFUS is a non-invasive technique currently gaining increased use in select cases.

8.3 Where to Place the Ports?

In both laparoscopic and robotic surgery, planning camera port location is important, especially so in robotic surgery since once docked, it is very difficult to change trocar positions with the standard daVinci Si system (Intuitive Surgical Inc., Sunnyvale, CA). The newer Xi systems are more flexible and allow introduction of the camera in any port; likewise, the robotic arms and instruments are far less bulky. The Senhance (TransEnterix, Research Triangle Park, NC) allows use of standard laparoscopic trocars, so at any given time the surgical assistant at the table can intervene laparoscopically or can use additional laparoscopic instruments through additional trocars.

The size of the uterus plays a great role in determining initial port placement in endoscopic myomectomy. The umbilicus is optimal both for cosmetic reasons and since it can be widened for morcellators or incision expanders when removing the myoma. Palmer's point (left upper quadrant, LUQ) can be utilized initially in those cases where adhesions are suspected or assessment of uterine size is needed. In some cases, an LUQ camera can be used throughout the procedure, particularly if a 30° scope is used which will allow visualization of the right side of the uterus more easily. Optimally, a distance of around 15–20 cm is needed between the lens and fundus of the uterus. Non-bulky uteri with small-sized myomas can be operated using the umbilicus. In cases of large uteri reaching up to the umbilicus or where there is suspicion of adhesions, placing a

supraumbilical port a few centimetres cephalad facilitates vision and accessibility [14, 15] Thirty-degree angled scopes are more popular in Europe and should be available in case the zero-degree scope does not allow proper vision with low anterior wall or broad ligamentary myomas. An additional three instrument ports are placed in the usual positions for myomectomy: two left lower quadrant ports, namely left and right side medial to the anterior superior iliac spines, and another 5 or 10 mm port is placed 10–13 cm lateral to the umbilicus. The larger the uterus the higher these should be. The port lateral to the umbilicus is usually used for insertion of a myoma screw or additional instrumentation.

When deploying the third arm in case of daVinci robotics, a single-tooth tenaculum forceps or Cobra grasper (Intuitive Surgical Inc., Sunnyvale, CA) can be utilized. It is worth noting that utilization of the third operative robotic arm in the 4-arm robot-assisted laparoscopic myomectomy technique accounted for a significant decrease in operative time [16]. To save costs, a regular trocar for the assistant can be used instead of using the third arm. In case of robotic-assisted surgery, particularly when used the older Si systems, it is best to use a side-docking method to free up space between the patient's legs. Right-sided docking allows the assistant to use his or her dominant hand and frees up space.

From personal experience docking can, with time, be cut down to less than 5 minutes. The type of trocars used is mainly down to surgeon preference. A 12 mm umbilical trocar can be beneficial if a similar-sized morcellator is passed through it and a 5 mm camera is placed in an accessory port. In very obese patients, it is imperative that longer trocars be used.

Three-D cameras, while not essential in laparoscopic myomectomy, can be beneficial, as shown by their use in robotic surgery. Two-D laparoscopy is marred by the lack of depth perception and increases the strain on the surgeon, compromising the safety of laparoscopy. Research shows that 3D cameras shorten the learning curve for laparoscopists considerably, to much less than that of robotic surgery [17] and will enhance the skills of a good surgeon and shorten the learning curve of a novice surgeon, ultimately shortening the surgical time [18]. Single-site laparoscopy showed 86% increased efficiency for beginners and 100% in case of expert surgeons in phantom exercises in urological skills [19]. The current drawbacks of bulky headsets and glasses are being overcome with new glassless type 3D systems [20]. I believe that in the future, the merging of glassless 3D systems and instruments with more freedom of motion – such as the previously mentioned totally mechanical FlexDex (FlexDex Inc., Brighton, MI) – will allow the continued flourishing of laparoscopy.

8.4 Controlling Bleeding

Myomectomy is a bloody procedure, and as a result hysterectomy was always a more popular treatment. When Victor Bonney introduced his famous clamp in 1922, he gave life to a relatively unpopular procedure. Many techniques have been utilized since then, including the use of tourniquets. Contrary to popular belief, myomas have a network of blood vessels supplying them. During development of a leiomyoma, the pre-existing blood vessels undergo regression and new vessels invade the tumour peripherally where intense angiogenesis, probably promoted by growth factors secreted by the tumour, leads to the formation of a 'vascular capsule' responsible for supply of blood to the growing tumour [21]. Recent arterial spin labelling MRI studies have shown increased perfusion of myometrium on the myoma-positive areas that is significantly higher than that of the myoma-negative areas [22]. Other investigators studying the effect of myomas on IVF by 3D power Doppler showed that intramural myomas >4 cm significantly increase endometrial vascularity [23].

The uterus receives the majority of its blood supply via the uterine arteries, which are branches of the internal iliac artery. Additional blood supply arrives via the ovarian ligaments and the round ligaments. Extensive anastomoses occur between the uterine arterial supply and the ovarian supply on either side of the uterus which culminate in the arcuate arteries traversing the myometrium. Any method of decreasing the flow during myomectomy will provide diminished intraoperative blood loss and reduce morbidity. Upfront control of vascular supply, prior to further dissection of tissue, may be beneficial in minimizing blood loss during difficult gynaecological procedures [24].

Since this chapter deals with instrumental techniques, I will not expound on the most common method of controlling bleeding: the use of vasopressin. Vasopressin, a synthetic analogue of the posterior pituitary hormone – antidiuretic hormone – is often injected into the uterus to reduce blood loss during surgery. To temporarily minimize bleeding in the surgical field, subserosal injection of dilute vasopressin (20–40 IU in 100 mL of normal saline) until visible vessels blanch is done. This practice is more effective than deep myoma or myometrial injection. Due to safety concerns about the cardiac effects of vasopressin, a recent randomized trial by Cohen et al. [25] looked at whether more dilute concentrations of the drug would be more effective than conventional dosing, while preserving safety. It failed to find any benefit in injecting diluted high-volume vasopressin as compared to low-volume concentrated hormone. These findings agree with the 2014 Cochrane review that showed moderate-quality evidence supporting use of vasopressin to decrease blood loss at the time of myomectomy but note that the optimal dosing and concentration has yet to be determined.

In the past decade, several groups have published their experiences with planned preoperative uterine artery embolization (PUAE), particularly with regard to large uterine myomas, to improve the surgical outcome of subsequent myoma enucleation and to reduce intraoperative blood loss [26–28]. Between 24 and 48 hours after performing UAE, the patients underwent operative myoma enucleation by laparoscopy or by laparotomy. These 'hybrid interventions' were meant to reduce the risk of hysterectomy and substantial intraoperative blood loss in women with individual or multiple very large myomas, but who wished for uterine preservation. In fact, this was the original intention of Ravina, who first published the technique in 1995 [29]. Against this is the additional cost/inconvenience of having two procedures.

Less costly and more practical is performing permanent or temporary bilateral uterine artery occlusion (BUAO) during the actual procedure. In women who have completed child bearing, permanent uterine artery occlusion at the origin of the uterine arteries retroperitoneally prior to myomectomy is best. Temporary occlusion is reserved for fertility-seeking patients. Laparoscopic bulldog clips and other vascular occlusion devices (e.g., Crafoord, Satinsky and DeBakey types) and the Hem-o-lok™ clip system (Weck Closure Systems, Research Triangle Pack, NC) are in wide used in laparoscopic partial nephrectomies and can also be used to temporarily (or permanently in the case of Hem-o-lok or titanium clips) ligate the uterine vessels at the time of surgery. Although this can be done using suture material, the difficulty in removing the knot in cases where fertility needs to be preserved means clips/clamps are an easier alternative.

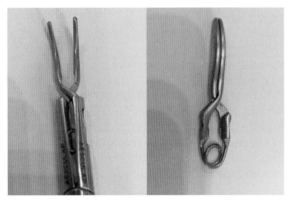

Figure 8.5 Titanium bulldog clamps used for uterine artery occlusion.

The bulldog clamp is a laparoscopic vascular clamp that may be used to decrease blood loss during surgical procedures. Made of titanium or stainless steel, it is a spring-loaded crossover clamp with serrated blades that effectively occlude vessels without slippage or significant crush injury. Several versions exist, depending on diameter and type of vessels to be occluded.

In my practice, I use 25 mm atraumatic curved arterial bulldog clips with DeBakey serrations (Aesculap AG, Tuttlingen, Germany). They are introduced via a special applier forceps and I recommend using one allowing angled application and removal since straight ones are sometimes difficult to reattach (Figure 8.5). When using a robotic platform the clips are introduced via a 5 mm × 12 mm accessory port. This was very beneficial in a case of cervical myomectomy that I performed robotically in a virgin (Figure 8.6 and Video 8.1), and has also been mentioned by others [30, 31]. As previously noted, the uterine artery may have a double c-shaped origin from the internal iliac, and in this case clamping both vessels or clamping the internal iliac artery before the bifurcation may be helpful in reducing uterine perfusion. It might be beneficial to also apply temporary clamps on the ovarian arteries in the infundibulopelvic ligaments in cases of very large fibroids.

Reperfusion occurs immediately after their removal and studies have shown no increased risk of embolization or irreversible uterine muscle damage with their prolonged use. Fibroids get their blood supply almost exclusively from the uterine arteries [32], whereas the uterine myometrium derives its blood supply from several vessels including the ovarian and round

Figure 8.6 Large cervical myoma in a 23-yr old virgin female.

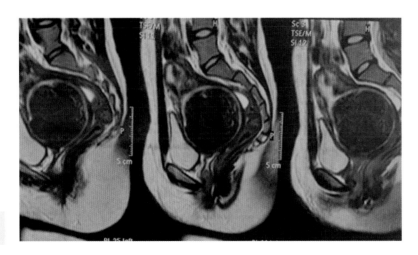

Video 8.1 Application of bulldog clamps to uterine arteries via a robotic approach.

ligament arteries. The temporary ischaemia caused by bilateral uterine artery occlusion affects the fibroid with little or no effect on the normal uterine myometrium [33–35]. This procedure usually adds anywhere between 15 and 30 minutes to operating time; with experience, the time is considerably reduced.

Advantages of uterine artery occlusion prior to myomectomy:

- The major advantage is that blood loss is considerably reduced.
- Studies show that there is shrinkage of very small fibroids that are not removed during the surgery.
- There is significant reduction in the recurrence rate of uterine fibroids. [32].

8.4.1 Approaches to Ligating the Uterine Arteries at their Origin

The techniques all involve securing the vascular supply at the uterine arteries as they branch from the hypogastric artery. A variant of normal anatomy exists where a double uterine artery arises in a C-shaped configuration from the internal iliac artery [36]. Three approaches are possible:

a. Anterior or paravesical approach. This is best utilized when dealing with bulky uteri with large posterior myomas or broad ligamentary myomas blocking access to the pelvic sidewalls and Douglas pouch. This is somewhat more difficult when the patient has had previous c-sections because of fibrosis. In some instances, such myomas displace the uterine vessels anteriorly and it may be easy to identify the arteries bordering the uterine cervix.

Anatomy of the paravesical space: laterally, the retropubic space is contiguous with the paravesical spaces, their point of separation being the medial umbilical ligaments (obliterated umbilical arteries). The paravesical space is bounded laterally by the obturator internus muscle and the obturator nerve, artery and vein. The posterior border is the endopelvic fascial sheath around the internal iliac artery and vein and its anterior branches, while the pubocervical fascia forms the floor.

The patient should be put in steep Trendelenburg to allow gravity to displace the uterus in a cephalad direction. The use of an intrauterine manipulator will greatly facilitate pushing the uterus cephalad and laterally to allow better access. One can proceed by opening the uterovesical fold of the peritoneum and then dissecting the bladder and pushing it caudad. This moves the ureters laterally and prevents them from being included in the bulldog/clip. The ascending uterine vessels are identified on either side and the bulldogs/clips are applied. The obliterated umbilical arteries can be utilized in identifying the arteries by pulling on them in the direction of the anterior abdominal wall. At the end of the procedure, the clamps can be removed.

b. The lateral approach. The landmark is the triangle between the round ligament, infundibulopelvic ligament and external iliac artery. The dissection is started by lifting the peritoneum between the round ligament and the infundibulopelvic ligament. The peritoneum is then incised immediately below the round ligament, parallel and medial to the external iliac vessels in a cephalad direction. The avascular space is dissected by blunt dissection. Too deep a dissection is not needed so the obturator nerve is not exposed. The ureter is identified and pushed medially. The anterior division of the internal iliac artery is then identified and the uterine artery is skeletonized at its origin from the internal iliac artery. The uterine artery is seen in between the ureter and obliterated umbilical ligament and can be identified by its tortuosity. Again, traction on the obliterated umbilical ligament will help identify the internal iliac. Apply clamps.

c. The posterior or pelvic approach. For the ligation of the uterine artery posteriorly to the uterus and medially to the pelvic infundibulum, the ureter should be first identified coursing under the peritoneum. A good uterine manipulator allowing anteversion such as the Rumi (Cooper Surgical, Trumbull, CT) or Tintara (Karl Storz, Tuttlingen, Germany) greatly helps in visualizing the pelvic sidewall. This needs to be done quickly while the peritoneum is still transparent. Grasping and pulling upwards on the obliterated umbilical artery allows the movement of the umbilical artery to be seen at the ovarian fossa perpendicular to the ureter. Incising the peritoneum just above and parallel to the ureter over the bulge of the umbilical artery is then done. The ureter is gently

71

retracted medially and the umbilical artery is dissected until the bifurcation is seen. The uterine artery can be identified at the bifurcation and clips/bulldogs are then applied [37].

8.5 Incision and Enucleation

Traditionally, a vertical incision was used to eliminate the need to incise vascular areas and avoid the injury of the interstitial portion of the fallopian tube. Many surgeons prefer a transverse uterine incision because it runs parallel to the arcuate vessels of the myometrium, leading to less bleeding, in their opinion. But myomas apparently disrupt the normal uterine blood flow and change the spatial positioning of the arcuate arteries within the uterine wall, the anatomy of which has been well detailed in previous studies [38]. This can induce vascular congestion and venous engorgement leading to an abnormal vascularization and bleeding pattern. This has implications for the incision into the uterus since transverse incisions should potentially have less bleeding.

An important and often overlooked fact is the ergonomics of wound closure. With improper positioning of the needle holders, the laparoscopic surgeon may have difficulty suturing the deep areas of the myoma bed, leading to postoperative bleeding. Many surgeons like a transverse incision since it facilitates closure from the lateral ports. Vast experience with caesareans verified that low transverse scar wound rupture in subsequent pregnancy is far less than with a vertical incision. But an oblique incision has been proposed by some when dealing with an anterior myoma and lateral ports. A vertical incision and a suprapubic placement of the needle holder is suggested to be more ergonomic for fundal and posterior wall myomas [24]. Broad ligamentary myomas require careful observation of the course of the ureters and large blood vessels. Depending on the location of the myoma, an incision is made on the anterior or posterior leaf of the broad ligament.

Tinelli et al. have described the myoma fibroneurovascular pseudocapsule and the importance of identifying and sparing as much as possible of it [39]. Their intracapsular approach to myomectomy helps preserve the integrity of the remaining uterine muscle and promotes better healing and functionality.

Laparoscopically, the incision can be made with a simple monopolar knife electrode with pure cutting current (40–60 W) to minimize damage to adjacent myometrium and decrease subsequent risk of rupture [40]. Better, if available, ultrasonic shears can be used (Harmonic scalpel; Ethicon Endosurgery, Cincinnati, OH or Thunderbeat, Olympus). Some surgeons who have CO_2 lasers available in the OR utilize them for a bloodless incision. Scalpel holders are available that allow the use of a #11 scalpel, and this can also be used, especially if vasopressin has been injected.

In robotic-assisted cases, it is best to use the tip of one blade of the sharp monopolar scissors (HotShears) with low wattage pure cutting current, or to use an ultrasonic shear (Harmonic Ace, Intuitive Surgical Inc., Sunnyvale, CA). The da Vinci permanent cautery hook is a monopolar instrument that is very effective and likewise should be used on a pure cut. Because robotic instruments have a fixed number of uses, surgeons should choose an instrument they can use for both incising and assisting in dissection of the myoma, to minimize changing and increasing costs.

A prior MRI or ultrasound will allow the surgeon to assess the depth of the initial incision. Not reaching the proper plane and capsule will be cause for difficult dissection and extraction. The incision should extend as close as possible to the width of the myoma in view to allow easy extraction.

Once the shiny pseudocapsule is reached, either a myoma screw is inserted for traction (through an accessory port in case of robotic-assisted) or a claw or tenaculum forceps is applied. The edges of the wound can then be grasped by atraumatic forceps or similar and gradually spread apart while simultaneously pulling on the myoma. This works well with bulging myomas or broad ligamentary ones: the overlying myometrium is thin enough to be stripped away. When dealing with deep intramural myomas, this approach is more difficult; a very useful technique is to extract the fibroid by applying generous traction with the tenaculum and counter-traction with an atraumatic grasper and suction device. Alternatively, using scissors in one hand the surgeon can, as in open surgery, open the blades and dissect gently between capsule and myometrium while applying traction on one side of the wound with the other hand and helped by an assistant pulling on the myoma screw. This use of sharp dissection can sometimes help dislodge a myoma in patients pretreated with GnRh. Repositioning the tenaculum or myoma screw regularly at the border of the myoma and myometrium allows better traction. In this fashion, total enucleation of the myoma from its pseudocapsule is achieved.

If vasopressin has been used it helps to inject a large quantity in the plane of the capsule, which greatly facilitates enucleation. Low-wattage bipolar coagulation to stop bleeding should be kept at a minimum. Haemostatic agents such as SurgiFlo (Ethicon Inc.) can help minimize usage of electrical coagulation. If proper haemostatic techniques are utilized then most blood encountered will be accumulated blood within the venous sinuses of the myometrium. If active bleeding is encountered then either inject more vasopressin or think of temporary uterine artery/ovarian artery ligation.

Enucleation of degenerated myomas can be difficult due to their friability. Placing an endobag around or under the uterus is beneficial to catch any pieces of myoma that might be ripped off during the unlodging of the tumour from its bed. Myoma screws should be of the 10 mm variety to allow better traction. Sharp dissection of the myoma from its bed is oftentimes helpful. Pedunculated fibroids are usually easily removed. The broad base of the pedicle can be bisected close to the myoma and the defect sutured in two layers.

In the past decade, several authors have reported using a hybrid technique variation in robotic myomectomy where a conventional laparoscopic enucleation of the myoma is followed by reconstruction with the da Vinci robot. They justified it by noting preservation of tactile sensation while separating very large tumour masses from delicate reproductive structures, and allowing the use of a rigid (not articulated) tenaculum that was capable of exerting significant pull at every angle with the benefit of haptic feedback and without risk of equipment damage [41, 42]. Gaining more experience in both laparoscopic and robotic-assisted myomectomy will allow the surgeon to choose a single method rather than this very wasteful and expensive method.

8.6 Suturing

Uterine Repair –– Suturing has been one of the main factors dividing laparoscopists into average and above average. Advances in instrumentation over the past decade have helped surgeons become more efficient. Suturing devices such as the Endostitch (Covidien), facilitators such as Laparotie (Ethicon, Somerville, NJ) and the newer intuitive needle holders such as the Flexdex are allowing more surgeons to perform more technically difficult suture procedures.

Traditionally, synthetic absorbable polyglactin sutures have been used for closure of the defect, but over the past decade barbed sutures have become very popular. These knotless sutures have either uni- or bi-directional cuts made into their surface during manufacture. The resulting 'barbs' anchor into the tissue at multiple points, locking the suture and preventing slippage. Pulling on the stitch serves to further pull and compress the opposing sutured edges. Examples include QUILL™ (Angiotech Pharmaceuticals, Inc., Vancouver, BC, Canada), the V-Loc™ (Covidien, Mansfield, MA) and STRATAFIX™ (Ethicon Inc.). Available in many sizes, the advantages include the complete absence of knots, the even distribution of tissue strength along the wound, decreased blood loss and great reduction in operative time especially for suture-challenged surgeons.

The technique and number of suture layers is not fixed but should vary according to the location/depth of the myoma. One, two and even three layers may be needed. In case of a superficial subserosal myoma and a shallow incision, bed closure is mandatory, but only one suture layer is needed. Separate single sutures of absorbable regular suture material (Vicryl 0, or 00) or continuous barbed sutures (V-Loc or STRATAFIX) are used for proper re-approximation of the edges. With a very shallow bed, the defect can be closed with a running non-locking imbricating 'baseball stitch' suture. In case of barbed suture material, it is important to cut the suture flush to the surface of the uterus to prevent bowel adhesions.

With deep intramural myomas, closure in several layers is important to prevent dead spaces and haematoma formation. Barbed suture (2-0 or 0) is best used as a continuous running suture for the deep bed. The final superficial layer can be closed with 2-0 baseball-type stitching. If properly done, then the barbed suture is hidden within the depths of the stitching. If the endometrial cavity is inadvertently entered (easily noticed by seeing the balloon of the uterine manipulator or sudden appearance of gas bubbles), the defect can be closed with a 3-0 Monocryl or Vicryl suture, taking special care not to pass the suture into the endometrial cavity. Overlapping sutures in the overlying myometrium cover the defect.

Tinelli and Malvasi [39] believe that the defect should be closed by simply introflecting muscle edges and approximating in one or two layers. They are of the opinion that proper technique of myoma intracapsular enucleation and preservation of the neurovascular capsule will allow for better healing with less foreign stitch material.

73

8.7 Extraction of the Myoma

Over the last 20 years, leiomyomas were usually removed with a power morcellator. Many devices have been marketed and one review documented 11 different types available as recently as 2014 [43]. Power morcellation of the uterus and uterine tumours permits the extraction of large tissue masses through small laparoscopic incisions in a very short time and became extremely popular. However, open power morcellation is associated with an increased risk of dispersing benign myoma tissue and occult malignant leiomyosarcoma tissue throughout the abdominal cavity. Donnez et al. [44] described the risk of uterine fragment dispersion with the subsequent appearance of parasitic leiomyomas. But since their first publication, Donnez no longer encountered this complication in a subsequent series of 400 laparoscopic hysterectomies when caution was exercised and extensive lavage used [45].

A lengthy debate started after the Food and Drug Administration (FDA) warning in 2014 about the use of electromechanical power morcellation, and clinical practice changed as a result. The FDA's latest [46] white paper suggests the prevalence of uterine sarcoma in women undergoing surgery for presumed fibroids to be in the range of approximately 1 in 225 to 1 in 580, and that for leiomyosarcoma (LMS) to be approximately 1 in 495 to 1 in 1,100, based on an analysis of 23 studies.

These numbers are at odds with other studies. In a series of 10,731 uteri morcellated for myomas during laparoscopic hysterectomy, the prevalence of sarcoma was just 0.06% [47]. A similar low incidence (1/2,000) was observed in a meta-analysis by Pritts et al. [48] and in a retrospective study including 4,791 women in Norway [49]. In my opinion, the debate on the use of electric morcellation has probably been overstated due to emotional and medicolegal reasons.

Gynaecologic surgeons should try, whenever possible, to reduce the use of open power morcellation. Several alternatives have emerged in a bid to minimize the risk of inadvertent tissue spread. Some gynaecologists propose vaginal removal through the cul-de-sac of Douglas or mini-laparotomy to avoid the risk of dispersing tissue fragments during sarcoma morcellation. Others have promoted the use of bags to contain the specimens. Many of the companies previously producing morcellators have stopped manufacture/recalled their products due to multiple law suits.

Alternative methods of safer morcellation were devised as a result of the decrease in use of power morcellation.

Power morcellation within a containment bag. The Lahey bag (Becton Dickinson, Franklin Lakes, NJ) is also known as an 'isolation' bag. Cohen, in 2014, reported a technique for the use of power morcellation within an insufflated Lahey bag [50]. The Lahey bag measures 45 cm × 45 cm and is sufficiently large to hold large uterine fibroid tumours. The bag is rolled up and inserted through an open single port cannula, the cannula recapped, the fibroid inserted in the bag, opening the port to bring the opening of the bag up through the port, recapping the port cannula, insufflating the bag and performing power morcellation within the bag. Power morcellation in the bag should thus reduce the risk of spreading tumour pieces throughout the abdominal cavity.

Serur et al. [51] reported on 5 years of their experience with a **manual morcellation technique** for all uteri >500 g at laparoscopic hysterectomy that can be also used for myomas. In this technique, once the uterus is separated from its vascular and supporting structures, an Endo Catch II 15 mm polyurethane specimen pouch (Covidien Surgical, Mansfield, MA) is inserted through an abdominal port or vaginally. The bag is opened and the uterus is placed inside it. An abdominal port incision is then enlarged to 20–30 mm so that the opening edge of the bag can be brought out through the incision to the skin surface. Clamps are used to hold the uterus against the abdominal wall while it is circumferentially cored with a scalpel. The median duration of morcellation was 14.8 minutes (range, 4.5–21.6 minutes) for the abdominal route and 11.7 minutes (range, 5.2–16.8 minutes) for the vaginal route. Occult malignancy was identified in two patients. There were no complications related to the morcellation technique or gross bag rupture. A simple technique but it can be time-consuming with very large myomas.

A recent study compared contained manual morcellation (n = 38) versus contained power morcellation (n = 62) in robotic-assisted myomectomies. A significant decrease in operating time was noted with manual technique, together with no difference in postoperative narcotic usage and discharge time compared to power morcellation [52].

Technical difficulties. Techniques that use morcellation in a bag are currently plagued by a number of technical difficulties. It can be very difficult to place a large tumour in a floppy bag. Current advances in bag technology use a deployable rigid bag opening that probably will help to overcome this difficult step.

Pulling the bag up through a port site or cannula requires an incision in the range of 30 mm – larger than the incision currently employed in many laparoscopic operations. The larger incision is likely associated with more pain and greater time to full postoperative recovery.

Calcified fibroids are very difficult to morcellate. Preferably, they should be extracted through a posterior colpotomy or via a min-laparotomy incision. Coring during extraction will require frequent changes of scalpel blades, which dull quickly on these myomas.

Natural orifice morcellation. Transvaginal placement of an Alexis retractor (Applied Medical, Rancho Santa Margarita, CA) can facilitate the process of vaginal coring, as reported by Kho et al. [53]. Coring or bivalving the large uterus has a small risk of spreading small bits of tissue into the vagina and near the vaginal apex, but this is much less than the risk of open power morcellation of a uterine tumour because the uterine serosa is pulled tightly against the vagina, reducing the spread of tissue into the peritoneal cavity.

Favero and colleagues have an alternative approach that involves placement of the fibroid within a bag and bringing the opening of the bag out through the vagina and performing hand morcellation of the tumour in the bag via the vagina [54]. A polyurethane bag with polypropylene draw strings (Lapsac, Cook Medical, Bloomington, IA) is inserted into the abdominal cavity through the vagina. The specimen is inserted into the bag and the drawstrings are pulled to close the bag. The surgeon pulls the strings and opening of the bag out to the vaginal introitus. The bag is opened and two narrow retractors are placed in the vagina to protect the vaginal tissue, urethra, bladder and rectum. Lahey clamps are placed on the uterine cervix and the uterus is morcellated using a cold-knife. Bivalving a small uterus will facilitate its removal through the vagina. Coring of the uterus may be preferred for very large uterine tumours.

This method is a modification of the original *laparoscopic-assisted vaginal myomectomy* reported by Pelosi and Pelosi [55] and later by Goldfarb and Fanarjian [56]. Their technique is best for posterior wall fibroids and greatly depends on a wide patulous vagina to pull down the uterus and enucleate, then sew the defect. Goldfarb considers this better than mini-laparotomy since the acute angulation of uterine blood vessels affords minimal blood loss.

Laparoscopic-assisted Myomectomy. First reported by Nezhat et al. in 1994 [57], this method enables conventional multi-layer suturing. After laparoscopic myomectomy, a mini-laparotomy can be made either suprapubically or by widening the umbilical port and the uterus or uterine tumour can be pulled up to the skin surface and removed by coring the tissue with a scalpel. An Alexis retractor (Applied Medical) is usually inserted. As with vaginal coring, although the process does not occur in a bag, the risk of spreading tumour tissue into the abdominal cavity is reduced compared with open power morcellation. However, using this technique, tissue may be spread into the abdominal incision, resulting in the postoperative growth of small nodules of endometrium or fibroids in the incision. But a plus to this technique is that proper suturing of the uterine myoma bed can be done through the mini-lap incision.

References

1. Sirkeci RF, Belli AM, Manyonda IT. Treating symptomatic uterine fibroids with myomectomy: current practice and views of UK consultants. *Gynecol Surg* 2017;**14**(1):11. doi: 10.1186/s10397-017-1014-4.

2. Bortoletto P, Hariton E, Gargiulo AR. The evolution of myomectomy: from laparotomy to minimally invasive surgery. *BJOG* 2018 Apr;**125**(5):586. doi: 10.1111/1471-0528.14936.

3. Semm K. New methods of pelviscopy (gynecologic laparoscopy) for myomectomy, ovariectomy, tubectomy and adenectomy. *Endoscopy* 1979;**11**(2):85–93.

4. Advincula AP, Song A, Burke W, Reynolds RK. Preliminary experience with robot-assisted laparoscopic myomectomy. *J Am Assoc Gynecol Laparosc* 2004 Nov;**11**(4):511–18.

5. Griffen FD, Sugar JG. The future of robotics: a dilemma for general surgeons. *Bull Am Coll Surg* 2013 Jul;**98**(7):9–15.

6. Zayed M, Fouda UM, Zayed SM, Elsetohy KA, Hashem AT. Hysteroscopic myomectomy of large submucous myomas in a 1-step procedure using multiple slicing sessions technique. *J Minim Invasive Gynecol* 2015;**22**(7):1196–202.

7. Reyes DA, Tang B, Cuschieri A. Minimal access surgery (MAS)-related surgeon morbidity syndromes. *Surg Endosc* 2006 Jan;**20**(1):1–13.

8. Brunk D. Robotic surgery is here to stay. *Surgery News* 2013;9(2):1

9. Alletti SG, Rossitto C, Cianci S, et al. The Senhance™ surgical robotic system ('Senhance') for total hysterectomy in obese patients: a pilot study. *J Robotic Surg* 2018;**12**(2):229–34.

10. Wang T, Tang H, Xie Z, Deng S. Robotic-assisted vs. laparoscopic

and abdominal myomectomy for treatment of uterine fibroids: a meta-analysis. *Minim Invasive Ther Allied Technol* 2018 Feb;**28**:1–16. doi: 10.1080/13645706.2018.1442349 [Epub ahead of print].

11. Bhave Chittawar P, Franik S, Pouwer AW, Farquhar C. Minimally invasive surgical techniques versus open myomectomy for uterine fibroids. *Cochrane Database Syst Rev* 2014 Oct 21;(10): CD004638.

12. Chandra V, Nehra D, Parent R, et al. A comparison of laparoscopic and robotic assisted suturing performance by experts and novices. *Surgery* 2010 Jun;**147** (6):830–9.

13. Zaghloul AS, El-Minawi AM, ElKordy MA, et al. First experience of the Egyptian National Cancer Institute using the robot-assisted laparoscopic approach in radical hysterectomies for cervical cancer. *J Egypt Natl Canc Inst* 2018 Jun;**30** (2):61–7. doi: 10.1016/j.jnci.2018.03.003.

14. Gingold JA, Gueye N-A, Falcone T. Minimally invasive approaches to myoma management. *J Minim Invasive Gynecol* 2018 Feb;**25** (2):237–50.

15. Granata M, Tsimpanakos I, Moeity F, Magos A. Are we underutilizing Palmer's point entry in gynecologic laparoscopy? *Fertil Steril* 2010;**94**:2716–19.

16. Sanderson D, Sanderson R, Ghomi A. Robot-assisted laparoscopic myomectomy: a comparison of techniques. *J Gynecol Surg* 2016;**32**(6):329–34. doi: 10.1089/gyn.2016.0058.

17. Sinha R, Sundaram M, Raje S, et al. 3D laparoscopy: technique and initial experience in 451 cases. *Gynecol Surg* 2013;**10**:123–8.

18. Sinha RY, Raje SR, Rao GA. Three-dimensional laparoscopy: principles and practice. *J Minim Access Surg* 2017;**13**(3):165–9. doi: 10.4103/072-9941.181761.

19. Vilaça J, Leite M, Correia-Pinto J, et al. The influence of 3D in single-port laparoscopy surgery: an experimental study. *Surg Laparosc Endosc Percutan Tech* 2018 Aug;**28**(4):261–6. doi:10.1097/SLE.0000000000000536.

20. Gu D, Jiang J, Li J, Yan Z. Design and implementation of the glasses-free three dimensional laparoscopy system. *Zhongguo Yi Liao Qi Xie Za Zhi* 2017 Sep 30;**41** (5):317–21. doi: 10.3969/j.issn.1671-7104.2017.05.002.

21. Walocha JA, Litwin JA, Miodonski AJ. Vascular system of intramural leiomyomata revealed by corrosion casting and scanning electron microscopy. *Hum Reprod* 2003;**18**(5):1088.

22. Takahashi N, Yoshino O, Hiraike O, et al. The assessment of myometrium perfusion in patients with uterine fibroid by arterial spin labeling MRI. *SpringerPlus* 2016;**5**(1):1907. doi:10.1186/s40064-016-3596-0.

23. Kamel A, El-Mazny A, Ramadan W, et al. Effect of intramural fibroid on uterine and endometrial vascularity in infertile women scheduled for in-vitro fertilization. *Arch Gynecol Obstet* 2018 Feb;**297**(2):539–45. doi: 10.1007/s00404-017-4607-2 [Epub 14 Dec 2017].

24. Landi S, Minelli L. Chapter 12: Technique of laparoscopic myomectomy. In: Mencaglia L, Minelli L, Wattiez A, editors, *Manual of Gynecological Laparoscopic Surgery*, 2nd ed. Tuttlingen, Germany: Endo Press GMBH; 2012:139–50.

25. Cohen SL, Senapati S, Gargiulo AR, et al. Dilute versus concentrated vasopressin administration during laparoscopic myomectomy: a randomised controlled trial. *BJOG* 2017 Jan;**124**(2):262–8.

26. Goldman KN, Hirshfeld-Cytron JE, Pavone M-E, et al. Uterine artery embolization immediately preceding laparoscopic myomectomy. *Int J Gynecol Obstet* 2012;**116**:105–8.

27. Schnapauff D, Russ M, Kröncke T, et al. Analysis of presurgical uterine artery embolization (PUAE) for very large uterus myomatosus; patient's desire to preserve the uterus; case series and literature review. *Fortschr Röntgenstr* 2018;**190**:616–22.

28. Dumousset E, Chabrot P, Rabischong B, et al. Preoperative uterine artery embolization (PUAE) before uterine fibroid myomectomy. *Cardiovasc Intervent Radiol* 2008 May–Jun;**31** (3):514–20.

29. Ravina JH, Herbreteau D, Ciraro-Vigneron N, et al. Arterial embolisation to treat uterine myomata. *Lancet* 1995;**346**:671–2.

30. Donat LC, Menderes G, Tower AM, Azodi M. A technique for vascular control during robotic-assisted laparoscopic myomectomy. *J Minim Invasive Gynecol* 2015 May–Jun;**22**(4):543. doi: 10.1016/j.jmig.2015.02.003 [Epub 11 Feb 2015].

31. Javadian P, Juusela A, Nezhat F. Robotic-assisted laparoscopic cervicovaginal myomectomy. *J Minim Invasive Gynecol* 2018 Mar 28;pii:S1553-4650(18)30167-5. doi: 10.1016/j.jmig.2018.03.014 [Epub ahead of print].

32. Pelage JP, Le Dref O, Soyer P, et al. Arterial anatomy of the female genital tract: variations and relevance to transcatheter embolization of the uterus. *Am J Roentgenol (AJR)* 1999;**172**:989–94.

33. Wang CJ, Yuen LT, Han CM, et al. A transient blocking uterine perfusion procedure to decrease operative blood loss in laparoscopic myomectomy. *Chang Gung Med J* 2008 Sep–Oct;**31**(5):463–8.

34. McGovern PG, Noah R, Koenigsberg R, Little AB. Adnexal torsion and pulmonary embolism: case report and review of literature. *Obstet Gynecol Surv* 1999;**54**:601–8.

35. Oelsner G, Cohen SB, Soriano D, et al. Minimal surgery for the twisted ischaemic adnexa can preserve ovarian function. *Hum Reprod* 2003;**18**:2599–602.

36. Peters A, Stuparich MA, Mansuria SM, Lee TT. Anatomic vascular considerations in uterine artery ligation at its origin during laparoscopic hysterectomies. *Am J Obstet Gynecol* 2016 Sep;**215** (3):393.

37. dos Santos Martin RL, Zomer MT, Hayashi R, Ribeiro R, Kondo W. How do I perform temporary occlusion of the uterine arteries during laparoscopic myomectomy? *Gynecol Obstet (Sunnyvale)* 2015;**5**:278. doi: 10.4172/2161-0932.1000278.

38. Farrer-Brown G, Beilby JO, Tarbit MH. The vascular patterns in myomatous uteri. *J Obstet Gynaecol Br Commonw* 1970;**77**:967–75.

39. Tinelli A, Hurst BS, Hudelist G, et al. Laparoscopic myomectomy focusing on the myoma pseudocapsule: technical and outcome reports. *Hum Reprod* 2012;**27**(2):427–35.

40. Parker WH, Einarsson J, Istre O, Dubuisson JB. Risk factors for uterine rupture after laparoscopic myomectomy. *J Minim Invasive Gynecol* 2010 Sep–Oct;**17** (5):551–4. doi: 10.1016/j. jmig.2010.04.015 [Epub 29 Jun 2010]. Review. Erratum in: *J Minim Invasive Gynecol* 2010 Nov–Dec;**17**(6):809.

41. Robinson NL, Srouji SS, Gargiulo, AR. Laparoscopic myomectomy: a hybrid approach utilizing the da Vinci robot. *Fertil Steril* 2008;**90**: S446.

42. Quaas AM, Einarsson JI, Srouji S, Gargiulo AR. Robotic myomectomy: a review of indications and techniques. *Rev Obstet Gynecol* 2010;**3**(4):185–91.

43. Driessen SRC, Arkenbout EA, Thurkow AL, Jansen FW. Electromechanical morcellators in minimally invasive gynecologic surgery: an update. *J Minim Invasive Gynecol* 2014; **21**(3):377–83.

44. Donnez O, Jadoul P, Squifflet J, Donnex J. Iatrogenic peritoneal adenomyoma after laparoscopic subtotal hysterectomy and uterine morcellation. *Fertil Steril* 2006 Nov;**86**(5):1511–12.

45. Donnez O, Donnez J. A series of 400 laparoscopic hysterectomies for benign disease: a single centre, single surgeon prospective study of complications confirming previous retrospective study. *BJOG* 2010 May;**117** (6):752–5.

46. FDA. Updated Assessment of the Use of Laparoscopic Power Morcellators to Treat Uterine Fibroids. December 2017; www .fda.gov/media/109018/download Accessed 10 Jan 2020.

47. Bojahr B, De Wilde RL, Tchartchian G. Malignancy rate of 10,731 uteri morcellated during laparoscopic supracervical hysterectomy (LASH). *Arch Gynecol Obstet* 2015 Sept; **292**(3):665–72.

48. Pritts EA, Vanness DJ, Berek JS, et al. The prevalence of occult leiomyosarcoma at surgery for presumed uterine fibroids: a meta-analysis. *Gynecol Surg* 2015;**12**(3):165–177.

49. Lieng M, Berner E, Busund B. Risk of morcellation of uterine leiomyosarcomas in laparoscopic supracervical hysterectomy and laparoscopic myomectomy, a retrospective trial including 4791 women. *J Minim Invasive Gynecol* 2015 Mar–Apr; **22**(3):410–4.

50. Cohen SL, Einarsson JI, Wang KC, Brown D, Boruta D, Scheib SA, Fader AN, Shibley T. Contained power morcellation within an insufflated isolation bag. *Obstet Gynecol.* 2014 Sep;**124**(3):491–7.

51. Serur E, Zambrano N, Brown K, Clemetson E, Lakhi N. Extracorporeal manual morcellation of very large uteri within an enclosed endoscopic bag: our 5-year experience. *J Minim Invasive Gynecol* 2016; **23**(6):903–8.

52. Sanderson DJ, Sanderson R, Cleason D, Seaman C, Ghomi A. Manual morcellation compared to power morcellation during robotic myomectomy. *J Robot Surg* 2019 Apr 15;**13**(2):209–14 doi: 10.1007/s11701-018-0837-y.

53. Kho KA, Shin JH, Nezhat C. Vaginal extraction of large uteri with the Alexis retractor. *J Minim Invasive Gynecol* 2009 Sep-Oct; **16**(5):616–7.

54. Favero G, Miglino G, Köhler C, Pfiffer T, Silva e Silva A, Ribeiro A, Le X, Anton C, Baracat EC, Carvalho JP. Vaginal morcellation inside protective pouch: a safe strategy for uterine extration in cases of bulky endometrial cancers: operative and oncological safety of the method. *J Minim Invasive Gynecol.* 2015 Sep-Oct; **22**(6):938–43.

55. Pelosi III M, Pelosi M. Laparoscopic-assisted transvaginal myomectomy. *J Am Assoc Gynecol Laparosc* 1997;**4**:241–6.

56. Goldfarb HA, Fanarjian NJ. Laparoscopic-assisted vaginal myomectomy: a case report and literature review. *J Soc Laparoendosc Surg* 2001 Jan–Mar;**5**(1):81–5.

57. Nezhat C, Nezhat F, Bess O, Nezhat CH, Mashiach R. Laparoscopically assisted myomectomy: a report of a new technique in 57 cases. *Int J Fertil Menopausal Stud* 1994;**39**:39–44.

Principles and Technique of Laparoscopic Myomectomy

Ephia Yasmin and Ertan Saridogan

9.1 Introduction

Uterine fibroids are the most common benign neoplasms of the female reproductive tract with an estimated incidence of 25–30% at reproductive age [1]. They are detected by ultrasound in about 70–80% of women by the age of menopause [2]. About 30% of fibroids produce symptoms such as abnormal uterine bleeding (AUB) which may result in anaemia, pain or pressure effects on contiguous structures such as urinary incontinence, urinary frequency, urinary outflow obstruction, hydronephrosis, constipation and tenesmus. Fibroids may also be associated with subfertility, and with adverse pregnancy outcomes such as miscarriage and fetal malpresentation [3]. The symptoms associated with fibroids are known to compromise quality of life [3].

9.2 Indications for Myomectomy

The surgical interventions for fibroids include myomectomy and hysterectomy, and these are considered when conservative management fails to control symptoms, when intractable bleeding induces iron deficiency anaemia or when quality of life is adversely affected [4]. The association between fibroid and subfertility, and the potential benefit of myomectomy for subfertility, continue to be a matter of debate. Systematic reviews on the effect of fibroids on reproductive outcome (both spontaneous and following medically assisted conception) suggest that submucosal and intramural fibroids are associated with adverse pregnancy outcomes and lower clinical pregnancy, and implantation rates with an increased rate of miscarriage, while subserosal fibroids do not seem to exert a detrimental effect on fertility or pregnancy outcome [5, 6]. Myomectomy is indicated when there is a desire to preserve the uterus.

Two systematic reviews examining the outcome of assisted reproductive techniques (ART) in the presence of fibroids demonstrated conflicting results.

Sunkara *et al.,* showed reduced clinical pregnancy and live birth rates in the presence of fibroids even when not distorting the cavity [7], while the Cochrane review by Metwally *et al.* demonstrated that presence of intramural fibroids did not appear to change live birth or miscarriage rates, although clinical pregnancy rates appeared to be lower in the presence of fibroids [8]. The role of myomectomy in otherwise asymptomatic women purely for purposes of fertility enhancement remains controversial. On the basis of current evidence, a lower threshold for treating certain fibroids, such as submucosal fibroids and intramural fibroids distorting the endometrial cavity, seems justifiable. At the other extreme, subserosal fibroids do not generally warrant treatment unless they are associated with symptoms such as menorrhagia or pain [3].

The approach for myomectomy is hysteroscopic for submucosal fibroids, open or laparoscopic for intramural and subserosal fibroids [9]. Laparoscopic myomectomy (LM) has been found to be associated with less postoperative pain, lower rates of postoperative fever and shorter hospital stay but longer operating times in comparison to traditional open myomectomy [10]. Other potential advantages of the laparoscopic approach include a quicker recovery time with a more rapid return to normal daily activities. Therefore LM is seen to be more advantageous to the patient than laparotomy.

9.3 Factors to Consider Prior to Surgery

Preoperative assessment and planning are crucial in choosing patients appropriately and minimizing risks of LM. Prior to considering LM, the number, size and location of fibroids must be mapped. This not only helps determine the feasibility of a laparoscopic approach over an open approach but also identifies submucosal fibroids which are generally better treated hysteroscopically [11, 12]. However, because of the potential for heavy bleeding and incomplete resection, some large submucosal myomas may be more effectively treated by the laparoscopic route, especially if resection is likely to result in significant endometrial loss/scarring or leave only a thin residual myometrial layer. A very thin myometrial layer may increase the risk of uterine rupture in subsequent pregnancy [12, 13].

There is no absolute restriction on the number and size of fibroids that can be removed laparoscopically, and this is often determined by the surgeon's experience and expertise [13]. However, the risk of conversion to laparotomy, blood loss and surgical duration increase with fibroid size and number, and with accompanying adenomyosis [14]. Whilst there is no consensus, some authors consider LM to be appropriate for a maximum of three or four myomas whose sizes do not exceed 8 cm [14], whereas others believe in individual choice based on surgical skill [15].

9.4 Preoperative Imaging

Preoperative fibroid mapping is of paramount importance prior to LM. It is crucial to know the fibroid location during LM, as there is no opportunity to palpate the uterus intraoperatively.

9.4.1 Ultrasound

Clinical examination and transvaginal ultrasound or a combination of transvaginal and transabdominal ultrasound is often employed for evaluating fibroids preoperatively. The advantages of ultrasound are accessibility and cost. The quality of imaging will depend on the expertise and experience of the operator. Key information to be derived from ultrasound assessment include fibroid dimensions, subtype (submucosal, intramural or subserosal) location (anterior wall, posterior wall, cervical or broad ligament extension) and the presence of adenomyosis [16]. Three-dimensional ultrasound (3D USS) and saline infusion sonohysterography may also assist in identifying submucosal fibroids and may be particularly useful when there is significant uterine distortion from several other fibroids [16].

9.4.2 Magnetic Resonance Imaging (MRI)

When ultrasound findings are atypical or unclear, or if the presence of multiple fibroids makes ultrasound assessment difficult, magnetic resonance imaging

(MRI) may be more reliable. In patients with more than six myomas and a voluminous uterus, MRI as a second-level examination may be particularly helpful [17]. MRI may also help in differentiating fibroids from adenomyosis [6]. The distinction between fibroid and adenomyosis is important as adenomyosis presents an added challenge during laparoscopy owing to the lack of a clearly defined dissection plane. The ureters and renal system need to be evaluated in the presence of large broad ligament fibroids or a very large uterus pressing on the pelvic sidewalls, because of the risk of ureteral obstruction.

It is worth noting that neither ultrasonography nor MRI can diagnose malignancy with any certainty [18]. While MRI findings can suggest a diagnosis of sarcoma, there is currently no reliable form of preoperative testing which can definitively rule it out [19].

In spite of meticulous preoperative evaluation, the final decision as to whether LM is feasible may only be possible at the time of surgery leading to a decision to convert to an open approach on the basis of the initial laparoscopic findings.

9.5 Pretreatment with Medical Agents

The medical treatments that are used to reduce size of fibroids, increase feasibility of a laparoscopic approach and reduce operating time are gonadotrophin hormone-releasing hormone agonists (GnRHa), selective progesterone receptor modulators (SPRM) and aromatase inhibitors. Of these, GnRHa is most widely used. More recently, four SPRMs investigated in clinical trials are mifepristone, asoprisnil, ulipristal acetate (UPA) and telapristone acetate [20]. All were shown to decrease leiomyoma size and reduce uterine bleeding in a dose-dependent manner. Some follow-up studies have raised concerns about unopposed estrogenic activity and liver toxicity with mifepristone [21]. UPA has shown promising results in terms of efficiency and safety. UPA was compared to a placebo and to leuprolide acetate (a GnRH agonist) in two randomized trials [22, 23], which concluded that control of uterine bleeding in more than 90% of patients receiving a 3-month course of UPA, and the median times to control bleeding, were shorter in the UPA group (5–7 days) than in the GnRH agonist group (21 days).

Studies examining the use of the aromatase inhibitor letrozole have shown that the total operative time, the time required to close uterine incision and intra-operative blood loss significantly decrease after pre-operative treatment with letrozole [24].

There are pros and cons to the use of size-reducing agents prior to LM. The main advantages include correction of anaemia, attenuation of blood loss, reduced uterine and fibroid size, and less adhesion formation [25]. The reduction of fibroid size may increase the feasibility of laparoscopic surgery and also the retrieval of the fibroids. The downsides include added cost and side effects. In addition, these agents increase the difficulty in identifying surgical dissection planes, which may lead to increase in surgical time and risk of conversion to laparotomy [26]. Preoperative GnRH agonists have also been reported as a risk factor for fibroid recurrence, presumably because smaller fibroids shrink and are overlooked at surgery only to regrow when the analogue's effects wear off [25].

Overall, given that medical therapies prior to surgery may increase the risk of recurrence, the routine use of these agents is not justified. This is especially so since other agents such as intraoperative vasopressin do not increase surgical intricacy and are of proven efficacy in reducing intraoperative bleeding [27, 28]. Therefore, the trade-off between reduction of volume and vascularity of fibroids and the ease of finding surgical planes must be considered prior to the use of GnRHa or UPA.

9.6 Correction of Anaemia

Anaemia is not uncommon in women having LM, owing to heavy menstrual bleeding (HMB). Preoperative intervention is required to resurrect the haemoglobin concentration to anaesthetically safe levels and to reduce postoperative morbidity. As already mentioned, GnRH analogues constitute one effective means for achieving this by temporarily avoiding heavy periods in the run-up to surgery. Some authors advocate recombinant erythropoietin, with evidence from an Italian prospective study showing a significant increase in haemoglobin concentrations before and after gynaecologic surgery (which included hysterectomy for large symptomatic fibroids) after using recombinant human erythropoietin for 8–16 days [29]. Women with borderline haemoglobin levels should also be advised on the use of oral iron therapy.

Regardless of the preoperative haemoglobin level, it should be ensured that cross-matched blood is readily accessible at the time of surgery.

9.7 Consent

The consent procedure for laparoscopic myomectomy should include discussion of the possibility of conversion to laparotomy and of the rare need for hysterectomy in addition to other standard complications associated with laparoscopic surgery. It is good practice to include a discussion on morcellation due to the additional risk of injury to vessels, bowel and other organs with the morcellator as well as the small risk of upstaging occult uterine sarcoma. According to a review carried out by the European Society for Gynaecological Endoscopy, prevalence of uterine sarcoma in fibroids is about 0.14% based on meta-analysis of retrospective trials [30]. It also appears to be age-related, with a lower risk in women <45 years [31]. However, current data on age and prevalence make it difficult to present an accurate risk.

9.8 Surgical Technique

9.8.1 Preparation in Operating Theatre

Under general anaesthesia, the abdomen is examined for size and mobility of the uterus and to plan placement of trocars. The Lloyd-Davies position with arms at the sides allows good movement and manoeuvrability of the surgeon and assistants. The cervix is grasped with a vulsellum forceps and a uterine manipulator placed. The vulsellum and uterine manipulator are useful for manipulating the uterus and exerting counter-traction during fibroid enucleation and suturing, and for methylene blue dye instillation if tubal patency testing is required. If there is any uncertainty from preoperative imaging regarding the presence and/or type of submucosal fibroids, a diagnostic hysteroscopy can be undertaken prior to laparoscopy and transcervical resection of fibroid carried out if required.

9.8.2 Trocar Placement

Trocar placement is at the surgeon's discretion and should facilitate fibroid enucleation and suturing. The choice of pneumoperitoneum depends on surgeon's preference. With large fibroids, a Palmer's point entry may be preferred with the 10 mm trocar placed under vision. This may sometimes be better when placed higher than the umbilicus for improved vision of large fibroids. The Palmer's point entry may also be preferred where periumbilical adhesions are anticipated as a result of prior surgery [32]. The authors' preference is to use three further ports: two 5 mm high lateral ports placed lateral to the epigastric vessels and a 11–12 mm suprapubic port (Figure 9.1a and b). The suprapubic port facilitates insertion of needles, sutures and 10 mm claw graspers or myomectomy screws. This port is later enlarged for the morcellator. Surgeons who perform ipsilateral suturing will place both 5 mm ports ipsilaterally.

As an initial step, it is important to carefully survey the pelvis and reassess whether the laparoscopic approach remains feasible. For deeper sited fibroids, that may not be readily evident on inspection. Sometimes, an intraoperative ultrasound evaluation may compensate for the lack of tactile evaluation, but the pneumoperitoneum may pose a challenge to image quality [33].

9.8.3 Minimizing Intraoperative Bleeding

Before the serosa is incised, a dilute solution of Pitressin® (20 U/mL; Goldshield Pharmaceuticals, Croydon, UK), a synthetic vasopressin, is injected. We dilute 20 U of Pitressin® (Argipressin) in 20 mL of saline and administer it using an 18-gauge spinal needle placed directly through the abdominal wall. Pitressin® is instilled bilaterally into the broad ligament just inferior to the round ligaments and subserosally over the fibroid in the plane that allows the solution to 'spread' over the fibroid (Video 9.1), accompanied by blanching (Figure 9.2a and b). Vasopressin causes rapid constriction of vascular smooth muscle and may cause untoward cardiovascular

> ▶ **Video 9.1** Initial assessment and argipressin injection.

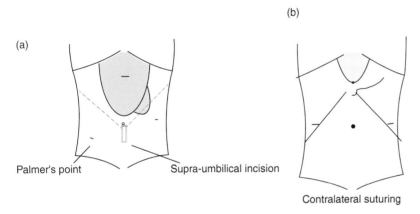

Figure 9.1 (a) Port placement for laparoscopic myomectomy. (b) Use of ports for contralateral suturing.

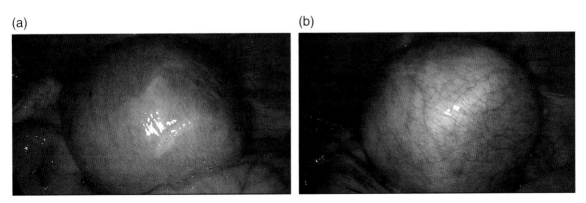

Figure 9.2 (a) An enlarged uterus due to fundal/anterior wall fibroids. (b) Blanching of the uterus after argipressin injection.

81

complications, making it important to forewarn the anaesthetist prior to its instillation. Pitressin® use in myomectomy is an off-label use of the drug. A recent meta-analysis affirms the efficacy of vasopressin in reducing intraoperative bleeding during myomectomies. Other agents used to reduce intraoperative bleeding are vaginal misoprostol, intravenous tranexamic acid or a combination of 0.25% bupivacaine and adrenaline [27, 28].

9.8.4 Uterine Incision

An incision is made in the uterine serosa overlying the fibroid. The surgeon can choose the monopolar hook or scissors with unmodulated high-wattage current (50 W or more) along with a smoke extractor to maintain a clear operative field. Alternatively, an ultrasonic Harmonic Scalpel® (Johnson & Johnson, New Brunswick, NJ, USA) or Thunderbeat® (combination of bipolar and ultrasound, Olympus) may be used (Video 9.2). The latter instruments are more expensive but have the advantages of limiting thermal damage, reducing the need for smoke evacuation and potentially less blood loss [34]. RCT data cite additional benefits for the harmonic scalpel over electrosurgical approaches, including reduced postoperative pain and reduced operative times [35].

The direction of the incision depends on fibroid location and must take into account avoidance of tubal injury and ease of suturing. The repair of horizontal incisions is easier with ipsilaterally placed ports whereas when ports are sited contralaterally, vertical incisions are more amenable to suturing [36]. Horizontal incisions may risk inadvertent extension into the cornua and interstitial portions of the tubes. Some advocate the use of elliptical as opposed to linear incisions to enable resection of some of the overlying myometrium and to reduce redundant tissue, thereby facilitating closure.

9.8.5 Fibroid Dissection and Enucleation

Identification of the correct plane helps fibroid extraction. The incision is carried through the serosa, the myometrium, the pseudocapsule and into the myoma itself. So-called onion-skinning allows the myometrium to retract and the fibroid to progressively become extruded, thereby allowing the correct plane to declare itself. This plane, which tends to be avascular, is often deeper than is commonly recognized (Video 9.2).

 Video 9.2 Uterine incision and enucleation of the fibroid.

Primary traction on the exposed fibroid is applied with a claw grasper or myoma screw placed through the 11–12 mm suprapubic port. A blunt probe along with a grasper such as a Manhes forceps to hold the myometrial/serosal edge via the paraumbilical ports is used to push the myometrial edge off the fibroid. This enables the space along the pseudocapsule to be gradually extended circumferentially. Tension on the fibroid by use of the suprapubic 10 mm claw forceps with simultaneous counter-traction from the blunt probe and/or Manhes forceps and the uterine manipulator, aided by division of more stubborn bands using the energy device, progressively coaxes the fibroid from its uterine bed. Once removed, the fibroid can be placed in the pouch of Douglas. Larger fibroids may be placed in the upper abdomen, but it would be better to keep smaller fibroids in the pelvis to avoid difficulty in locating them later in the upper abdomen among the loops of bowel and the omentum (Figure 9.3a–d).

9.8.6 Haemostasis and Repair of the Myometrial Defect

It is often felt that a distinct primary vascular pedicle will be found at the fibroid base. However, this is not supported by vascular studies which demonstrate that the vascular supply completely surrounds the fibroid as a dense vascular capsule [37]. Electrocautery to wide areas should be avoided. Individual bleeding vessels should be isolated and cauterized to limit thermal spread and tissue charring. Extensive cautery leads to poor healing of tissue and is implicated in the risk of uterine rupture [38]. Use of a vasoconstrictor may maintain a bloodless field to allow prompt suturing without recourse to diathermy. Two studies have reported on pregnancies following LM during which electrocoagulation was avoided and haemostasis secured by suturing; no uterine ruptures were observed in 111 deliveries in one study [39] and 106 deliveries in the other [40].

Difficulty encountered with suturing is a major cause of conversions to laparotomy [41]. The uterine defect can be closed using conventional laparoscopic needle drivers and delayed absorbable sutures. Knot tying may be either intra- or extracorporeal. Care should be taken to identify any breach of the

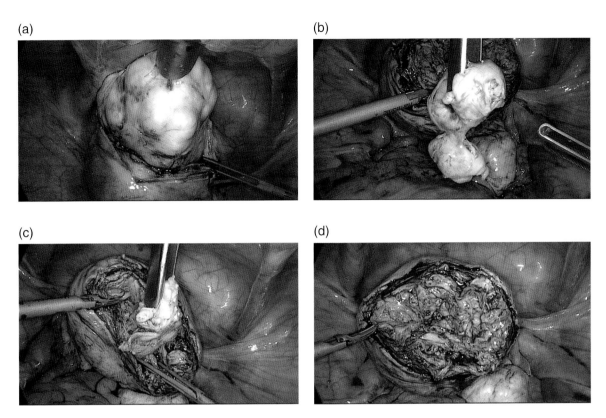

Figure 9.3 (a) Enucleation of an intramural fibroid through an anterior wall oblique incision. (b) Removal of two further smaller fibroids located deep in myometrium. (c) Removal of a fourth fibroid. (d) The myometrial defect after enucleation of fibroids.

endometrial cavity. If the endometrial cavity is breached, the endometrium should be closed separately with interrupted 3-0 monofilament polyglactin. The myometrium is closed using large curved needles swaged to 1-0 or 0 polyglactin in one or two continuous running layers depending on the depth of fibroid invasion and the thickness of myometrium to be approximated. Continuous sutures are associated with a significantly smaller drop in haemoglobin levels [42]. Suturing is made more convenient with an anchoring suture placed on the proximal end of the defect on which the assistant exerts traction so as to bring the target into a favourable position for placing the running suture, which is commenced at the distal end. A separate layer of 0 or 2-0 monofilament polyglactin is used to close the serosa.

Technological innovations such as self-righting needle drivers that snap the needle into place with the correct orientation and barbed sutures that obviate the need for knot tying may simplify suturing and make the procedure expeditious [43, 44] (Video 9.3). The barbs in barbed sutures face either in one

 Video 9.3 Suturing of the myometrial defect.

direction with a needle swaged to one end (V-Loc™ Device; Covidien, MA, USA; Stratafix™, Johnson & Johnson, USA) or in opposite directions from the midpoint with needles at either end (Quill™ SRS; Angiotech Pharmaceuticals, Inc. Vancouver BC, Canada). The barbed suture distributes tension more uniformly along the length of the uterine incision and self-anchors (Figure 9.4).

9.8.7 Fibroid Removal and Anti-adhesion Agents

The fibroid is usually removed using a single-use or reusable electromechanical morcellator. The 10 mm suprapubic trocar is removed and the skin incision extended to accommodate a 12 or 15 mm morcellator. The fibroid is drawn into the morcellator via a heavy grasper and the morcellator is activated, taking

83

(a)

(b)

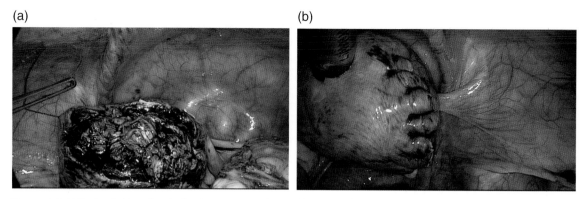

Figure 9.4 (a) Uterine incision after the first layer myometrial repair. (b) Serosal closure.

extreme care that its tip is free of the abdominal wall and in a pocket of pneumoperitoneum having proper 360-degree clearance from bowel and adjacent structures to minimize potential risk of damage to vessels and organs. The morcellator blade is kept retracted except when actively morcellating the fibroid. Morcellation injuries, if they happen, can be fatal. After the main bulk of the fibroid is removed, meticulous inspection of the abdominopelvic cavity and removal of fibroid fragments is imperative, as morcellated fragments of fibroid have been implicated in the development of disseminated peritoneal leiomyomatosis [45].

Following the concerns of morcellation of undiagnosed leiomyosarcoma, two statements by the FDA (United States Food and Drug Administration) in April and November 2014 discouraged the use of electromechanical morcellation in the majority of women due to the potential risk of spreading occult uterine sarcoma. Morcellation in a bag has been proposed to diminish the risk of vessel and organ injury, prevent scattering of the fragments and also minimize upstaging occult uterine sarcoma. Several techniques of in-bag morcellation of fibroids have been proposed to avoid many of the reported morcellation complications (Video 9.4). However, not all risks have been addressed such as spillage from the content of the bag in the abdomen, especially if the bag is punctured. Small series of in-bag morcellation have been published with good results [46, 47]. Vaginal morcellation in a bag has been also been described [48]. Possible drawbacks are the need for a sufficient vaginal entry and the fact that only hysterectomy specimens are suitable for this technique. There is insufficient evidence for concrete recommendations on fibroid morcellation, but in-bag morcellation appears to be an option that requires further evaluation.

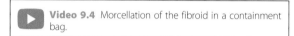

Video 9.4 Morcellation of the fibroid in a containment bag.

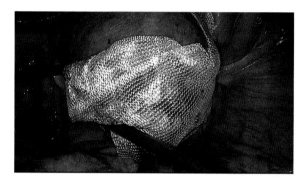

Figure 9.5 Uterine incision covered with a barrier anti-adhesion measure after the repair.

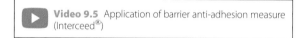

Video 9.5 Application of barrier anti-adhesion measure (Interceed®)

Another option for fibroid removal is via a colpotomy incision, which may be faster than morcellation [34]. However, colpotomy leaves the woman with a vaginal incision, may increase the risk of infection and cannot be used for very large fibroids unless the fibroids are reduced.

After removal of the fibroid, the uterus is irrigated and haemostasis confirmed.

Barriers to adhesion may be used upon completion of suturing (Figure 9.5 and Video 9.5). A Cochrane review found that oxidized regenerated cellulose (Interceed®; Johnson & Johnson, New Brunswick, NJ, USA) reduces adhesions following laparoscopy and that expanded polytetrafluoroethylene (Gore-Tex®;

WL Gore and Associates, Newark, DE, USA) surgical membrane may be superior to Interceed®, although its usefulness is limited by the need for suturing and later removal [49]. No evidence of effectiveness for sodium hyaluronate/carboxymethylcellulose (Sepra-film®; Genzyme, Cambridge, MA, USA) and Fibrin sheet (Tacho Comb, Tokyo, Japan) in preventing adhesion formation was found [49]. As yet, however, there is no substantial evidence that any of these agents improve fertility, reduce pain or decrease the incidence of postoperative bowel obstruction [50].

Finally, when closing the abdominal wall incisions, it is important to repair the rectus sheath defect within the 15 mm suprapubic incision to avoid later herniation. Closure can be effected with either a J-shaped needle or a suture passer needle.

9.9 Complications

Surgeons require training and appropriate skills to perform laparoscopic myomectomy. Initial concern about increased risk of complications has been replaced by the focus on early recovery [14, 51–53]. In 2007, a large prospective study of 2050 LM procedures undertaken in four Italian referral centres reported an overall complication rate of 11.1%, of which 9.1% were considered minor and 2% major [15]. Intraoperative bleeding occurred in 0.68% of women and serious secondary haemorrhage in 0.1%. One of these required laparoscopic hysterectomy. Failure to complete the planned surgery occurred in 0.34% of instances; conversion to laparotomy occurred in the other seven women (one due to bleeding, three due to anaesthetic problems, one because of a suspected sarcoma and two women because of insufficient space limiting mobilization for very large myomas). In this series, only one woman suffered a bowel injury. One woman had an unrecognized episode of prolonged hypotension resulting in acute kidney failure, which resolved after 2 days of dialysis, and two women had an unexpected sarcoma. Among 386 women who became pregnant, one woman had uterine rupture at week 33 of gestation; this woman had had an 8 cm adenomyoma.

The most common complications included unexplained transient pyrexia (105 of 2050 women; 5.1%) and urinary tract infections (70 of 2050 women; 3.4%). There were 12 (0.6%) episodes of uterine manipulator injury. Overall, the mean drop in haemoglobin was approximately 1.6 g/dL and hospital stay was about 2 days [15].

Complications correlate positively with fibroid number and size [54]. It should be remembered that compared with open myomectomy, LM is a relatively new procedure that is still evolving. Furthermore, some of the skills needed for LM are not readily transferable from more routinely performed procedures as might be the case for open myomectomy. As such, many operators are still on their learning curve and as their repertoire of laparoscopic skills continues to be honed, complication rates will undoubtedly fall. Furthermore, new innovations in laparoscopic equipment to aid suturing and fibroid removal have made LM easier. In a very insightful study, some of these authors appraised their own practice over a 13-year period. They found that as their dexterity improved and they supplemented their practice with electro-mechanical morcellation and vasoconstrictive agents, they could cope with considerably larger fibroids while at the same time decreasing their operating times and blood loss [55]. Our own case series of 514 LMs reported successful completion of the procedure in 512 women with 18/514 (3.5%) women suffering significant complications: blood loss >1000 mL (n = 15), bowel injury (n = 1), bladder injury (n = 1), small bowel obstruction secondary to port site hernia (n = 1). Two cases were converted to open surgery, one because of suspected uterine malignancy and another due to bowel injury at initial entry, and there were no cases of undiagnosed uterine malignancies following morcellation of fibroids [56].

9.9.1 Robot-Assisted Laparoscopic Myomectomy

Computer-assisted or robotic technology is increasingly being applied to LM [57]. Robot-assisted laparoscopic myomectomy (RALM) is still in its nascent stage as there are no randomized controlled trials that compare RALM and LM. One retrospective matched-control study found similar blood loss, postoperative complication rates and hospital stay for RALM and LM but significantly longer operating times for RALM [58]. Another retrospective analysis found that RALM did not significantly increase surgical time and advocated robotic technology as a means for enabling a laparoscopic approach in cases that would otherwise require open surgery due to larger fibroid size or a difficult location [59]. It remains to be seen how benefits offered by RALM such as a 3-dimensional image, superior instrument articulation, absence of tremor, downscaling of movements and increased comfort for the surgeon compare with its downsides such as bulkiness, cost of equipment and lack of haptic feedback.

9.10 Laparoscopic Myomectomy versus Open Myomectomy

Reduced pain and bleeding are consistent features after laparoscopy, identified in several studies. Randomized controlled data from two studies also support reduced febrile morbidity following laparoscopy and a shorter duration of postoperative ileus [55, 60]. Although the lack of a tactile component during laparoscopy could possibly allow smaller fibroids to be missed, this does not seem to be of any clinical consequence [60].

Owing to the technical challenges of laparoscopic suturing and the time taken for removal of fibroids from the abdominal cavity, laparoscopic myomectomy would be expected to be a longer procedure. However, major differences in operating times are not consistently apparent from RCTs. Increasingly acceptable operating times for LM probably reflect refinement of laparoscopic skills along with access to better surgical equipment. The large Italian multicentre study reported a mean operating time of 107.7 minutes for 2050 LM procedures [15].

One of the major criticisms levelled against LM has been that the integrity of uterine repair is inferior to that attainable following open myomectomy; however, in many instances, suboptimal operative technique may have contributed to poor outcome. It is hard to establish how the risk of uterine rupture following LM compares with that following open surgery. It is clear from recent series that when good surgical discipline is maintained, dehiscence rates well below 1% can be expected [15].

The outcomes in terms of cumulative pregnancy, live birth and miscarriage rates among the women with unexplained infertility were similar regardless of the surgical approach used [40]. Interestingly, however, reproductive parameters were significantly better following LM among women with symptomatic fibroids. As a group, women having LM had significantly higher pregnancy and live births per cycle and a shorter time to first conception [40]. Thus, there is a suggestion that fertility prospects might improve with the laparoscopic approach. One mechanism by which LM could be advantageous to fertility is through reduced adhesion formation [50].

9.11 Conclusions

Modern LM is the result of years of refinement, often in response to weaknesses highlighted by adverse effects, combined with key advances such as the development of intraoperative vasoconstrictors, barbed sutures and electromechanical morcellation. The end result is a technique with impressive efficacy and safety profiles. Although there are no preset restrictions, surgeons must be pragmatic in matching their skill to fibroid burden, opting for a laparotomy approach when fibroids are too many or too large. In such circumstances, laparoscopic-assisted myomectomy (LAM) may be of value. Compared with conventional myomectomy, apart from its obvious aesthetic superiority, LM is consistently associated with reduced rates of pain, bleeding, febrile morbidity and ileus, shorter hospital stay and faster recovery. Importantly, recent evidence indicates that with careful attention to surgical detail, the rate of uterine rupture in pregnancy following LM is low and operating times are not dissimilar to open surgery. Moreover, in terms of reproductive outcome in subsequent pregnancy LM is superior to uterine artery embolization and may offer advantages over the open approach.

References

1. Ryan GL, Syrop CH, Van Voorhis BJ. Role, epidemiology and natural history of benign uterine mass lesions. *Clin Obstet Gynecol* 2005;**48**:312–24.

2. Baird D, Dunson DB, Hill MC, Cousins D, Schectman JM. High cumulative incidence of uterine leiomyoma in black and white women: ultrasound evidence. *Am J ObstetGynecol* 2003;**188**:100–7.

3. Klatsky PC, Tran ND, Caughey AB, Fujimoto VY. Fibroids and reproductive outcomes: a systematic literature review from conception to delivery. *Am J Obstet Gynecol* 2008;**198** (4):357–66.

4. Parker WH. Uterine myomas: management. *Fertil Steril* 2007;**88** (2):255–71.

5. Pritts EA, Parker WH, Olive DL. Fibroids and infertility: an updated systematic review of the evidence. *Fertil Steril* 2009;**91**:1215–23.

6. Dubuisson JB, Fauconnier A, Deffarges JV, Norgaard C, Kreiker G, Chapron C. Pregnancy

outcome and deliveries following laparoscopic myomectomy. *Hum Reprod* 2000;**15**(4):869–73.

7. Sunkara S, Khairy M, El-Toukhy T, Khalaf Y, Coomarasamy A. The effect of intramural fibroids without uterine cavity involvement on the outcome of IVF treatment: a systematic review and meta-analysis. *Hum Reprod* 2010;**25**(2):418–29.

8. Metwally M, Cheong YC, Horne AW. Surgical treatment of fibroids for subfertility. *Cochrane Database Syst Rev* 2012;(11):CD003857. doi: 10.1002/14651858.CD003857.pub3.

9. Saridogan E. Surgical treatment of fibroids in heavy menstrual bleeding. *Women's Health (Lond)* 2016;**12**:53–62.

10. Bhave Chittawar P, Franik S, Pouwer AW, Farquhar C. Minimally invasive surgical techniques versus open myomectomy for uterine fibroids. *Cochrane Database Syst Rev* 2014;**10**:CD004638.

11. Hurst BS, Matthews ML, Marshburn PB. Laparoscopic myomectomy for symptomatic uterine myomas. *Fertil Steril* 2005;**83**(1):1–23.

12. Saridogan E, Cutner A. Endoscopic management of uterine fibroids. *Hum Fertil (Camb)* 2006;**9**(4):201–8.

13. Sinha R, Hegde A, Mahajan C, Dubey N, Sundaram M. Laparoscopic myomectomy: do size, number, and location of the myomas form limiting factors for laparoscopic myomectomy? *J Minim Invasive Gynecol* 2008;**15**(3):292–300.

14. Dubuisson JB, Fauconnier A, Fourchotte V, Babaki-Fard K, Coste J, Chapron C. Laparoscopic myomectomy: predicting the risk of conversion to an open procedure. *Hum Reprod* 2001;**16**(8):1726–31.

15. Sizzi O, Rossetti A, Malzoni M et al. Italian multicenter study on complications of laparoscopic myomectomy. *J Minim Invasive Gynecol* 2007;**14**(4):453–62.

16. Lindheim SR, Adsuar N, Kushner DM, Pritts EA, Olive DL. Sonohysterography: a valuable tool in evaluating the female pelvis. *Obstet Gynecol Surv* 2003;**58**(11):770–84.

17. Battista C, Capriglione S, Guzzo F et al. The challenge of preoperative identification of uterine myomas: is ultrasound trustworthy? A prospective cohort study. *Arch Gynecol Obstet* 2016 Jun;**293**(6):1235–41. doi: 10.1007/s00404-015-3937-1.

18. Stewart EA. Clinical practice. Uterine fibroids. *N Engl J Med* 2015;**372**:1646–55.

19. Lin G, Yang LY, Huang YT et al. Comparison of the diagnostic accuracy of contrast-enhanced MRI and diffusion-weighted MRI in the differentiation between uterine leiomyosarcoma/smooth muscle tumor with uncertain malignant potential and benign leiomyoma. *J Magn Reson Imaging* 2015;**10**:1002.

20. Whitaker LH, Williams AR, Critchley HO. Selective progesterone receptor modulators. *Curr Opin Obstet Gynecol* 2014;**26**:237–42.

21. Tristan M, Orozco LJ, Steed A, Ramírez-Morera A, Stone P. Mifepristone for uterine fibroids. *Cochrane Database Syst Rev* 2012;**8**:CD007687.

22. Donnez J, Tatarchuk TF, Bouchard P et al. Ulipristal acetate versus placebo for fibroid treatment before surgery. *N Engl J Med* 2012;**366**:409–20.

23. Donnez J, Tomaszewski J, Vázquez F et al. Ulipristal acetate versus leuprolide acetate for uterine fibroids. *N Engl J Med* 2012;**366**:421–32.

24. Leone Roberti Maggiore U, Scala C, Venturini PL, Ferrero S. Preoperative treatment with letrozole in patients undergoing laparoscopic myomectomy of large uterine myomas: a prospective non-randomized study. *Eur J Obstet Gynecol Reprod Biol* 2014 Oct;**181**:157–62. doi: 10.1016/j.ejogrb.2014.07.040.

25. Imai A, Sugiyama M, Furui T, Takahashi S, Tamaya T. Gonadotrophin-releasing hormones agonist therapy increases peritoneal fibrinolytic activity and prevents adhesion formation after myomectomy. *J Obstet Gynaecol* 2003;**23**(6):660–3.

26. Lethaby A, Vollenhoven B, Sowter M. Pre-operative GnRH analogue therapy before hysterectomy or myomectomy for uterine fibroids. *Cochrane Database Syst Rev* 2001;(2):CD000547. doi: 10.1002/14651858.CD000547.

27. Kongnyuy EJ, van den Broek N, Wiysonge CS. A systematic review of randomized controlled trials to reduce hemorrhage during myomectomy for uterine fibroids. *Int J Gynaecol Obstet* 2008;**100**(1):4–9.

28. Kongnyuy EJ, Wiysonge CS. Interventions to reduce haemorrhage during myomectomy for fibroids. *Cochrane Database Syst Rev.* 2014 Aug 15;(8):CD005355. doi: 10.1002/14651858.CD005355.pub5.

29. Sesti F, Ticconi C, Bonifacio S, Piccione E. Preoperative administration of recombinant human erythropoietin in patients undergoing gynecologic surgery. *Gynecol Obstet Invest* 2002;**54**(1):1–5.

30. Brölmann H, Tanos V, Grimbizis G et al. Options on fibroid morcellation: a literature review. *Gynecol Surg* 2015;**12**(1):3–15. Published online 2015 Feb 7. doi: 10.1007/s10397-015-0878-4

31. Leibsohn S, d'Ablaing G, Mishell DR Jr, Schlaerth JB. Leiomyosarcoma in a series of hysterectomies performed for presumed uterine leiomyomas. *Am J Obstet Gynecol* 1990 Apr;**162**(4):968–74; discussion 974–6.

32. Vilos GA, Ternamian A, Dempster J, Laberge PY, The Society of Obstetricians and Gynaecologists of Canada. Laparoscopic entry: a review of techniques, technologies, and complications. *J Obstet Gynaecol Can* 2007;**29**(5):433–65.

33. Lin PC, Thyer A, Soules MR. Intraoperative ultrasound during a laparoscopic myomectomy. *Fertil Steril* 2004;**81**(6):1671–4.

34. Ou CS, Harper A, Liu YH, Rowbotham R. Laparoscopic myomectomy technique. Use of colpotomy and the harmonic scalpel. *J Reprod Med* 2002;**47**(10):849–53.

35. Litta P, Fantinato S, Calonaci F *et al*. A randomized controlled study comparing harmonic versus electrosurgery in laparoscopic myomectomy. *Fertil Steril* 2010;**94**(5):1882–6.

36. Koh C, Janik G. Laparoscopic myomectomy: the current status. *Curr Opin Obstet Gynecol* 2003;**15**(4):295–301.

37. Walocha JA, Litwin JA, Miodonski AJ. Vascular system of intramural leiomyomata revealed by corrosion casting and scanning electron microscopy. *Hum Reprod* 2003;**18**(5):1088–93.

38. Hasbargen U, Summerer-Moustaki M, Hillemanns P, Scheidler J, Kimmig R, Hepp H. Uterine dehiscence in a nullipara, diagnosed by MRI, following use of unipolar electrocautery during laparoscopic myomectomy: case report. *Hum Reprod* 2002;**17**(8):2180–2.

39. Kumakiri J, Takeuchi H, Itoh S *et al*. Prospective evaluation for the feasibility and safety of vaginal birth after laparoscopic myomectomy. *J Minim Invasive Gynecol* 2008;**15**(4):420–4.

40. Seracchioli R, Manuzzi L, Vianello F *et al*. Obstetric and delivery outcome of pregnancies achieved after laparoscopic myomectomy. *Fertil Steril* 2006;**86**(1):159–65.

41. Nezhat F, Seidman DS, Nezhat C, Nezhat CH. Laparoscopic myomectomy today. Why, when and for whom? *Hum Reprod* 1996;**11**(5):933–4.

42. Rossetti A, Sizzi O, Chiarotti F, Florio G. Developments in techniques for laparoscopic myomectomy. *JSLS* 2007;**11**(1):34–40.

43. Einarsson JI, Vellinga TT, Twijnstra AR, Chavan NR, Suzuki Y, Greenberg JA. Bidirectional barbed suture: an evaluation of safety and clinical outcomes. *JSLS* 2010;**14**(3):381–5.

44. Einarsson JI, Chavan NR, Suzuki Y, Jonsdottir G, Vellinga TT, Greenberg JA. Use of bidirectional barbed suture in laparoscopic myomectomy: evaluation of perioperative outcomes, safety, and efficacy. *J Minim Invasive Gynecol* 2011;**18**(1):92–5.

45. Miyake T, Enomoto T, Ueda Y *et al*. A case of disseminated peritoneal leiomyomatosis developing after laparoscope-assisted myomectomy. *Gynecol Obstet Invest* 2008;**67**(2):96–102.

46. Cohen SL, Einarsson JI, Wang KC *et al*. Contained power morcellation within an insufflated isolation bag. *Obstet Gynecol* 2014 Sep**124**(3):491–7.

47. Einarsson JI, Cohen SL, Fuchs N, Wang KC. In-bag morcellation. *J Minim Invasive Gynecol* 2014 Sep–Oct;**21**(5):951–3.

48. Favero G. Tips and tricks for successful manual morcellation: a response to "vaginal morcellation: a new strategy for large gynecological malignant tumors extraction. A pilot study".

Gynecol Oncol 2013 Jan;**128**(1):151.

49. Ahmad G, O'Flynn H, Hindocha A, Watson A. Barrier agents for adhesion prevention after gynaecological surgery. *Cochrane Database Syst Rev* 2015; (4): CD000475. doi: 10.1002/14651858.CD000475.pub3.

50. Practice Committee of the American Society for Reproductive Medicine, Society of Reproductive Surgeons. Pathogenesis, consequences, and control of peritoneal adhesions in gynecologic surgery. *Fertil Steril* 2007;**88**(1):21–6.

51. Oktem O, Gökaslan H, Durmusoglu F. Spontaneous uterine rupture in pregnancy 8 years after laparoscopic myomectomy. *J Am Assoc Gynecol Laparosc* 2001;**8**(4):618–21.

52. Pelosi MA, Pelosi MA. Spontaneous uterine rupture at thirty-three weeks subsequent to previous superficial laparoscopic myomectomy. *Am J Obstet Gynecol* 1997;**177**(6):1547–9.

53. Harris WJ. Uterine dehiscence following laparoscopic myomectomy. *Obstet Gynecol* 1992;**80**(3 Pt 2):545–6.

54. Landi S, Zaccoletti R, Ferrari L, Minelli L. Laparoscopic myomectomy: technique, complications, and ultrasound scan evaluations. *J Am Assoc Gynecol Laparosc* 2001;**8**(2):231–40.

55. Malzoni M, Sizzi O, Rossetti A, Imperato F. Laparoscopic myomectomy: a report of 982 procedures. *Surg Technol Int* 2006;**15**:123–9.

56. Bean EMR, Cutner A, Holland T, Vashisht A, Jurkovic D, Saridogan E. Laparoscopic myomectomy: a single centre retrospective review of 514 patients. *J Minim Invasive Gynecol* 2017;**24**(3):485–93. doi: 10.1016/j.jmig.2017.01.008.

57. Quaas AM, Einarsson JI, Srouji S, Gargiulo AR. Robotic myomectomy: a review of indications and techniques. *Rev Obstet Gynecol* 2010;**3** (4):185–91.

58. Nezhat C, Lavie O, Hsu S, Watson J, Barnett O, Lemyre M. Robotic-assisted laparoscopic myomectomy compared with standard laparoscopic myomectomy – a retrospective matched control study. *Fertil Steril* 2009;**91**(2):556–9.

59. Barakat EE, Bedaiwy MA, Zimberg S, Nutter B, Nosseir M, Falcone T. Robotic-assisted, laparoscopic, and abdominal myomectomy: a comparison of surgical outcomes. *Obstet Gynecol* 2011;**117**(2 Pt 1):256–65.

60. Seracchioli R, Rossi S, Govoni F *et al.* Fertility and obstetric outcome after laparoscopic myomectomy of large myomata: a randomized comparison with abdominal myomectomy. *Hum Reprod* 2000;**15**(12):2663–8.

10

Uterine Fibroids
The Morcellation Debate

Jimena B. Alvarez and Charles E. Miller

10.1 Background

One of the risks of electronic power morcellation, central to the morcellation debate, is the concern of spread of malignant uterine tissue. Uterine cancer is the most common gynaecologic cancer in the United States with an estimated 49,560 cases and 8,190 deaths in 2013. Uterine sarcomas arise from the mesodermal tissues of the uterine body and account for 3% of all uterine cancers, and represent 3.3 cases per 100,000 women [1]. Leiomyosarcoma (LMS) represents 40% of all uterine sarcomas, and 2% of all uterine malignancies, and the annual incidence has been estimated to be 0.64 per 100,000 women [2]. It can present at any age, but most commonly between 45 and 55 years old, and its prevalence increases by 10% in patients over 60 years old.

While 15% of all leiomyosarcoma can be diagnosed preoperatively with endometrial biopsy or dilation and curettage, the majority of cases are incidentally diagnosed after hysterectomy [1]. Moreover, leiomyosarcoma is difficult to distinguish clinically from benign leiomyomas, especially degenerating leiomyomas. A prospective imaging study by Goto et al. published in 2002 studied 130 women with degenerating leiomyomas and 10 women with leiomyosarcoma to evaluate the diagnostic accuracy of conventional MRI and dynamic MRI with or without serum measurement of lactate dehydrogenase (LDH) levels and LDH isoenzymes [3]. Their results indicated 100% specificity, positive and negative predictive values, as well as diagnostic accuracy for the combined MRI and LDH panel group including LDH isoenzyme 3. Unfortunately, these findings have not been replicated and hence have not been widely integrated into clinical practice.

Due to its haematogenous spread, leiomyosarcoma has a poor prognosis, even in early-stage disease and even when removed intact from the body [2]. Hence, distant metastasis could be present during early-stage disease, but this is unpredictable in cases of incidental diagnosis via postoperative pathologic diagnosis.

10.1.1 The Role of Minimally Invasive Surgery in the Treatment of Uterine Fibroids

Hysterectomies and myomectomies, when done via a minimally invasive surgery (MIS) approach, have been shown to have far fewer complications. The benefits of MIS are well documented and include faster postoperative recovery including shorter hospital stay and shorter recovery time at home leading to faster return to work, less pain, and reduced risk of perioperative complications. A Cochrane systematic review by Nieboer et al. in 2009 evaluated 27 randomized controlled trials comparing total abdominal hysterectomies, laparoscopic hysterectomies, and vaginal hysterectomies performed for benign causes and reported that vaginal hysterectomy has the best outcomes and should be performed when possible. The review also recommended that although laparoscopic hysterectomy may be associated with longer operating times and higher rates of urinary tract injury, laparoscopic hysterectomy has advantages over total abdominal hysterectomy, including faster return to normal activity, shorter duration of hospital stays, lower intraoperative blood loss, and fewer wound infections [4]. Furthermore, a retrospective cohort study of 465,798 women by Wiser et al. evaluated outcomes of women who underwent abdominal and laparoscopic hysterectomies, and found a three times higher mortality risk for abdominal hysterectomy compared to laparoscopic hysterectomy (0.03% vs. 0.01%, OR 0.48 (0.24–0.95), respectively) [5].

Following the results published by Nieboer et al., the American College of Obstetricians and Gynecologists (ACOG) published a committee opinion [6] supporting the recommendations made by the Cochrane review. The AAGL followed with a position statement recommending that most hysterectomies for benign disease should be performed either vaginally or laparoscopically and that continued efforts should be taken to facilitate these approaches. Moreover, surgeons without the training and skills required for the safe performance of vaginal hysterectomy or laparoscopic hysterectomy should request the aid of colleagues who do, or refer patients requiring hysterectomy to such individuals capable of performing the procedure via a minimally invasive route, for their surgical care [7].

Given such emphasis on minimally invasive hysterectomies, gynaecology practice has seen significant changes in trends of modes of hysterectomy. Among approximately 600,000 hysterectomies performed every year in the United States, 63% were performed via laparoscopy in 2012, compared to 30% in 2002 [7]. Symptomatic uterine leiomyomas are the indication for 210,000 hysterectomies and 50,000 myomectomies annually [8]. Thus, it comes as no surprise that 50,000–150,000 patients with large-size specimens undergo power morcellation to maintain a minimally invasive approach [9]. This highlights the importance of the morcellation procedure avoiding extension of small laparoscopic incisions in order to allow completion of minimally invasive procedures and to optimize perioperative outcomes by avoiding exploratory laparotomy and its inherent risks.

10.2 History of Morcellation

While morcellation has been widespread in various gynaecologic procedures for decades, its beginnings date back to 1949 when Allen published the first use of manual morcellation during vaginal hysterectomy [10].

Since then, manual morcellation was performed routinely in gynaecology during both vaginal and open surgery for hysterectomy and myomectomy. Hasson et al. subsequently published a report in 1992 on laparoscopic myomectomy, indicating that traditional morcellation was used initially but was abandoned because of long operating time [11]. A year later, Steiner et al. introduced the concept of electrical power morcellation into the literature, describing a cylinder placed inside the trocar with a coning knife at its intra-abdominal end, rotated by an electrical micro-engine attached to the trocar [12].

The first intracorporeal power morcellator for gynaecologic use received approval from the Food and Drug Administration (FDA) in 1995 under the 510K process, and was categorized as an intermediate-risk device. The procedure was performed without a containment bag system. In 1997, Carter and McCarus presented for the first time a cost analysis reporting significant time and financial savings with the use of the electronic power morcellator as compared with the manual technique [13].

10.2.1 Timeline of the Debate

Since the initial use of electronic power morcellation, a variety of articles have been published referencing dissemination of benign and malignant tissue after uterine and fibroid morcellation, suggesting the possibility of worsening prognosis. In 1997, Schneider published the first case report of an undetected adenocarcinoma of the uterus after morcellation [14]. The article stated that malignant cells could have been detected via preoperative curettage, and recommended this diagnostic procedure be performed routinely prior to laparoscopic hysterectomy with planned morcellation. A more recent retrospective study by Siedman et al. in 2012, reviewing 1,091 cases of laparoscopic uterine morcellation, reported that the rate of unexpected sarcomas in women undergoing power morcellation was 0.09%, suggesting a nine times higher risk of spreading undetected cancer than previously suspected [15]. While these outcomes were acknowledged to be concerning, the gynaecologic community accepted them as a rare occurrence, with an overall balance favouring morcellation due to the markedly decreased perioperative morbidity and mortality rates of laparoscopic versus abdominal surgery.

However, the opposition to morcellation increased after the care of Amy Reed, MD, an anaesthesiologist at Beth Israel Hospital, in Boston, who underwent a laparoscopic hysterectomy in October 2013 for presumed benign uterine fibroids utilizing electronic power morcellation. The unfortunate final pathologic report was consistent with leiomyosarcoma. Given that electronic power morcellation was used during this procedure – thus leading to possible peritoneal dissemination of sarcomatous tissue – the possibility of increased staging and potentially worsening prognosis was a strong concern.

Within the same month, the Society of Gynecologic Oncology (SGO) released a position statement asserting that morcellation is generally contraindicated when there exists a high suspicion of malignancy or documented malignancy. The document also stated that less than 1 in 1,000 women undergoing hysterectomy for fibroids have an underlying malignancy. Further, the SGO acknowledged that while there is no reliable method to differentiate benign from malignant myomas before resection, leiomyosarcoma and endometrial stromal sarcoma have an extremely poor prognosis even when specimens are removed intact. They recommended informed consent to allow patients to make an informed decision to accept or decline the option of morcellation [16]. In an additional statement, the SGO added that hysterectomies are done to treat benign uterine fibroids in the majority of cases, and that since intracorporeal morcellation benefits thousands of women, it would be a disservice to deny these women this option [17].

A Safety Communication was issued in April of 2014 by the FDA, discouraging the use of laparoscopic electronic power morcellation during hysterectomy or myomectomy for uterine fibroids, based on their review of literature showing a prevalence of 1 in 352 of unsuspected uterine sarcoma and 1 in 498 of unsuspected leiomyosarcoma [18, 19]. Since then, the concern for dissemination of tumour cells at the time of electronic power morcellation has led many hospitals and hospital systems in the United States to ban the use of electronic power morcellation, thus by necessity leading to the conversion of several cases to a laparotomy. Nevertheless, the debate has remained contentious due to further review of literature, revealing a much smaller risk of sarcoma and the decreased risks of minimally invasive surgery as compared to laparotomy.

As a response to the evidence published in the FDA Safety Communication report, a number of opinion papers by several medical societies have been written recommending the use of electronic power morcellation in the appropriate patients only after proper informed consent. Other medical institutions issued new policies advocating the use of a morcellation bag to attempt containment of the specimen and decrease the risk of spread of pathology into the peritoneal cavity.

In response to the FDA statements and reaction by the medical community, the AAGL assembled a Task Force to evaluate electronic power morcellation for tissue extraction [20], recommending that electronic power morcellation should be avoided in postmenopausal patients, and in the setting of known malignant or pre-malignant conditions. The Task Force further recommended that consideration of electronic power morcellation should be granted for patients with reassuring preoperative evaluation, including cervical cytology and endometrial biopsy. Moreover, alternatives to morcellation, including laparotomy, should be considered in cases of a non-reassuring evaluation. Finally, the importance of informed consent and the further investigation of morcellation within the specimen retrieval bag containment system was stressed. Lastly, the group concluded that since there is no single method of tissue extraction that can protect all patients, all current methods should remain available.

An expert panel convened by the FDA met in July 2014 to discuss the options for morcellation including status quo, black box warning, and a ban on electronic power morcellation; no consensus was reached. During the meeting, and later published in the *Journal of Minimally Invasive Gynecology* (JMIG) [9], Dr Jubilee Brown stated that there is limited data available on the risk of undetected uterine malignancy at time of hysterectomy with power morcellation, estimates ranging from 1:360 to 1:7,400. Dr Brown cautioned against eliminating a beneficial technology based on scant and imprecise data regarding the risk of undetected uterine malignancy prior to hysterectomy with planned electronic power morcellation, and further emphasized the limited data on the risk of upstaging, or worsening prognosis, of a leiomyosarcoma after power morcellation. Dr Brown further stated that 'the elimination of power morcellation would result in conversion to open procedures; the risks of power morcellation would have to exceed the benefits of MIS in order for that to be justified'.

Ultimately, the FDA updated their Safety Communication in November 2014, and issued a black box warning against power morcellation stating that the use of laparoscopic electronic power morcellators during fibroid surgery may spread cancer and decrease the long-term survival of patients [21]. The report also established contraindications for laparoscopic electronic power morcellation used for removal of uterine tissue with suspected or known malignancy as well as tissue containing suspected fibroids in peri- or postmenopausal women or women who are candidates for en bloc tissue removal (i.e. vaginal extraction or via mini-laparotomy). It is interesting that criteria for perimenopause were not defined.

Following these recommendations, in a study by Siedhoff et al., a decision tree model was created to evaluate outcomes of a hypothetical cohort of 100,000 premenopausal women undergoing hysterectomy for presumed fibroids. Outcomes included postoperative complications, incidence of leiomyosarcoma, death related to leiomyosarcoma, and procedure-related death. The analysis predicted fewer overall deaths with laparoscopic hysterectomy compared to abdominal hysterectomy (98 vs. 103 per 100,000). While more deaths from leiomyosarcoma followed laparoscopic hysterectomy (86 vs. 71 per 100,000), increased deaths related to the open procedure were predicted with abdominal hysterectomy (32 vs. 12 per 100,000). Morbidity results for the laparoscopic group included lower rates of transfusion (2,400 vs. 4,700 per 100,000), wound infection (1,500 vs. 6,300 per 100,000), venous thromboembolism (690 vs. 840 per 100,000), and incisional hernia (710 vs. 8,800 per 100,000), but a higher rate of vaginal cuff dehiscence (640 vs. 290 per 100,000) [22].

In response to the updated FDA statement, a Leiomyoma Morcellation Review Group expressed disagreement with the methodology used by the FDA to calculate the prevalence of leiomyosarcoma among women with suspected benign fibroids and which led to their severely restrictive recommendations against the use of electronic power morcellators [8]. Based on their review, the FDA estimated that 1 out of 458 women undergoing surgery for presumed fibroids would have an occult leiomyosarcoma. To perform their search, the FDA used the words 'uterine cancer' and 'hysterectomy or myomectomy'. Since the search required to look for 'uterine cancer', studies where cancer was not diagnosed or discussed were not identified. Out of nine studies, eight were retrospective, one was a non-peer-reviewed letter to the editor, and another was an abstract from an unpublished study. In addition, three of the leiomyosarcoma cases identified by the FDA did not meet pathologic criteria for cancer, and would not be classified as benign atypical leiomyomas. Excluding the data from the non-peer-reviewed letter and the three cases of atypical leiomyomas, the Leiomyoma Morcellation Review Group identified eight cases of leiomyosarcoma among 12,402 women who underwent surgery for suspected leiomyomas, with a prevalence of 1 in 1,550 (0.064%) [8]. The review group described two additional studies by Pritts and Bojahr who did not limit their

methodologies to literature written in English, which reported a prevalence of 1 in 1,960 (0.051%) [23] and 2 in 8,720 (0.023%) [24], respectively.

On the basis of the above review of the literature, the review group asked the FDA to modify its guidance and to promote patient participation in the decision-making process by promoting informed consent that would empower patients to make informed decisions regarding the use of morcellation in their medical care. Lastly, the group suggested the following clinical recommendations:

- The risk of leiomyosarcoma is higher in older postmenopausal women, and greater caution should be exercised before recommending morcellation procedures for these women.
- Preoperative consideration of leiomyosarcoma is important, and women aged 35 years or older with irregular uterine bleeding and presumed leiomyomas should have an endometrial biopsy, which occasionally may detect leiomyosarcoma before surgery. Women should have normal results of cervical cancer screening.
- Ultrasonography or magnetic resonance imaging findings of a large irregular vascular mass, often with irregular anechoic (cystic) areas reflecting necrosis, may cause suspicion of leiomyosarcoma.
- Women wishing minimally invasive procedures with morcellation, including scalpel morcellation through the vagina or mini-laparotomy, or power morcellation using laparoscopic guidance, should understand the potential risk of decreased survival should leiomyosarcoma be present. Open procedures should be offered to all women who are considering minimally invasive procedures for 'leiomyomas'.
- After morcellation, careful inspection for tissue fragments should be undertaken and copious irrigation of the pelvic and abdominal cavities should be performed to minimize the risk of retained tissue.
- Further investigations of a means to preoperatively identify leiomyosarcoma should be supported. Likewise, investigation into the biology of leiomyosarcoma should be funded to better understand the propensity of tissue fragments or cells to implant and grow. With that knowledge, minimally invasive procedures could be avoided for women with leiomyosarcoma and women choosing minimally invasive surgery could be reassured that they do not have leiomyosarcoma.

Interestingly, the authors of this study were disappointed that the review group's recommendations

93

did not include the use of containment systems. Not surprisingly, following the FDA statement recommending against morcellation in perimenopausal women, and despite the declarations by the Leiomyoma Morcellation Review Group and articles by Siedhoff [22], Pritts [23], and Bojahr [24], the most recent trends in the mode of hysterectomy across the country have been observed to favour a decrease in laparoscopic hysterectomies or myomectomies and an increase in abdominal hysterectomies or myomectomies. A retrospective cohort study by Harris et al. reported their trends in mode of hysterectomy, including abdominal, laparoscopic, and vaginal, as well as postoperative complications from the 15 months preceding the initial FDA safety communication discouraging the use of power morcellation through the 8 months following the FDA statement. A decrease in laparoscopic hysterectomy rates by 4.1% (p = 0.005) was noted, and abdominal and vaginal hysterectomies increased by 1.7% (p = 0.112) and 2.4% (p = 0.012), respectively. A significant rise in major surgical complications excluding blood transfusions was noted, with an overall increment of 2.2–2.8% (p = 0.015) and an increased rate of hospital readmission within 30 days from 3.4% to 4.2% (p = 0.025) [25].

Another retrospective analysis by Barron et al. demonstrated a significant decrease in the proportion of minimally invasive hysterectomies and myomectomies following the initial FDA statement. Proportions of minimally invasive surgery cases including laparoscopic, robotic-assisted, and vaginal cases were compared between an 8-month period before and after the FDA statement. The study found an overall downtrend in minimally invasive hysterectomies after the FDA warning statement, from 85.7% before to 79.9% (1,451/1,694 vs. 1,350/1,690; p = 0.001) after the statement. When oncology cases were excluded, a downtrend was again observed, from 90.2% before to 81.5% (985/1,092 vs. 834/1,023; p = 0.001) after the statement. A similar decline was seen in myomectomies, with 62.7% procedures prior to the FDA statement versus 43.7% (64/102 vs. 38/87; p = 0.009) in the 8 months afterwards [26].

Lastly, a more recent retrospective review by Wright et al. in 2016 evaluated trends of abdominal, minimally invasive, and vaginal hysterectomies before and after the FDA advisory [27]. Between the last quarter of 2013 and the first quarter of 2015, the study showed an increase of abdominal hysterectomy rates from 27.1% to 31.8% (p = 0.004), and a decline in minimally invasive hysterectomy rates from 59.7% to 56.2% (p < 0.001), as well as a declining trend in vaginal hysterectomy. Additionally, a marked decline was noted in electronic power morcellation use within the minimally invasive group; a remarkable downtrend from 13.5% in the first quarter of 2013 to 2.8% in the first quarter of 2015 (p < 0.001). The study once again showed the markedly lower risk of complications in the minimally invasive surgery group.

The studies above illustrate the increasing trends of abdominal procedures versus laparoscopic procedures, despite an increase in complication rates. Furthermore, these results underscore the need for further research to investigate methods to improve data collection on postoperative diagnosis of occult uterine malignancy, the diagnosis of pathology preoperatively, and safe ways to perform morcellation in an effort to improve the safety of methods for specimen retrieval.

10.3 Options for Tissue Extraction

Since the statement made by the FDA, there have been significant changes made to a number of tissue extraction methods. Current options for minimally invasive tissue extraction include the following: electronic power morcellation with or without use of a containment system, mini-laparotomy with hand morcellation with or without use of a containment system, and manual vaginal morcellation with or without a containment system.

Laparoscopic intracorporeal morcellation allows the removal of large specimens through incisions no more than 25 mm in length and requires the use of a power morcellator. The power morcellation procedure involves dividing a large specimen into small pieces with the use of a rotary device with a blade that slices the specimen into pieces of smaller diameter that can be extracted through the morcellator's trocar, allowing tissue extraction via a small incision. Since the statement made by the FDA against power morcellation, this procedure has been modified by our MIS team and others to be performed within a containment system using a bag. The multi-port and single-site methods were first described by Cohen et al. [28]. At our institution, we perform laparoscopic intracorporeal, contained power morcellation via two techniques: laparoscopic hysterectomy and myomectomy, both performed via a 12 mm port at the umbilicus and two 5 mm ports placed laterally. Once the hysterectomy or myomectomy is completed, except for specimen removal, the Espiner 2,300 cc bag is placed through the 12 mm umbilical port into the abdomen. The specimen is placed into the bag. The mouth of the containment system is then brought out the umbilicus and the 12 mm port placed through the mouth of the containment system into the abdominal cavity. As the abdominal cavity is deflated, the bag is insufflated. Once insufflation is complete, the laparoscope is placed through the 12 mm port using one of the lateral incisions, and a 5 mm inflatable balloon trocar with a sharp-tip obturator is used to enter the bag laterally with direct visualization. Ultimately, the laparoscope is placed through this 5 mm port and the 12 mm port at the umbilicus replaced by the 12–15 mm power morcellator.

Our minimally invasive gynaecologic surgery (MIGS) team also has utilized a simple port technique at the umbilicus so that the bag is not compromised. In this case, we have used the GelPOINT Mini, a 30° laparoscope and a 12 mm morcellator. Recently, a single-port system, the Olympus bag, has received FDA approval.

In regards to outcomes using a multi-port intracorporeal power morcellation technique, a retrospective chart review from our MIGS team by Steller et al. studied a group of 187 patients who underwent either hysterectomy or myomectomy using this method, and had no bag rupture after inspection post-use, or bag failures, and minimal complications. The study reported a postoperative admission rate of 12.3%, the majority due to nausea and urinary retention, and 20 patients in total (10.7%) who developed postoperative complications, most of which were minor, including wound cellulitis, postoperative fever, one patient with pulmonary embolism, labial haematoma, corneal abrasion, vaginal infection, urinary tract infection. Overall, the study showed that this procedure is feasible, reliable, and reproducible even for large specimens [29].

In addition, Cohen et al. described the outcomes of their retrospective analysis of 73 cases. They reported no cases of conversion to laparotomy, no cases of bag failure or rupture after inspection postoperatively, no readmissions, and a 78% rate of discharge on the day of surgery. Postoperative complications included four patients who required treatment for respiratory infection, ileus, and pain [28].

Manual morcellation via a mini-laparotomy incision, an alternative to power morcellation, was described by Seidman et al. in 2001. This technique uses a transverse midline 5 mm puncture for the initial part of the procedure that is enlarged to 4–5 cm after myomectomy. Using a corkscrew manipulator, the specimen is raised to the incision to be shelled sequentially with a scalpel and morcellated gradually while exposing new areas until complete removal of the leiomyoma [30]. Their morbidity outcomes described in another article by the same group reported one case of pneumonia and one incisional hernia at the mini-laparotomy site, and most women resumed normal activity within 3 weeks [31].

Serur et al. described an approach to morcellation via mini-laparotomy and vaginal approach using a bag containment system. This retrospective study reviewed a total of 104 women with a uterine weight of >500 g undergoing laparoscopic hysterectomy. Two 10 mm incisions, one umbilical and one suprapubic, and two 5 mm accessory ports were made in the abdomen to perform the hysterectomy, after the specimen bag was inserted followed by extension of the umbilical 10 mm incision to 20–30 mm, and the edges of the specimen bag were elevated through the incision, bringing the specimen to the level of the abdomen and grasping the specimen with Lahey clamps. The scalpel was then used to circumferentially core the portion that had been exteriorized, elevating it above the abdominal incision. An abdominal manual morcellation approach was achieved in 58.7% of the patients, and vaginal manual morcellation was done in the remaining 41.3% of patients. Perioperative complications included one patient with severe blood loss up to 1,200 cc due to bleeding from a myoma requiring uterine artery ligation, eight patients requiring blood transfusions, with a mean number of units of packed red blood cells transfused of 2.25 units, and a mean length of hospital stay of 1.38 days with three patients requiring 4-day-long admissions due to postoperative ileus and medical comorbidities. There were no complications related to the morcellation technique via either approach and no instance of visually noted bag rupture or specimen spillage. Unfortunately, two patients (1.9%) were noted to have occult malignancy – uterine sarcoma and endometrial adenocarcinoma – diagnosed postoperatively, with no diagnosis based on preoperative workup. There is no indication of the morcellation approach for these two patients [32].

10.4 Potential Complications of Morcellation

As with any medical procedure, there are risks associated with morcellation. Risks vary from morcellator-related trauma to organs nearby including solid organs or vessels, potentially leading to significant perioperative morbidity and possibly death, to the widely recognized risk of spread of uterine pathology throughout the peritoneal cavity, with dissemination of uterine cancer tissue being the most dangerous.

The spread of uterine tissue leading to ectopic implantation on abdominal organs or the peritoneum – benign leiomyomatosis – can involve benign uterine pathology such as leiomyomas, endometriosis, and adenomyosis. But more important to this discussion is the spread of uterine malignancy. In regards to the spread of LMS, it is noteworthy to mention that the possibilities of upstaging, need for more invasive treatment, and decreased survival remain unclear. As mentioned above, the haematogenous nature of its spread allows metastasis even in early stages of the disease. Furthermore, four studies previously used to examine survival after morcellation were analysed by the ACOG Leiomyoma Morcellation Review Group, and it was found that a remarkable minority used power morcellation. Park et al. reported that in a group of patients who underwent morcellation, only 1 out of 25 patients had power morcellation [33], while in the study by Perri et al., none of the patients underwent power morcellation [34]. In the article by Morice et al., there was no difference in recurrence rates or overall and disease-free survival at 6 months [35], similar to Oduyebo et al., who reported no difference in outcomes for 10 patients who underwent power morcellation [36]. Finally, a life table analysis of these studies showed no difference in survival between morcellation methods.

10.5 Improvement Measures

For women who desire to pursue minimally invasive surgery for uterine fibroids, regardless of the route (laparosopic, mini-laparotomy, vaginal), informed consent is a cumbersome, yet necessary, step that allows full disclosure of risks and benefits of the procedure to the patient, invites clear communication between the patient and the surgeon, and empowers the patient to take an active role in the decision-making of her own medical care. For patients who choose laparoscopic power morcellation, the risks specific to power morcellation mentioned above should be fully discussed.

Meanwhile, the gynaecologic community has encouraged further investigation for diagnosis of LMS in the preoperative setting as well as the biology of this malignancy to further understand its nature with the hope to prevent unnecessary intervention for women in the future. Investigative efforts have also focused on assessing the safety and feasibility of power morcellation within a containment system in an attempt to avoid spread of uterine tissue. Technical difficulties that have been associated with the bag containment system include proper visualization inside and outside the bag, ability to fit variable uterine sizes and shapes, and risk of bag perforation. Several studies are currently investigating containment systems and their associated challenges at multiple institutions, including our MIGS group. Lastly, the gynaecologic community has also encouraged the creation of a nationwide registry including data on gynaecologic devices used, quality of outcomes, and complications in order to equip providers with reliable data for patient selection and monitoring of devices to allow well-informed clinical management decisions [37].

10.6 Conclusion

Although the debate has created a strain on the availability of morcellation in a large number of hospitals across the country, it has promoted a deep analysis of the current evidence as well as a search by the medical community for avenues to improve the use of morcellators for the benefit of patients. While data remain limited on the question of worsened prognosis for LMS diagnosed after power morcellation of fibroids, and evidence to support reliable preoperative diagnostic tools for LMS is also lacking, small- and large-scale studies are currently being performed to find answers to these important questions. Meanwhile, another important question relevant to the morcellation debate is whether the risk of using power morcellation in the rare case of a patient with occult LMS is greater than the risk of undergoing laparotomy instead of a minimally invasive surgery. Given the low reported rates and limited data, the AAGL has cautioned against abandoning morcellation based on the evidence currently available. Instead, we are encouraged to improve power morcellation, and advised that power morcellation with appropriate informed consent should remain available to appropriately screened, low-risk women.

References

1. Benoit M, Williams-Brown MY, Edwards, C. *Gynecologic Oncology Handbook: An Evidence-Based Clinical Guide.* Demos Medical Publishing, LLC; 2013.

2. American Cancer Society. *Uterine Sarcoma.* Atlanta, GA: American Cancer Society; 2013.

3. Goto A, Takeuchi S, Sugimura K, Maruo T. Usefulness of Gd-DTPA contrast-enhanced dynamic MRI and serum determination of LDH and its isozymes in the differential diagnosis of leiomyosarcoma from degenerated leiomyoma of the uterus. *Int J Gynecol Cancer* 2002;12(4):354–61.

4. Nieboer TE, Johnson N, Lethaby A, et al. Surgical approach to hysterectomy for benign gynaecological disease. *Cochrane Database Syst Rev* 2009;(3): Cd003677.

5. Amir Wiser A, Holcroft C, Tulandi T, Abenhaim H. Abdominal versus laparoscopic hysterectomies for benign diseases: evaluation of morbidity and mortality among 465,798 cases. *Gynecol Surg* 2013;**10** (2):117–22.

6. American College of Obstetricians and Gynecologists. Choosing the route of hysterectomy for benign disease. Committee Opinion No. 444. *Obstet Gynecol* 2009;**114**:1156–8.

7. AAGL, Advancing Minimally Invasive Gynecology Worldwide. AAGL position statement: route of hysterectomy to treat benign uterine disease. *J Minim Invasive Gynecol* 2011;**18**(1):1–3.

8. Parker WH, Kaunitz AM, Pritts EA, et al. U.S. Food and Drug Administration's guidance regarding morcellation of leiomyomas: well-intentioned, but is it harmful for women? *Obstet Gynecol* 2016;**127**(1):18–22.

9. Brown J. AAGL advancing minimally invasive gynecology worldwide: statement to the FDA on power morcellation. *J Minim Invasive Gynecol* 2014;**21** (6):970–1.

10. Allen E. Vaginal removal of the uterus by morcellation. *Am J Obstet Gynecol* 1949;**57** (4):692–700.

11. Hasson HM, Rotman C, Rana N, Sistos F, Dmowski WP. Laparoscopic myomectomy. *Obstet Gynecol* 1992;**80**(5): 884–8.

12. Steiner RA, Wight E, Tadir Y, Haller U. Electrical cutting device for laparoscopic removal of tissue from the abdominal cavity. *Obstet Gynecol* 1993;**81**(3):471–4.

13. Carter JE, McCarus SD. Laparoscopic myomectomy. Time and cost analysis of power vs. manual morcellation. *J Reprod Med* 1997;**42**(7):383–8.

14. Schneider A. Recurrence of unclassifiable uterine cancer after modified laparoscopic hysterectomy with morcellation. *Am J Obstet Gynecol* 1997;**177** (2):478–9.

15. Seidman MA, Oduyebo T, Muto MG, et al. Peritoneal dissemination complicating morcellation of uterine mesenchymal neoplasms. *PLoS One* 2012;**7**(11):e50058.

16. Society of Gynecologic Oncology. SGO Position Statement: Morcellation. 2013. Available at: www.sgo.org/newsroom/position-statements-2/morcellation/. Accessed 1 Dec 2016.

17. Goff BA. SGO not soft on morcellation: risks and benefits must be weighed. *Lancet Oncol* 2014;**15**(4):e148.

18. FDA Safety Communication. Laparoscopic uterine power morcellation in hysterectomy and myomectomy. Apr 2014. Available at: www.fda.gov/MedicalDevices/Safety/AlertsandNotices/ucm393576.htm. Accessed 1 Dec 2016.

19. FDA. Quantitative assessment of the prevalence of unsuspected uterine sarcoma in women undergoing treatment of uterine fibroids. Apr 2014. Available at: www.fda.gov/downloads/MedicalDevices/Safety/AlertsandNotices/UCM393589.pdf. Accessed 1 Dec 2016.

20. AAGL Advancing Minimally Invasive Gynecology Worldwide. AAGL practice report: morcellation during uterine tissue extraction. *J Minim Invasive Gynecol.* 2017;**21**(4):517–30.

21. FDA Safety Communication. Updated laparoscopic uterine power morcellation in hysterectomy and myomectomy. Nov 2014. Available at: www.fda.gov/MedicalDevices/Safety/AlertsandNotices/ucm424443.htm. Accessed 1 Dec 2016.

22. Siedhoff MT, Wheeler SB, Rutstein SE, et al. Laparoscopic hysterectomy with morcellation vs abdominal hysterectomy for presumed fibroid tumors in premenopausal women: a decision analysis. *Am J Obstet Gynecol* 2015;**212**(5):591.e591–8.

23. Pritts EA, Vanness DJ, Berek JS, et al. The prevalence of occult leiomyosarcoma at surgery for presumed uterine fibroids: a meta-analysis. *Gynecol Surg* 2015;**12**(3):165–77.

24. Bojahr B, De Wilde RL, Tchartchian G. Malignancy rate of 10,731 uteri morcellated during laparoscopic supracervical hysterectomy (LASH). *Arch Gynecol Obstet.* 2015;**292** (3):665–72.

25. Harris JA, Swenson CW, Uppal S, et al. Practice patterns and postoperative complications before and after US Food and Drug Administration safety communication on power morcellation. *Am J Obstet Gynecol* 2016;**214**(1):98.e91–98.e13.

26. Barron KI, Richard T, Robinson PS, Lamvu G. Association of the

U.S. Food and Drug Administration morcellation warning with rates of minimally invasive hysterectomy and myomectomy. *Obstet Gynecol* 2015;**126**(6):1174–80.

27. Wright J, Chen L, Burke W, et al. Trends in use and outcomes of women undergoing hysterectomy with electric power morcellation. *JAMA* 2016;**316**(8):877–8.

28. Cohen SL, Einarsson JI, Wang KC, et al. Contained power morcellation within an insufflated isolation bag. *Obstet Gynecol* 2014;**124**(3):491–7.

29. Steller C, Miller C, Sasaki K, Cholkeri-Singh A. Review and outcome of electromechanical power morcellation using an innovative contained specimen bag system. *J Minim Invasive Gynecol* 2015;**22**(6):S100–1.

30. Seidman DS, Nezhat CH, Nezhat F, Nezhat C. The role of laparoscopic-assisted myomectomy (LAM). *J Soc Laparoendosc Surg* 2001;**5**(4):299–303.

31. Nezhat C, Nezhat F, Bess O, Nezhat CH, Mashiach R. Laparoscopically assisted myomectomy: a report of a new technique in 57 cases. *Int J Fertil Menopausal Stud* 1994;**39**(1):39–44.

32. Serur E, Zambrano N, Brown K, Clemetson E, Lakhi N. Extracorporeal manual morcellation of very large uteri within an enclosed endoscopic bag: our 5-year experience. *J Minim Invasive Gynecol* 2016;**23**(6):903–8.

33. Park JY, Park SK, Kim DY, et al. The impact of tumor morcellation during surgery on the prognosis of patients with apparently early uterine leiomyosarcoma. *Gynecol Oncol* 2011;**122**(2):255–9.

34. Perri T, Korach J, Sadetzki S, et al. Uterine leiomyosarcoma: does the primary surgical procedure matter? *Int J Gynecol Cancer* 2009;**19**(2):257–60.

35. Morice P, Rodriguez A, Rey A, et al. Prognostic value of initial surgical procedure for patients with uterine sarcoma: analysis of 123 patients. *Eur J Gynaecol Oncol* 2003;**24**(3–4):237–40.

36. Oduyebo T, Rauh-Hain AJ, Meserve EE, et al. The value of re-exploration in patients with inadvertently morcellated uterine sarcoma. *Gynecol Oncol* 2014;**132**(2):360–5.

37. Kho KA, Nezhat CH. Evaluating the risks of electric uterine morcellation. *JAMA* 2014;**311**(9):905–6.

Total Laparoscopic Hysterectomy for the Fibroid Uterus

Alpha K. Gebeh and Mostafa Metwally

11.1 Introduction

Hysterectomy is one of the most common major gynaecological procedures and has been reported in early Greek manuscripts as early as 50 BC and AD 120, though proof that it was performed is limited. However, it was not until the 1800s that the first planned vaginal hysterectomy was recorded [1]. Traditionally, hysterectomy is done either by an open abdominal approach via a midline or transverse incision, or by a vaginal approach. The first laparoscopic hysterectomy was described by Harry Reich and colleagues in 1989 [2]. With advances in technology, development of new instruments and standardization of surgical techniques, the laparoscopic approach has fast gained popularity across gynaecological practice and has become an independent alternative treatment option [3–6]. Performance of a hysterectomy through the laparoscopic route has clear advantages to the patient from the point of view of recovery and return to normal activity. Open hysterectomy is now often reserved for very large uteri or in settings where the appropriate expertise is not available. Laparoscopic hysterectomy includes total laparoscopic hysterectomy (TLH) and laparoscopic subtotal hysterectomy (LASH). The presence of fibroids can present a technical challenge to performing laparoscopic hysterectomy, but with knowledge of these challenges and how to address them, performing a laparoscopic hysterectomy even in the presence of relatively large or numerous fibroids can be made feasible. These challenges will be covered in this chapter.

11.2 Indications and Contraindications

The indications for laparoscopic hysterectomy are similar to other forms of hysterectomies and include leiomyoma, abnormal uterine bleeding, adenomyosis, gynaecological cancers and pelvic organ prolapse. Laparoscopic hysterectomy for a large fibroid uterus

(>500 g) can be associated with a longer operating time, higher intraoperative blood loss, high risk of conversion to laparotomy and longer hospital stay [7]. These challenges mean that a laparoscopic hysterectomy for a fibroid uterus merits special tips and tricks to facilitate safe surgery and reduce morbidity. The fibroid uterus is usually large, and the upper limit for a safe and successful laparoscopic approach is dictated to a large extent by the skill of the surgeon, the location of uterine bulk/fibroid, the patient's medical comorbidities, and ease of access to uterine vasculature, and to some extent it depends on the nature of the pathology being treated. Examples of situations where a laparoscopic approach is contraindicated include known cases of gynaecological cancer where the specimen may not be removed intact by a laparoscopic approach, or patients with significant cardiopulmonary disease with associated intolerance to increased intra-abdominal pressure or deep Trendelenburg position which in turn may limit visualization of pelvic anatomy, or where the skill of the surgeon is inadequate.

11.3 Procedure and Complications

The surgical steps may have minor variations between surgeons, but the detailed procedure is outside the scope of this chapter. In general, the steps include uterine manipulation, laparoscopic entry, round ligament transection, preparation of the vesicouterine space and development of the bladder flap, securing and dividing the upper and lower pedicles, colpotomy and removal of uterus and finally colporrhaphy. The risk of minor and major complications with laparoscopic hysterectomy is generally low (<2%) but can be higher in the presence of large uterine fibroids that add to the technical difficulty of the case. Recognized complications include infections (wound, urinary tract, infected haematoma, peritonitis), bleeding, bowel injury, vaginal vault complications (haematoma, dehiscence), urinary tract injuries (ureters, bladder), venous thromboembolism, conversion to laparotomy, anaesthetic risks and rarely nerve injury [8, 9].

Complications are therefore directly related to the skill of the surgeon. Surgeons still at the early stages of training to preform laparoscopic hysterectomy, needless to say, need to carefully select cases within their skill limit. With more experience, technically challenging cases such as those with uterine fibroids can be tackled with relative ease. The key is to know the challenges and how to pre-emptively avoid them. The surgeon should also have a diversity of techniques and the flexibility to switch from one technique to the other as the case dictates.

11.4 Challenges Associated with Laparoscopic Hysterectomy for Fibroids

11.4.1 Preoperative Challenges

A thorough and meticulous preoperative assessment and obtaining a thorough clinical history is vital in all patients for a successful operative and postoperative course. Management options include the following:

a. *Optimization of anaemia and shrinkage of fibroid volume*: a common problem of fibroid uterus is anaemia from heavy menstrual bleeding which requires correction before surgery. Options include iron therapy for iron deficiency anaemia and preoperative blood transfusion in selected cases. Another approach is to concurrently minimize menstrual blood loss or induce amenorrhoea and shrink fibroid volume, e.g. by use of GnRH analogues or selective progesterone receptor modulators (SPRMs), i.e. ulipristal acetate. These approaches minimize the likelihood of requiring postoperative blood transfusion, and the shrinkage in fibroid volume will facilitate laparoscopic hysterectomy by aiding visualization, reduce the likelihood of intraoperative blood loss and reduce operating time. There is good evidence from a Cochrane review that the use of GnRH analogues for 3–4 months before hysterectomy is associated with reduced fibroid volume, improvement in preoperative and postoperative haemoglobin and haematocrit when used prior to surgery, reduction in intraoperative blood loss and

reduced risk of vertical abdominal incision. These benefits translate into reduced operating time and decreased hospital stay [10], though their use is associated with adverse side effects from pituitary down-regulation including hot flashes, night sweats, vaginal dryness, low mood and loss of bone mineral density after prolonged use [11, 12]. Ulipristal acetate has become more widely available and evidence from trials suggests that a 3-month course results in approximately 50% reduction in fibroid volume. Recent preliminary data, however, required monitoring of liver function before and during treatment due to reported rare but severe cases of liver failure with the use of ulipristal. This amount of volume reduction in the context of TLH may provide similar benefits to those seen with GnRH analogues.

b. *Preoperative imaging*: a pelvic ultrasound scan should be undertaken to assess the location, size and number of fibroids to help plan the surgical approach. There is a possibility that a myomectomy will need to be performed during the surgery to facilitate the procedure, and for this reason performing an MRI has clear advantages over ultrasound scan by helping to differentiate between fibroids and adenomyomas which are not amenable to surgical enucleation. Furthermore, although MRI scans cannot diagnose malignancy, they can provide some useful information regarding potential malignancy and therefore pre-empt the surgeon to consider an open rather than a laparoscopic approach where performing a myomectomy or morcellating the specimen may carry the risks of disseminating a malignancy.

c. *Concurrent pelvic pathology*: where concurrent pathology is expected, e.g. significant endometriosis or bowel adhesions from previous surgery, appropriate measures should be put in place, e.g. ensuring assistance from a colorectal surgeon is available where bowel adhesions is anticipated.

d. *Enhanced recovery after surgery (ERAS)*: women with large uteri are at risk of prolonged surgery and longer operative stay and are therefore suitable for ERAS protocols. ERAS protocols aim to reduce the physical and psychological impact of elective gynaecological surgery on patients and should be undertaken for women having laparoscopic hysterectomy for large uteri. The basic components of enhanced recovery include patient education, modifying standard oral feeding, drinking policies, carbohydrate loading, avoiding dehydration, eliminating bowel preparation requirements, avoiding open procedures and using minimally invasive surgical techniques when possible, minimizing use of surgical drains, minimizing intravenous fluid infusion intraoperatively, modified analgesia intraoperatively and postoperatively, aggressive prophylaxis of perioperative nausea and vomiting and early postoperative oral nutrition [13]. ERAS provides multiple benefits including faster recovery, increased patient satisfaction and decreased healthcare costs without additional risks to women.

11.4.2 Intraoperative Challenges

a. *Port placement*: the most important step is planning correct port placement. Good versus poor port placement is the key difference between an easy and a difficult laparoscopic hysterectomy. Every surgeon will have a preferred port configuration when performing a laparoscopic hysterectomy but this needs to be modified when performing the procedure for a large fibroid uterus.

The first step is to perform an examination in theatre by the primary operating surgeon. The size of the uterus will determine the position of the ports. To make a large uterus smaller, the surgeon will need to move the primary port away from the uterus. Even a few millimetres can make a large difference to visibility during the procedure. Operating with the laparoscope close to the uterus makes the procedure extremely difficult. Occasionally, even the Palmer's point can be used for the primary port. Similarly, having the secondary ports close to the uterus leaves very little room for manoeuvrability of the surgical instruments. The surgeon can therefore retain the normal port configuration but shift the ports cephalad in proportion to the size of the uterus. Care of course must be taken to avoid injury to upper abdominal viscera, particularly the stomach and transverse colon.

The authors usually use a supraumbilical primary port, taking care to ensure the stomach

has been emptied using a nasogastric tube. Secondary ports normally placed in the left and right iliac fossae are instead placed in a higher position and a third right paraumbilcal port can also be valuable to provide an additional port for the assistant and for suturing, but care needs to be taken to avoid damage to the inferior epigastric vessels.

b. *Assessment of pelvic anatomy*: the next step is thorough assessment of the size and anatomical position of the fibroids. Fibroids are unique in that they can vary in number and size and no two cases are exactly the same. It is important to note fibroids that may significantly alter the anatomy or preclude safe completion of the procedure, at which stage the procedure can be converted to a laparotomy if the procedure is found to be beyond the skill level of the surgeon. The following fibroids are of particular relevance:

i. *Lateral or broad ligament fibroids*: these can complicate safe access to the uterine vessels and also significantly alter the course of the ureter, increasing the risk of ureteric damage. Given that the surgeon has the skills to perform a laparoscopic myomectomy, these fibroids can be first removed to facilitate securing of the uterine vessels and also allow the ureter to move back to its normal position before securing the uterine vessels. The authors use 5–10 units of intramyometrial vasopressin prior to performing a laparoscopic myomectomy to minimize bleeding. Vasopressin, however, is a potentially dangerous drug and should only be used with adequate experience regarding its effects, side effects and pharmacokinetics. An alternative method is to secure the uterine vessels at their origin from the internal iliac artery. Again, this requires considerable expertise in retroperitoneal dissection. The surgeon should also have the skill to identify and dissect the ureter. When the anatomy in the lower pelvis is distorted due to the fibroid, it is best to identify the ureter at the pelvic brim and follow it down. The ureter is easily identified as the first retroperitoneal structure seen medial to the infundibulopelvic ligament at the pelvic brim.

ii. *Low corporeal fibroids*: these fibroids may significantly hinder access to the lower pelvis

101

and make colpotomy more difficult. Even if the surgeon decides to resort to a laparoscopic subtotal hysterectomy, the presence of a low corporeal fibroid can make safe separation of the uterine body from the cervix more difficult. A low corporeal anterior wall fibroid can stretch the bladder and increase the risk of bladder injury. Low corporeal fibroids may therefore be removed in order to facilitate colpotomy. In cases of anterior fibroids, the uterovesical pouch needs first to be carefully dissected to minimize risk of damage to the bladder. If these fibroids need to be removed, it is better to postpone until the uterine vessels have been secured to minimize the risk of bleeding and avoid the need for vasopressin or similar measures.

c. *Ergonomics*: to ensure the correct ergonomics, the surgeon may stand on a footstep or lower the table as much as possible to ensure an adequate arm reach across the operating table. In addition, a tilt of the operating table towards the primary surgeon during laparoscopic suturing may be useful. These measures could help reduce the surgeon's muscle fatigue and strain, and facilitate a more ergonomic position. Another recognized challenge with laparoscopic pelvic surgery is the mobilization of bowels during the colpotomy. In such a situation, a deep Trendelenburg position would facilitate adequate exposure to the pelvic anatomy, especially in cases where colpotomy is anticipated to be difficult.

d. *Removal of uterus*: removal of the uterus is arguably sometimes the biggest challenge with laparoscopic hysterectomy for fibroids. This is influenced by uterine size and location of the fibroids. Options include enucleation of a few fibroids first to decrease the uterine size, allowing

it to be removed vaginally. The uterus can also be bisected laparoscopically, vaginally or using a combination of both techniques. Fibroids can also be enucleated vaginally.

Fibroids that have been separated from the uterus can be removed with the specimen vaginally or by morcellation. The procedure of morcellation has been subject to extensive debate recently and is covered in detail in other areas of this book. A laparoscopic subtotal hysterectomy (LASH) can often be considered, particularly if the colpotomy is found to be difficult. The technique is particularly suitable for patients who mainly suffer from pressure symptoms and where the fibroids are mainly limited to the uterine body. Performing a LASH will cure the pressure symptoms with minimal risk. In women with significant bleeding problems, however, a small proportion will continue to experience bleeding from retained endometrial tissue with the cervix. The endocervix should, therefore, always be ablated using electrosurgical energy. It is also important that there is no significant cervical abnormality, so the patient should have had up-to-date normal cervical smears prior to performing a LASH. Another approach is to perform a LASH in the first instance, thus facilitating the colpotomy and removal of the cervix separately.

11.5 Conclusion

Laparoscopic hysterectomy for fibroid uterus has significant technical challenges, but with adequate training, thorough preoperative planning and modifications to the standard procedure, these technical challenges can be managed appropriately. Patient safety is paramount, and where continuing with a laparoscopic approach will increase the patient's morbidity, alternatives operative options should be considered.

References

1. Baskett TF. Hysterectomy: evolution and trends. *Best Pract Res Clin Obstet Gynaecol* 2005;**19**(3):295–305.
2. Reich H, Decaprio J, Mcglynn F. Laparoscopic hysterectomy. *J Gynecol Sur* 1989;**5**(2):213–16.
3. Mikhail E, Salemi JL, Wyman A, et al. National trends of bilateral salpingectomy during vaginal hysterectomy with and without laparoscopic assistance, United States 1998–2011. *J Minim Invasive Gynecol* 2015;**22**(6S):S85.
4. Kroft J, Li Q, Saskin R, et al. Trends over time in the use of laparoscopic hysterectomy for the treatment of endometrial cancer. *Gynecol Oncol* 2015;**138**(3):536–41.
5. Lee EJ, Park, HM. Trends in laparoscopic surgery for hysterectomy in Korea between 2007 and 2009. *J Obstet Gynaecol Res* 2014;**40**(6):1695–9.
6. Gante I, Medeiros-Borges C, Águas F. Hysterectomies in Portugal (2000–2014): what has changed? *Eur J Obstet Gynecol Reprod Biol* 2017;**208**:97–102.

7. Fiaccavento A, Landi S, Barbieri F, et al. Total laparoscopic hysterectomy in cases of very large uteri: a retrospective comparative study. *J Minim Invasive Gynecol* 2007;**14**(5):559–63.

8. Donnez O, Jadoul P, Squifflet J, Donnez J. A series of 3190 laparoscopic hysterectomies for benign disease from 1990 to 2006: evaluation of complications compared with vaginal and abdominal procedures. *BJOG* 2009;**116** (4):492–500.

9. Donnez O, Donnez J. A series of 400 laparoscopic hysterectomies for benign disease: a single centre, single surgeon prospective study of complications confirming previous retrospective study. *BJOG* 2010;**117**(6):752–5.

10. Lethaby A, Vollenhoven B, Sowter M. Pre-operative GnRH analogue therapy before hysterectomy or myomectomy for uterine fibroids. *Cochrane Database Syst Rev* 2001; (2):CD000547.

11. Donnez J, Donnez O, Matule D, et al. Long-term medical management of uterine fibroids with ulipristal acetate. *Fertil Steril* 2016;**105**(1):165–73.e4.

12. Donnez J, Hudecek R, Donnez O, et al. Efficacy and safety of repeated use of ulipristal acetate in uterine fibroids. *Fertil Steril* 2015;**103**(2): 519–27.e3.

13. Mukhopadhyay D. Enhanced recovery programme in gynaecology: outcomes of a hysterectomy care pathway. *BMJ Qual Improv Rep* 2015; **4**(1):2.

Hysteroscopic Resection of Submucosal Fibroids

Rudi Campo, Cristine Di Cesare and S. Gordts

12.1 Introduction

Fibroids represent an extremely common benign uterine pathology, being a major cause of abnormal uterine bleeding disorders. Although most myomas are of benign origin, it is important to have a correct diagnostic procedure prior to endoscopic myoma resection. Preoperative imaging techniques as well as histological criteria have to be taken into account. The true prevalence of uterine sarcoma in presumed fibroids is not known, given the wide range of prevalence (0.014–0.45%) from meta-analyses mainly based on retrospective trials. Age and certain imaging characteristics are associated with a higher risk of uterine sarcoma, although the risks remain low [1, 2].

The incidence of myomas increases with age, and although the association between uterine myoma and infertility is still controversial, evidence exists that subserosal myomas do not impair pregnancy rate in IVF, whereas submucosal myomas significantly decrease implantation rate. Unfortunately, the effect of intramural myomas upon reproduction outcomes remains unknown and, until now, no adequate diagnostic and therapeutic guidelines have been established.

Recently, magnetic resonance imaging (MRI) has contributed greatly to the correct anatomical and functional mapping of myomas. Functionally, MRI differentiates the muscle layer into the junctional zone (JZ) myometrium, where the cells are responsible for the implantation and growth of the placenta. The outer myometrium, normally contributing two-thirds of the diameter, provides the muscular power for the delivery. Submucosal fibroids (SF), originating from the JZ myometrium, differ also from subserosal fibroids that originate from the outer myometrium because they have fewer cytogenetic abnormalities and the expression of sex steroid hormone receptors are more responsive to GnRH analogue treatment, providing fewer recurrences after surgery [3].

Junctional zone myomas are responsible for abnormal uterine bleeding disorders and reproductive failure. The physiological pathway to access the JZ myometrium is the hysteroscopic approach, and as such hysteroscopy plays a major role in the diagnosis and treatment of symptomatic myomas.

Since 1976, when Neuwirth and Amin reported the first five cases of excision of submucosal myomas [4], several techniques have been developed in order to render hysteroscopic myomectomy a safe and effective procedure.

This chapter will demonstrate the newest techniques of hysteroscopic diagnosis, the therapy of submucosal and intramural myomas, as well as the new instrumentation and tips and tricks to prevent complications.

12.2 Diagnosis and Preoperative Treatment

12.2.1 Classification

Several classification systems are proposed, but the most frequently used are the FIGO [5] and the European Society of Gynaecological Endoscopy (ESGE) classifications [6].

Figure 12.1 shows the different myoma locations according to the FIGO classification accessible for hysteroscopic treatment.

Type 0 defines a pedunculated myoma into the cavity, while type 1 myoma has a significant intramural portion, but the largest diameters into the cavity. The type 2 myoma, on the other hand, is recognized with a small portion into the cavity, but with its largest diameter in the myometrium. Type 3, only referred to in the FIGO classification, does not have a portion into the cavity, but originates from the JZ myometrium and has sufficient security zone towards the uterine serosa. Today, with the help of concomitant ultrasound, that myoma also can be removed using hysteroscopic techniques.

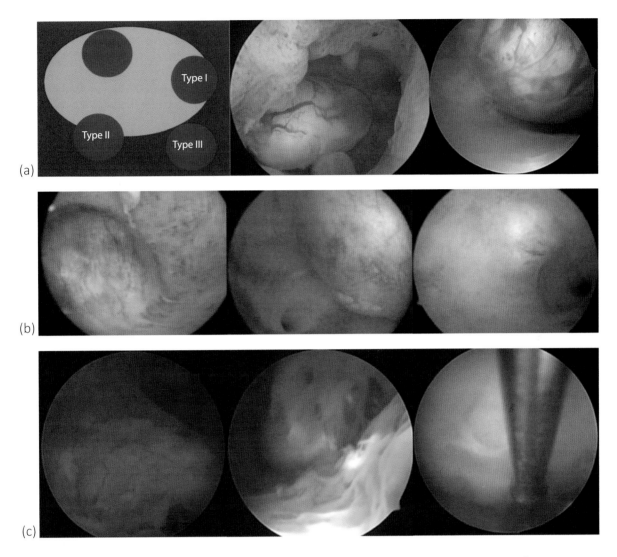

Figure 12.1 Different myoma locations. (a) Different locations accessible for hysteroscopic surgery, hysteroscopic view of a type 0 myoma, with detail view on the base. (b) Type 1 myoma – more than 50% is in the cavity, type 2 myoma – more than 50% is intramural but myoma is visible in the cavity. (c) Type 3 myoma – only bulging of the endometrial line visible, capsula identification with overlying endometrium; intramural part is dissected with the 5 Fr. instrument.

12.2.2 MRI

A study on inter-observer reproducibility in MRI versus transvaginal ultrasonography (TVS), hysteroscopy (HSC) or hysterosalpingography (HSG) demonstrated that the agreement on evaluation of myomas was significantly greater by magnetic resonance imaging (MRI) than by any other technique [3].

Unlike ultrasound, MRI demonstrates that the non-pregnant myometrium is not a homogeneous smooth muscle mass, but consists of two different structural and functional entities. The myometrium adjacent to the endometrium is a hormone-dependent different uterine compartment called junctional zone (JZ) myometrium, and it is seen as a smaller central zone of increased density due to its higher nuclear/cytoplasm ratio, decreased extracellular matrix and lower water content. The JZ is an entity functionally important in reproduction and it is ontogenetically related to the endometrium. Indeed, cyclic changes in sex steroid hormone receptor expression in the JZ mimic those of the endometrium. Highly specialized

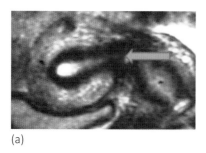
(a)

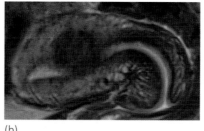
(b)

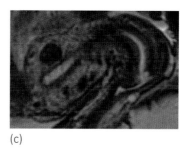
(c)

Figure 12.2 MRI T2 image in sagittal plane. (a) Submucosal myoma originating from the JZ myometrium. (b) Normal JZ myometrium with several small myomas in the outer myometrium. (c) Normal functional differentiation in MRI, access to the JZ through HSC.

contraction waves originate exclusively from the JZ and participate in the regulation of diverse reproductive events, such as sperm transport and embryo implantation. Evidence exists that structural changes in the JZ also play an important role during pregnancy by regulating trophoblast invasion and the formation of a functional placenta [7].

The most commonly used classifications of myomas are related to their location, namely submucosal, intramural or subserosal. Based on the information gathered by MRI, it must be stated that the intramural myoma must be seen as a misnomer, and a myoma should be classified either as JZ myometrium or outer myometrium myoma (Figure 12.2).

In agreement with this evidence, the physiological pathway to access the JZ myometrium is obviously the hysteroscopic approach.

12.2.3 One-Stop Uterine Diagnosis by Combining Hysteroscopic and Ultrasound Exam

A one-stop uterine diagnosis includes a transvaginal ultrasound followed by a fluid mini-hysteroscopy using the vaginoscopic technique, and it concludes with a vaginal ultrasound, using the fluid of the hysteroscopy as contrast, to finally evaluate the uterus as a whole (Figure 12.3a).

Especially for the diagnosis of myoma, the combination of ultrasound and hysteroscopy is very beneficial; size and location can be defined correctly in this manner (Figure 12.3b).

The feasibility of ambulatory ultrasound has been greatly accepted, but even nowadays diagnostic hysteroscopy can be performed under the same conditions. The scientific evidence provided shows that small-bored 30° rigid scopes are needed, as well as saline as a distension medium, while employing the vaginoscopic approach [8–11].

Based on these findings, the CAMPO TROPHYSCOPE® was invented. The publication in *The Lancet* demonstrates that in 350 hysteroscopies performed in eight different centres in patients with failed IVF, no complication and no access failure occurred [11].

The CAMPO TROPHYSCOPE® consists of an all-in-one system, where the exam is started with the compact 2.9 mm atraumatic rigid 30° single-flow optic. If necessary, a second sheath can be forwarded by a visually controlled dilatation, without removing the scope (Figure 12.4a). This reduces the risk of discomfort, perforation or involuntarily lesion to the fragile endometrium.

The exam always starts with an instrument diameter of 2.9 mm and is increased to a diameter of 3.7 mm for the Continuous-Flow Examination Sheath and 4.4 mm for the Continuous-Flow Operating Sheath.

A very important feature of the CAMPO TROPHYSCOPE® is that, by removal of the scope, the Continuous-Flow Examination Sheath can be used to insert instruments like the TROPHY Curette or an endo–myometrial tissue sampler, like the Spirotome, to perform tissue sampling of the endo- and myometrium under ultrasound control.

In this way, correct anatomo-pathological examination of the endometrium and JZ myometrium is possible without the need for a speculum. Both ultrasound and post-sampling hysteroscopy control the correctness of the procedure.

With use of the Continuous-Flow Operating Sheath, the instrument diameter is visually enlarged to 4.4 mm, providing the possibility to enlarge the diagnostic procedure with minimally invasive actions, using the mechanical and bipolar 5 Fr. instruments (Figure 12.4b).

Combining ultrasound and hysteroscopy makes it possible to enlarge the diagnostic procedure with safe

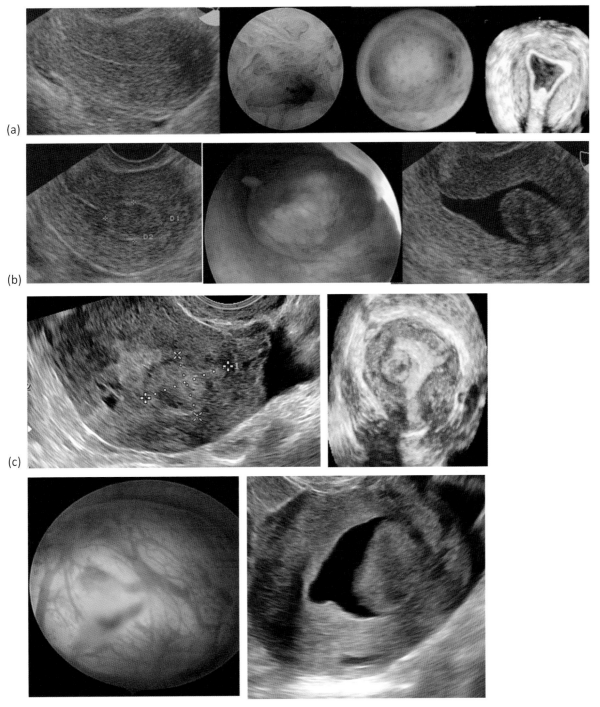

Figure 12.3 The one-stop diagnostic exam includes transvaginal ultrasound (2 or 3D) followed by hysteroscopy and contrast sonography of the uterine cavity. (a) Normal findings. (b) Intrauterine myoma type 0. (c) Combination ultrasound and HSC for type 1 myoma.

(a)

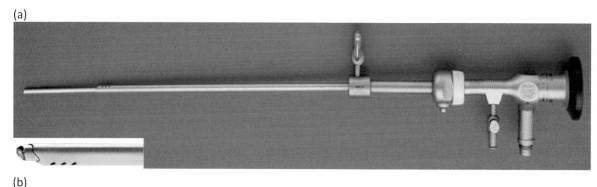

(b)

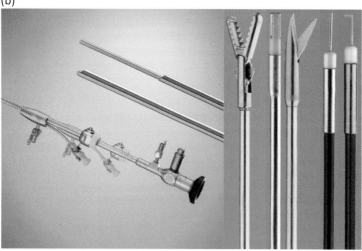

Figure 12.4 CAMPO TROPHYSCOPE®. (a) CAMPO TROPHYSCOPE® 30° rigid optic single flow of 2.9 mm in diameter with Continuous-Flow Examination Sheath in passive position, 7 cm from top of instrument. By forward movement it is possible to perform visually guided dilatation up to 3.7 mm, creating also the double flow function. (b) The Continuous-Flow Operating Sheath uses the same dilatation methodology and enlarges the diameter from 2.9 to 4.4 mm, giving access to 5 Fr. instrumentation for surgical action. (KARL STORZ SE & Co. KG, Germany)

and ambulatory tissue sampling, which is certainly an advantage if myoma dignity is questioned.

12.2.4 Myometrial Biopsy with the Spirotome® (Figure 12.5)

Today, uterine exploration in patients with infertility, abnormal uterine bleeding and pain should not be restricted to the visual exploration of only the uterine cavity, but should also include the exploration of the inner and outer myometrial structures. In case of suspicion of abnormality in the JZ myometrium or in case of myoma in a patient above 40 years of age with a suspicious image on ultrasound, a biopsy should be performed prior to hysteroscopic surgery (ESGE) [12, 13].

The Spirotome consists of a specially designed helix, which is turned clockwise under ultrasound

control to enter the target, then the sample is cut from the surroundings by turning the cutting cannula clockwise over the helix until the distal ends meet.

The TROPHY hysteroscopy offers the possibility to facilitate the introduction of the Spirotome into the uterine cavity. After the diagnostic hysteroscopy is performed, the 2.9 mm scope is removed and the atraumatic Continuous-Flow Examination Sheath remains in the uterine cavity. Under ultrasound guidance, the TROPHY Continuous-Flow Examination Sheath is positioned exactly towards the sonographic suspicious area.

Once the position is agreed on, the helix is introduced in the TROPHY Continuous-Flow Examination Sheath and, thanks to its specific navigation features under ultrasound control, a precise navigation and a correct direction and position of the helix point can be achieved. There tends to be minimal or

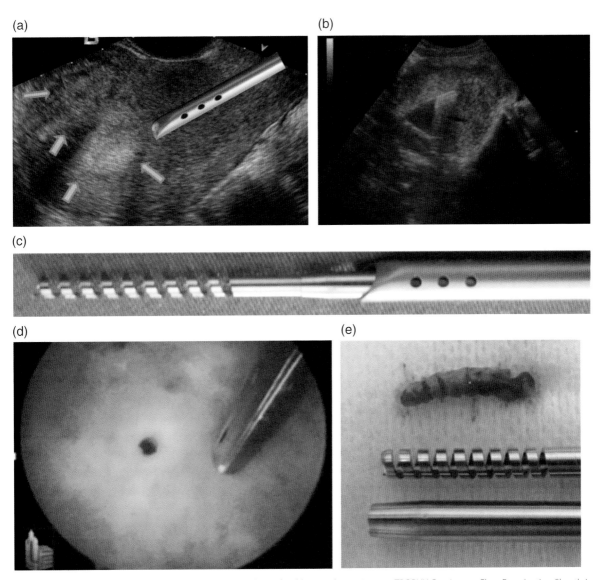

Figure 12.5 Spirotome biopsy. (a) 2D ultrasound image shows focal hyperechogenic zone; TROPHY Continuous-Flow Examination Sheath is used as atraumatic guide to insert the Spirotome. (b) Introducing the Spirotome in an enlarged (>2 cm) anterior uterine wall under ultrasound guidance. (c) Spirotome inserted in the TROPHY Continuous-Flow Examination Sheath. (d) Hysteroscopic view of the puncture place showing the atraumatic character. (e) Biopsy specimen, corkscrew and cutting device.

no bleeding during helix navigation and the (ultrasound) image remains unchanged without confounding by blurring, as it may otherwise occur in the event of bleeding. The sample is preserved inside the helix. In other words, it is as if the histology is untouched except for the spiral wire that traverses through the tissue.

Subsequently, the cutting cannula is turned clockwise and a sample of up to 20 mm in length can be taken.

During cutting, the sample is fixed by the contours of the helix and by the tissue fibres running through it. This means that the suspicious target tissue is cut at a stage when the sample is not dislocated by ballistics or aspiration. It is noteworthy that there is no need for additional cutting of the sample at the (open) distal end of the helix. The sample remains in the helix when retracted. This is achieved through the tissue fibres that run through the helix when exposed during navigation. This keeps the sample in the helix at the moment of

109

retraction. The Spirotome, also used in numerous other applications, claims to have the lowest possible risk of cell spreading by performing the biopsy [14, 15].

12.2.5 Preoperative Treatment

The increased size of a myoma exponentially increases surgical time, using the conventional resection technique with the resectoscope [16]. Surgery time correlates directly with operative risks. For this reason, it is advisable to pretreat large myomas to reduce their size prior to hysteroscopic resectoscopy. For the combined medical–surgical treatment, we administer long-acting GnRH analogue prior to menstruation, preventing a flare-up reaction, and surgery is planned following 10–12 weeks of treatment. Possible anaemia can be corrected during this period. It has been demonstrated that this treatment is effective in reducing operative times, fluid absorption and the difficulty of the procedure [17]. Although reports describe the removal of very large intrauterine myomas [18], we recommend individualizing the combined medical–surgical approach according to the size, location, amount of myoma and concomitant pathology.

GnRH preoperative treatment is recommended for single myomas type 0 larger than 4 cm, type 1 myomas larger than 3 cm and type 2 myomas larger than 2.5 cm. In case of multiple myomas, medical treatment is advised when the total diameter exceeds 4 cm. Concomitant pathology, like anaemia or adenomyosis, are arguments in favour of a combined therapy.

Ulipristal acetate (UPA) or progesterone is not as effective in reducing size, but can soften the hardness of the tissue and facilitate the use of the shaving procedure. Unlike the resectoscope, the shaver is not limited by size only, but additionally by the hardness of the tissue. In case of soft pathology, the shaver can remove more than 3 cm of tissue within a few minutes [19–21].

Experience today in the use of progesterone or UPA to prepare a myoma for appropriate shaver use is insufficient to draw up guidelines, and their application for this indication is limited to research.

12.3 Hysteroscopic Treatment of Myoma

12.3.1 Instrumentation

The newest generation of operative instruments has brought a revolution to the hysteroscopic surgical possibilities (Figure 12.6).

The most important evolution is the miniaturization of the different operative hysteroscopes to a similar diameter of 15–19 Fr. and the visual dilatation with the CAMPO TROPHYSCOPE®. This provides the possibility to make a diagnosis and perform therapy without the need for blind dilatation, use of tenaculum or speculum insertion. The operative hysteroscopes, such as the CAMPO TROPHYSCOPE®XL, 15 Fr. Office Resectoscope and 19 Fr. Intrauterine BIGATTI Shaver (IBS), can be interchanged depending on the individual needs of the surgery. Also, the newest-generation pump systems have improved safety and patient compliance.

The HYSTEROMAT E.A.S.I.® is an intelligent, pressure-controlled double roller pump that maintains a constant intrauterine pressure control, in contrast to conventionally used pump systems that work with a predefined extrauterine pressure [20].

12.3.2 Basic Principles for Surgical Strategy in Hysteroscopic Myoma Removal

The surgical strategy is related to the size, position and hardness of the myoma.

Large myoma:	Large myomas benefit from the use of the shaver, and a combined medical–surgical approach or a two-step procedure is recommended.
Intramural position:	For type 2 and type 3 myomas, the surgery starts with the dissection and liberation of the intramural part.
Hard myoma:	Calcified or hard myomas need the use of the resectoscope or bipolar needle.
Instrument interchange (Figure 12.6)	New operative instruments like CAMPO TROPHYSCOPE®, 15 Fr. Office Resectoscope and 19 Fr. Intrauterine BIGATTI Shaver (IBS®) have a similar diameter and, as such, interchange is possible, allowing the surgeon to choose the most appropriate instrument for each section of the surgery.

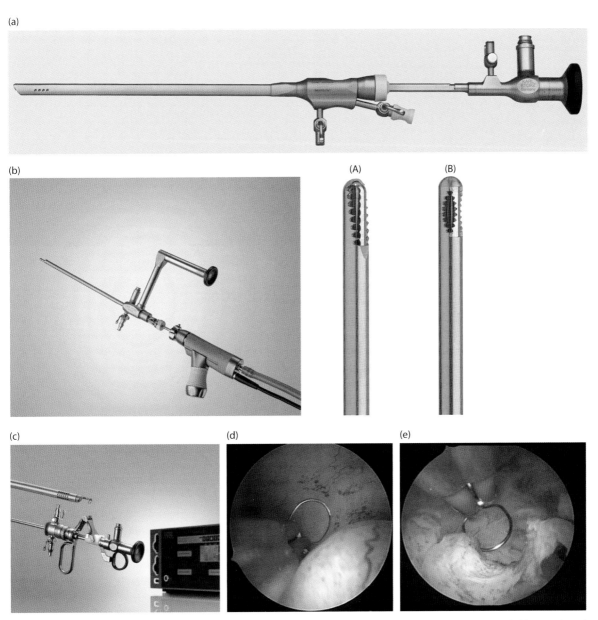

Figure 12.6 Newest hysteroscopic operative instrumentation for minimally invasive myoma removal. (a) 9–15 Fr. Optical dilatation CAMPO TROPHYSCOPE®, 30°, size 3.7 mm, length 22 cm, Continuous-Flow Operating Sheath, size 5.8 mm, length 16 cm, with channel for semi-rigid instruments 5 Fr. (KARL STORZ SE & Co. KG, Germany) (b) 19 Fr. Intrauterine BIGATTI Shaver (IBS®). Wide-angle straight, forward telescope 6°, with parallel eyepiece, length 20 cm, 19Fr., obturator, with integrated outflow channel with LUER-Lock connector replaceable with Shaver Blades (KARL STORZ SE & Co. KG, Germany). The blades have an opening of 25 mm² with either a flute beak shape (A) or an elliptically open shape, similar to shark jaws (B). (c) 15 Fr. Office Resectoscope, Straight Forward telescope 0°, diameter 2.9 mm, with bipolar and cold loop electrodes. 15 Fr. Office Resectoscope: Vascularized and dense pathology (KARL STORZ SE & Co. KG, Germany). The current runs between the active (d) and passive (e) electrode. The electrical pathway is local, reducing risk of adhesion formation and complications. To provide the necessary tissue, cutting firm tissue contact at the start is necessary.

12.3.3 Myoma Resection with the Resectoscope

Until recently, the resectoscope was the only and most frequently used instrument for removing intrauterine myomas, using the same technique of slicing as in prostate resection [22–24].

The uterine application, however, has the problem of tissue removal after resection and the uterus as an organ has a higher risk for fluid overload syndrome.

111

(a)

(b)

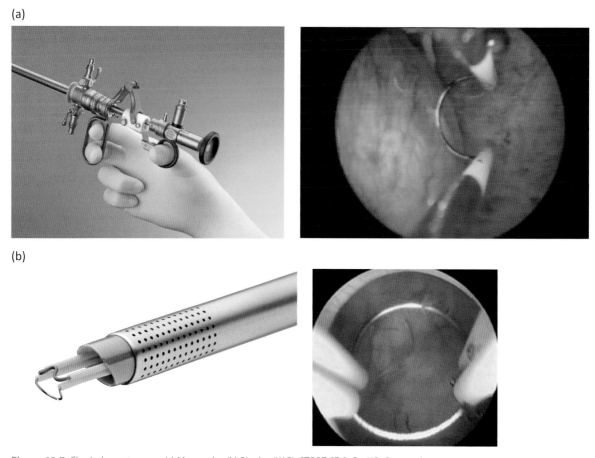

Figure 12.7 Classical resectoscope. (a) Monopolar. (b) Bipolar. (KARL STORZ SE & Co. KG, Germany)

Traditionally, the monopolar resectoscope was used for myoma resection, but nowadays, bipolar resectoscopes are used with ever-increasing frequency (Figure 12.7).

In order to prevent complications, it is recommended to choose either monopolar or bipolar current in operative hysteroscopy, as both surgical handling and OR room organization are quite different for each technique.

12.3.3.1 Monopolar or Bipolar System

In the monopolar system, the body of the patient is integrated into the electrical circuit. The generator produces high-frequency current, which is conducted via the resectoscope into the uterine cavity. The 'active' electrode touches the surface of the pathology with a very small diameter. Therefore, current density is the highest at the tip of the 'active' electrode leading to maximum heat creation for cutting and

coagulation. The current disperses through the tissue 'myometrium'. The surrounding fluid may cool the electrode, but, as long as it is non-conductive, it acts as an insulator. Electrical current is only passing through the electrode and cannot spread through the fluid. The current is dispersed in the patient's body and wanders via the uterine wall, parametrium and connective tissue to the so-called neutral electrode. The neutral electrode should usually be placed on one of the patient's thighs. Monopolar electrosurgery needs non-conductive solutions; glycine or sorbitol–mannitol solutions are often used as distension medium. Ideally, the operation should not exceed 45 minutes and the fluid deficit should not be over 500–1,000 mL with a maximum of 6 L of glycine to avoid serum electrolyte alteration (fluid overload syndrome) [25–27]. The above drawbacks of the monopolar current are the main reasons for most users to change to bipolar surgery.

The bipolar system is one of the major achievements of the last years.

Also, in bipolar electrosurgery, we have heat created by alternating current. The only, but decisive, difference is that 'active' and 'neutral' electrodes are brought close together in one instrument and the distension fluid must be conductive. Current sparks from one electrode to the other and, when tissue is brought into this electric arc, it will be cut, coagulated or vaporized, dependent on the voltage. As current always searches for the easiest way, it is only spreading from one electrode to the other and not wandering through the patient's body. Therefore, a plate on the patient's thigh is not needed and it is possible to use saline solution as distension medium.

Overhydration becomes less dangerous and the amount of fluid loss that can be tolerated is less restrictive in bipolar surgery than with anionic solutions. It provides surgeons with a more comfortable environment and they will be able to finalize the interventions in a single step more frequently.

Not only is the distension medium of advantage, but also the localized current pathway in bipolar surgery decreases the risks of electrosurgical hazards and the overall surgical risk.

Some bipolar resectoscopes have a rather voluminous electrode design, where active and neutral electrodes are placed one in front of the other. Although this kind of electrode reduces the field of movements of the surgeon, it also obliges the surgeon to adapt surgical manoeuvres to this specific type of electrode and reduces the risk of involuntary electrical perforation of the uterine wall (Figure 12.7b).

12.3.3.2 Surgical Technique

The classical resectoscopic excision of an intracavitary fibroid is carried out by using the electric loop (monopolar or bipolar). Resection usually begins from the top of the fibroid, progressing in a uniform way towards the base, also in the case of a pedunculated fibroid [23, 28]. During the resection of the fibroid, particularly when it is large or the cavity is small, the fragments that are sectioned and then accumulated into the cavity may interfere with a clear vision. Thus, they must be removed from the uterine cavity by taking out the resectoscope after grasping the loose tissue elements with the loop electrode. Frequent in and out movement of the resectoscope is related with a risk of laceration of the cervical branch of the uterine artery and the risk of air

embolism. To minimize the risk of air embolism, it is recommended not to use speculum and tenaculum but the vaginoscopic approach of filling up the vagina with fluid.

When using monopolar current, mechanical forces must never be used and forward movements of the electrodes are not allowed while the current is activated. The loop should be in view at all times when the electrode is activated. Due to the absence of combined mechanical and electrical manoeuvres, J. Hamou proposed the technique of hydromassage to deal with the intramural part.

It is performed through rapid changes of intrauterine pressure, using an electronically controlled irrigation and suction device. Indeed, by interrupting and restarting the supply of distension liquid several times, myometrial contraction is stimulated, obtaining the maximum possible migration of the intramural component of the fibroid into the cavity. This technique developed starting from the observation that the intramural portion of a submucosal fibroid squeezes out of its base after contractions of the uterus during the removal of the intrauterine portion.

Using a bipolar resectoscope, the surgical technique to deal with the intramural part is different.

The conventional bipolar resectoscope has a stronger and more voluminous loop, which can combine mechanical and electrical energy; firm tissue contact is necessary prior to activation of the cutting current. The cutting procedure concentrates at first in the middle part of the myoma, removing as much tissue as possible toward the deepest part of the intramural location. As soon as sufficient volume has been removed, the sidewalls will collapse under gentle mechanical pressure (Figure 12.8a). Hydromassage is not necessary and the myoma can be resected totally by clear identification of the capsule due to the combined use of mechanical and electrical power.

12.3.3.3 Removal of the Intramural Part by the Cold Loop Resectoscope Technique

This surgical procedure uses a resectoscope with cold and electrical loops [29, 30, 31].

It is performed in a sequence of three steps.

The first step consists of the excision of the endocavitary component of the fibroid with the usual technique of slicing, using the angled cutting loop. The surgeon must stop the slicing at the level of the plane of the endometrial surface.

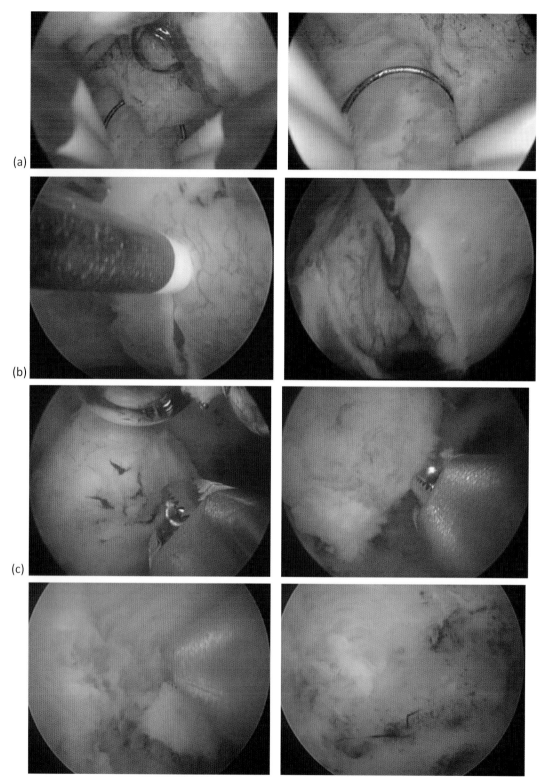

Figure 12.8 Myoma resection. (a) Bipolar resection. (b) Shaping with bipolar needle. (c) Shaver removal.

The second step consists of the enucleation of the intramural component of the myoma through traction and leverage manoeuvres with a non-electrical cold loop. Once the cleavage plane has been identified, the rectangular loop is inserted into the plane between the fibroid and myometrium and then used mechanically along the surface of the fibroid, thus achieving a progressive blunt dissection from the myometrial wall. The single tooth loop is then used to hook and lacerate the slender connective bridges that join the fibroid and the adjacent myometrium. During this phase of enucleation, electric energy must not be used in the thickness of the wall and the loop must be used in a cold manner.

Step three consists of the excision of the intramural component, which has been totally dislocated inside the uterine cavity with an angled cutting loop [24, 29, 30].

Concomitant transabdominal or transrectal ultrasound improves safety and the possibility of removing the intramural part of the myoma in one step. As such the permanent presence of an ultrasound machine, preferably integrated into the endoscopic tower, is highly recommended [32–34].

12.3.4 Myoma Resection with a Shaver

The 19 Fr. Intrauterine BIGATTI Shaver (IBS®) or TruClear shaver have the advantage that the tissue is suctioned, grasped, cut and simultaneously removed [35–39].

The 19 Fr. Intrauterine BIGATTI Shaver (IBS®) consists of two hollow reusable metal tubes fitting into each other. The inner tube, rotated within the outer tube, is connected to a handheld (DRILLCUT-X® II KARL STORZ SE & Co. KG) motor drive unit (UNIDRIVE® S III by KARL STORZ SE & Co. KG) and to a roller pump (HYSTEROMAT E.A.S.I.® KARL STORZ SE & Co. KG) controlled by a foot pedal.

The TruClear hard tissue shaver (Medtronic) is equipped with a rotation shaver blade, shielded by a sheath and connected to a suction system. Fragments are directly removed.

Inflow of distension medium is through the inflow channel of the scope and behind the shaving blade. This results in a fluid passage, which allows working in very narrow spaces, proving of advantage compared with the resectoscope. On the other hand, a performant fluid administration system is necessary for optimal shaver use. Inappropriate fluid pressure

management will result in cavity collapse and will provoke bleeding, disturbing the vision.

When the tissue is removed by the shaver, the surgery becomes very easy and fast. Unlike the resectoscope, the shaver is not really limited by the size of the pathology, but rather by the hardness of the tissue.

This approach does not introduce an electrical current inside the uterus and has no risk of potential thermal damage to healthy endometrium.

Bigatti has shown that the use of the 19 Fr. Intrauterine BIGATTI Shaver (IBS®) is less difficult than the use of a resectoscope. Based on his experience, the shaver should be recommended as the primary approach to intrauterine tissue

12.3.5 Myoma Removal with Mechanical Instruments and Bipolar Needle

Both dissections, as slicing of the myoma, can be performed with the mechanical and bipolar instruments. The intracavitary part of the myoma is first divided in long small slices and sectioned at the endometrial line. The slices are now easily removed through the cervical channel with the grasping forceps. In a second step, the myoma is dissected out of the capsule and sliced in the same way as the intracavitary part (Figure 12.8b).

12.3.6 Combined Approach to Myoma Resection

12.3.6.1 Intramural Dissection with the 5 French Instruments and CAMPO TROPHYSCOPE®

For type 1 to 3 myomas, the first step is the dissection of the myoma out of its capsule with the blunt microscissor using the CAMPO TROPHYSCOPE® or the cold loop technique of the resectoscope.

After localizing the myoma, an incision is made at the transition zone with the endometrium of a type 1 or type 2 myoma. For a type 3 myoma, the site of incision is determined under concomitant ultrasound control.

Once the capsule is identified, the incision is enlarged and the CAMPO TROPHYSCOPE® is inserted in the space between the myoma and myometrium, the capsule space (Figure 12.9).

The myoma is liberated from the surrounding myometrium by hydro dissection, mechanical dissection with the scope tip and section with the 5 Fr.

115

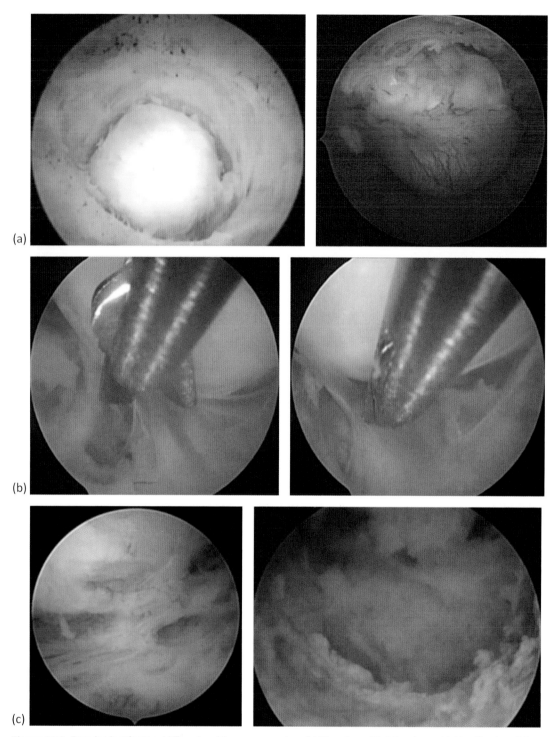

Figure 12.9 Capsule identification. (a) Type 3 and 2 myoma overview. (b) Dissection with 5 Fr. scissor with identification of the space of the capsula. (c) Identification and coagulation of the vascular steal; capsule after total resection of the myoma.

scissors. Pinpoint coagulation of vessels is performed with the bipolar probe to reduce bleeding and to improve visual conditions; this considerably facilitates the subsequent surgical procedure. It is important to perform the coagulation and section of the important afferent and efferent vessels prior to myoma resection.

The liberation of the myoma out of its surroundings is performed for 80% including the vascular steal. The myoma has to remain partially attached to the wall in order to facilitate the resection and removal.

The cold technique avoids myometrial stimulation or damage of the surrounding healthy myometrium and is to be preferred, especially in patients of childbearing age.

12.3.6.2 Resection and Removal

The myoma that is devascularized and still partially attached to the wall still has to be removed. Depending on the size, tissue hardness and position, the surgeon can choose amongst three options:

a. Continue with the 5 Fr. instruments and cut the myoma into long and small strips, which can easily be removed with the grasping forceps.
b. Insert the 19 Fr. Intrauterine BIGATTI Shaver (IBS®) and remove the myoma with the shaver. The success of this procedure depends on the hardness of the tissue. One can combine the above technique with the shaver to improve the accessibility of the shaver. As soon as the myoma is shaped with the bipolar resectoscope into small pieces, the shaver can be used to remove the chips (Figure 12.8c).
c. The 15 Fr. Office Resectoscope can be used to resect the avascular myoma in the typical way as described previously.

12.3.7 Complete Excision of Fibroid by a Two-Step Procedure

Classically, the technique consists of the following steps:

The surgery starts with the excision or incision of the intracavitary portion of the fibroid.

With the use of the bipolar resectoscope, the shaver or the bipolar needle, the myoma is progressively resected up to the endometrial line, then the surgery is stopped. The surgeon does not enter the intramyometrial part, but haemostasis must then be performed carefully.

A hysteroscopic reassessment is carried out 20–30 days after the operation or after the first menstruation to verify that the intracavitary migration of the residual intramural component of the fibroid has taken place; once this has been verified, the second operation can be done with complete excision, by means of slicing, of the residual component of the fibroid, which has now become a type 0 myoma.

Recently, several authors have described a new ambulatory surgical technique to prepare large (>1.5 cm) submucosal myomas with partially intramural development (G1 and G2) in an outpatient setting with miniaturized Office Hysteroscopes either using bipolar current [40] or the laser [41]. In a second phase approximately 4 weeks later, final excision of the myoma is performed. This technique consists of an incision into the endometrial mucosa and the pseudo-capsule that covers the myoma in the first step. Hereby, the myoma is pushed into the uterine cavity by the main force operated by the myometrial fibres and readied for final removal in a second step [40, 41].

12.4 Complications and their Management

12.4.1 Intraoperative Complications

12.4.1.1 Uterine Perforation

Uterine perforation most often occurs during cervical dilatation, hysteroscope insertion or intramyometrial tissue resection. It is more likely to occur in those with cervical stenosis, retroverted or anteverted uterus and in nulliparous or postmenopausal women. The danger of a uterine injury is especially great during the resection of intramural myoma components with the use of energy conductors; injury of organs behind the uterus, especially the intestine, may occur.

In the case of an electrical uterine perforation with the resectoscope, a diagnostic laparoscopy should be conducted for the exclusion of intra-abdominal injuries. With injuries of the intestine, an adequate surgical treatment should follow. It should be kept in mind that the zone of thermal necrosis can be bigger than the visible trauma. Even if there are no further injuries visible in the abdomen, an intensive surveillance of the patient should follow for the next few days to

(a) (b)

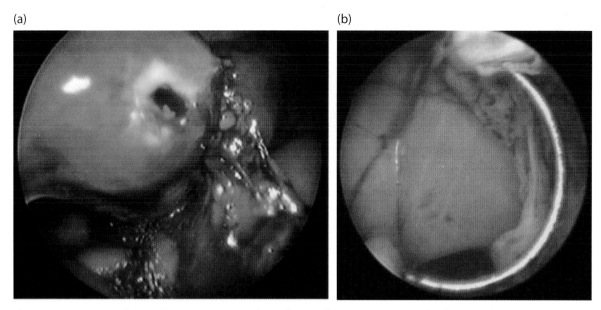

Figure 12.10 Uterine perforation. (a) Laparoscopic view after perforation. (b) Hysteroscopic view of perforation with the resectoscope with view on the peritoneum.

exclude an unidentified intestine lesion or a secondary necrosis (Figure 12.10).

In case of a mechanical perforation, a surgical approach is not necessary in most cases. Observation and perioperative antibiotic prophylaxis for prevention of inflammatory intra-abdominal processes is recommended. In case of longer postoperative pain, one should not make the mistake of attributing this to an ascending infection, using strictly conservative treatment. An intestine injury must be excluded by diagnostic laparoscopy.

To reduce the risk of perforation, the surgeon should start the surgery with a transvaginal ultrasound, measuring the myometrial thickness and checking the safety zone between the myoma border and the uterine serosa, which should be more than 5 mm. The endoscopic approach uses small instruments, allowing a vaginoscopic atraumatic entrance in the uterine cavity; further dilatation of the cervical canal can be achieved by forwarding the continuous-flow examination sheath under continuous supervision, reducing the risk of inadvertent perforation.

To avoid perforation during surgery, concomitant sonography is necessary. Preferentially, ultrasound is performed transabdominally, but intermittent transvaginal evaluation or concomitant transrectal exam are also used to make the risk calculation for a perforation [32–34].

As a surgical rule, one should only activate the electrode of the resectoscope when safe and sure orientation inside the uterine cavity is confirmed. In case of doubt, when the view is obscured by blood or by myometrial fragments, the operation should rather be abandoned and be repeated at a later date. The most vulnerable areas are the area of the tubal angle (the thinnest part of the uterus) and the fundus uteri.

12.4.1.2 Fluid Overload Syndrome

Intravasation of anionic fluid used to distend the uterine cavity in monopolar surgery is a very dangerous complication. Fluid absorption occurs through the open veins of the fibroid, the fallopian tubes and transperitoneally. Fluid overload may cause electrolyte imbalance and the patient may then suffer from nausea, vomiting, headache and confusion. In serious cases, pulmonary and brain oedema may occur [6]. Guidelines indicate that fluid intravasation of 750 mL during surgery requires planned termination of the operation and the intervention must immediately be stopped as soon as the balance exceeds 1,000 mL. Management of this risk relies on close monitoring of the fluid balance and interruption of the procedure before excessive fluid absorption occurs.

The use of normal saline combined with bipolar energy reduces the risk of hyponatraemia, but an excessive intravasation (>2,500 mL) still remains a risk and might cause cardiac overload [25–27].

During each hysteroscopy, distension fluid may get into the patient's circulation system via the lymphatic vessels and small uterine veins. The amount of the absorbed fluid depends on the intra-uterine pressure and the duration of the operation. Even with an intact endometrium, fluid is absorbed, not only with an operation and the opening of uterine veins. Let us, for example, remember the technique of hysterosalpingography, where with increased pressure application, we may immediately have a radiological picture of the pelvic venous system! With increased intravasal uptake of fluid, a hypotonic fluid overload may occur. In urology, this is known as transurethral resection of the prostate syndrome (TURP syndrome). In conscious patients, clinical signs are initially nausea, vomiting, dizziness, vision disorders and even reversible amaurosis followed by cramps, coma and death. The arterial and the central venous pressure rise. Bradycardia and arrhythmia occur. In the ECG, initial broadening of the QRS complex, followed by T-wave inversion, can be observed. The haematocrit, serum sodium and serum potassium values decrease. In serious cases, pulmonary or brain oedema can lead to a fatal ending.

The pathomechanism of the TURP syndrome works in two ways. Firstly, a relatively quick and excessive intake of fluid may lead to an acute cardiac decompensation with pulmonary oedema as a pure volume problem. Patients with cardiac disease have an increased risk. Secondly, the exuberant intake of electrolyte-free fluid starts a regulation mechanism inside the body, which may cause cerebral damage: due to the excess of free water, a hypotonic hyperhydration occurs. If the fluid is not eliminated quickly enough, the osmotic gradient, which has been formed between intracellular and intravascular compartment, leads to the passing of free fluid into the brain tissue because water passes the blood–brain barrier relatively fast. This can result in brain swelling with symptoms of crushing at the osseous skull. It is reckoned that this results from an increase of brain volume by about 5%. A volume increase of 10% is incompatible with life.

The overwhelming part of fluid intake happens directly via the uterine vascular and lymphatic system. The amount of fluid passing through the fallopian tubes is relatively small. Even in longer hysteroscopic operations, it must only be reckoned with a fluid

volume of about 50–100 mL. However, in the case of a uterine perforation, a larger volume may pass into the abdominal cavity at a relatively fast rate, where it can be absorbed secondarily via the peritoneum. This may lead to a delayed postoperative hypotonic hyperhydration. In these cases, the fluid should be emptied from the abdominal cavity under laparoscopic or sonographic control.

To avoid hyperhydration during the operation, the distension pressure should stay as low as possible and operation time should be kept as brief as possible. The distension pressure should stay between 90 and 120 mmHg. It does not make sense to reduce the distension pressure too much, as poor visual conditions only prolong the operation and increase the risk of uterine perforation. It is also important to ensure that, when using anionic distending fluids, the operation follows quickly after the diagnosis and that the phase of diagnosis and demonstration to other persons in the operating theatre is not prolonged unnecessarily.

Intraoperatively, the amount of intake and outflow has to be accounted for every 10–15 minutes. It is helpful to use a roller pump, especially designed for operative hysteroscopy, with an integrated fluid-balancing system. Another issue is the accountability of the non-measurable loss of rinsing fluids in the operation sheets and onto the floor under the operating table. It is important that all fluids flowing from the patient should be brought together in a container in order to account for the amount of outflow.

In case of a real loss account of 1,000 mL, serum sodium control should follow. In case of hyponatraemia or loss account of over 1,500 mL, the operation should be brought to an end as quickly as possible or should be abandoned. The individual situation of the patient has to be considered; an older patient with cardiac insufficiency can support less stress through volume than a younger, healthy patient.

In manifest hyperhydration, a urinary bladder permanent catheter must be placed. Diuresis should be stimulated with a fast-responding diuretic such as furosemide (Lasix) in a dose of 10–20 mg. This will be a sufficient treatment in most cases. In severe cases with sodium level below 120 mmol/L, a central venous catheter should be placed to control the central venous pressure and for the application of hypertonic electrolyte solutions. According to the amount of hyponatraemia, 20–40 mL of a 20–40% hypertonic saline solution should slowly be applied, while

119

simultaneously reducing the intake of other fluids. The hyponatraemia has to be balanced carefully and slowly. When sodium level reaches 130 mmol/L, further application should be stopped.

Severe cases of hyperhydration have to be treated in intensive care with diuretics, dopamine infusion and possible artificial ventilation.

In different studies, complication rates for fluid overload were reported in 0.14–6.0%.

The use of isotonic fluid in operative hysteroscopy is considered safer, as fluid absorption does not cause hyponatraemia. However, the exact volume of normal saline absorption that is safe is not known. In theory, this could be higher than hypotonic solutions [26].

However, even with normal saline, close vigilance to the fluid deficit is imperative as there are case series where large volumes of fluid have been absorbed, leading to excessive fluid overload and pulmonary oedema [42, 43].

The British and European Society for Gynaecological Endoscopy (BSGE/ESGE) safety guidelines recommend that a fluid deficit of more than 1,000 mL should be used as threshold to define fluid overload when using hypotonic solutions in healthy women of reproductive age.

A fluid deficit of 2,500 mL should be used as threshold to define fluid overload when using isotonic solutions in healthy women of reproductive age [27].

12.4.1.3 Bleeding

Major bleeding, occurring during a myoma resection, should be immediately dealt with by spot electrocoagulation. If coagulation fails to control the bleeding, the procedure may have to be abandoned and tamponade performed by inserting a Foley catheter and distending the balloon. Also, vasoconstrictive drugs can be administered to support the compression treatment. In case of heavy uterine bleeding, an intracervical injection of 10 mL Ornipressin solution (1 ampule a 2.5 I.E. diluted in 50 mL sodium solution) can be helpful. Strict care must be taken that the injection is applied extravascularly, as in the case of an intravascular injection, severe complications in the form of hypertonic crises may occur. Furthermore, bleeding can be reduced by oxytocin, secale alkaloids (Methergine) or prostaglandins (e.g. Sulpostron as a synthetic derivate) to incite a contraction of the uterus. Apart from this treatment, local gauze tampons drenched in Ornipressin or Sulpostron or a

Foley catheter blocked with 30–40 mL of fluid may be put into the uterine cavity in case of heavy postoperative bleeding.

The catheter should be left in situ for a few hours, after which the bleeding nearly always stops. Sometimes, these simple measures fail to control haemorrhage. This may occur if resection has been carried out too deep into the myometrium and a plexus of vessels has opened. In this case, other measurements, such as laparoscopy or embolization, may be necessary.

Heavy bleeding after removing the resectoscope can be caused by frequent in and out movement of the 26 Fr. resectoscope, causing laceration of the uterine arterial branch. To identify the site of bleeding and to control an immediate compression of the descending branch, the placement of a paracervical clamp at 3 or 9 hours can be performed. If bleeding continues after removal of the clamp, a 2-0 vicryl haemostatic suture is to be placed. Severe bleeding was reported in different studies in 0–3.6% of cases.

12.4.1.4 Burns through Use of Monopolar Current

With use of the monopolar resectoscope, specific complications are reportedly attributed to heat damage because of suspected current density concentration at uncontrollable regions far from the operating area. During recent years, many improvements have been developed in high-frequency technology. Through introduction of modern generators with automatic voltage control, a minimization of energy output has become possible. The experience has shown that the output of these appliances in operative hysteroscopy was between 30 and 60 W where these systems were used. As yet, it is not quite clear how to evaluate the usage of electrosurgical vaporization electrodes in the long run. Here, much higher voltages are used than in conventional operative hysteroscopy.

Through introduction of warning systems, other potential sources of disturbance may also be excluded. As in each medical use of monopolar current, special care has to be taken that the return plate is correctly applied near the operating area, preferably on the patient's thigh. The return plate has to have broad and tight skin contact and has to lie with the longer edge at a right angle to the expected current flow and must thus be glued diagonally and not longitudinally on to the thigh. A connection between the body and the conducting and grounded parts at and next to the operating table is to be avoided. Modern high-frequency generators help to avoid these complications by safety systems with automatic control of input and output and the registration of current leakage. Therefore, they are preferable in modern electrosurgery.

12.4.1.5 Air Embolism

Operative hysteroscopy is, as a rule, conducted in fluid distension media.

However, the occurrence of an embolism is possible by introducing air through the pump system by repeated introduction of the resectoscope with introduction or aspiration of air and through major production of bubbles during bipolar surgery.

To avoid the first situation, care must be taken at the beginning of each operative hysteroscopy to make sure that the tube system is completely filled with fluid before the hysteroscope is introduced into the uterus. Furthermore, no systems are to be used that allow an intraoperative inflow of air. The pneumatic compression of the distending fluids, as used in some types of laparoscopic fluid pumps, may not be applied for hysteroscopy, because the compressing air can get into the system relatively quickly when the fluid storage is being emptied. Systems of this kind have been available for some time and have already led to at least one documented case of death. The pump should be immediately turned off when the ingoing fluid bag is being emptied, so that the remaining air from the bag – even if it is only a small amount – is not forced into the uterus. Likewise, the pump system must be turned off while the infusion bag is being changed in order to ensure that no air gets into the tube system.

The second situation is possible in operations that are connected with repeated introduction and removal of the resectoscope; it is particularly worth mentioning the hysteroscopic myoma resection as well as the endometrium resection. To avoid this complication, intraoperative removal of fragments should be carried out using the vaginoscopic approach with the vagina filled with fluid. The use of speculum and tenaculum can create an increased risk of aspiration of room air due to a negative pressure gradient in the uterine veins during systole, while the resectoscope is being removed. Especially a head-down Trendelenburg position, with exposed opened cervix, should be avoided. When the scope is reintroducing, the fluid inflow and outflow tap should be open so that pressure in the uterine cavity does not increase suddenly and intracavitary air can escape via the outflow sheath.

Bipolar surgery can produce a major amount of air bubbles during surgery, which, if not aspirated correctly, can enter into the venous system and cause the same symptoms as a room air embolism.

An air embolism can be recognized first of all by a decrease of end-expiratory CO_2 saturation. This is caused by the decreasing perfusion of the lung as a result of air bubble formation in the right heart, which leads to ineffective contractions with the air bubble wobbling to and fro. Modern anaesthetic instruments conduct a continuous measurement of end-expiratory CO_2. During the course of an endoscopic operation, the anaesthesiologist has to react carefully in case of a CO_2-decrease. In the precordial region, a certain characteristic 'mill-wheel' murmur may be auscultated, which is caused by the contractions of the heart with the moving intracardial air bubble. Initially, tachycardia occurs, which may be followed by bradycardia up to an asystole. In case of an open foramen ovale or a septum defect, together with the air-caused occlusion of the outflow into the right heart chamber, passing of air into the left side of the heart may occur, causing arterial air embolisms, which can affect the brain.

In this case, the operation must be abandoned at once. The cervix should be closed to avoid further intake of air, i.e. by inserting a Hegar's dilator, and the vagina should be closed, maybe accompanied by a vaginal tamponade. Specula are to be removed. The patient should be brought to a right lateral position, so that the air bubble, following gravity, can be respirated via the pulmonary vessels into the lung. In very severe cases, there should be no hesitation in trying to remove the air from the heart chambers by intracardial puncture.

The occurrence of a fulminant air embolism is extremely rare, but each case is a complication that is very difficult to treat as the operating physicians must recognize the reason for it in a very short time, which should be followed by immediate, adequate therapeutic measures. Due to misinterpretation of the unexpected situation, deaths happen quite often through air embolisms. As the expiratory CO_2 decrease is mostly the first recognizable symptom, an intraoperative capnography should be standard in the course of operative hysteroscopies.

121

12.4.2 Postoperative Complications

12.4.2.1 Haemorrhage

Haemorrhage after hysteroscopic operations is extremely rare. After hysteroscopic myoma resection, the postoperative vaginal bleeding can last about 2–5 days. On the first day, it is heavier than period bleeding, then it adapts to period bleeding and ends in light spotting. As a rule, this bleeding is not painful. If the patient suffers from pain, an examination must be conducted and a postoperative infection should be excluded with the usual laboratory tests.

In isolated cases, heavier postoperative bleeding may occur, demanding a secondary intervention. Patients with acquired or therapeutic blood coagulation changes are more endangered than others. In case of heavy postoperative bleeding, the same measures can be taken as in intraoperative bleeding. A control of the blood clotting physiological parameter is strongly advised in order to be able to recognize the occurrence of a consumption coagulopathy in time during the course of heavy bleeding. Then it can be adequately treated with fresh plasma preparations or the exchange of coagulation factors.

Patients receiving warfarin treatment are often candidates for a hysteroscopic endometrial ablation as an alternative to hysterectomy. It is advisable to conduct the endometrial ablation only when a quick account of over 50% has been reached after ending the coumarin therapy. To avoid vein thrombosis, the patients should, as an alternative to coumarin treatment, be heparinized.

12.4.2.2 Infection

Post-hysteroscopic endometritis occurs in 1–5% of cases. Main risk factors are history of pelvic inflammatory disease, long operative procedure, repeated insertion and removal of hysteroscope through cervix and tissue fragments left in the uterus. Although prophylactic antibiotics have not been demonstrated to reduce the incidence of postoperative infection, a prophylactic antibiotic injection intraoperatively is often recommended.

12.4.3 Late Complications

12.4.3.1 Postoperative Intrauterine Adhesions (IUA)

The incidence of postoperative IUAs represents the major long-term complication of hysteroscopic myomectomy, ranging from 1% to 13% (14). Electrosurgical damage to the subendometrial myometrial layer should be avoided. Extensive coagulation, especially using monopolar current, results in major thermal damage, which can heal with major adhesion formation. The cold dissection of the intramural part of the myoma with pinpoint coagulation of the vessels must be recommended to avoid adhesion formation [16].

Especially with multiple myoma treatment, complete resection and minimal thermal damage to the myometrium is mandatory in order to prevent adhesion formation. Concomitant adenomyosis puts the patient at a higher risk for adhesion formation. In those cases, it is not recommended to treat opposite myomas in the same session.

Early second-look hysteroscopy, after any hysteroscopic surgery, is another effective preventive and therapeutic strategy. Several pharmacologic agents (conjugated oestrogen, levonorgestrel-releasing intrauterine devices) and barrier agents – including Foley catheter, hyaluronic acid gel and carboxymethylcellulose – have been used to reduce IUA development. The application of an adhesion barrier following surgery that may lead to endometrial damage significantly reduces the development of IUAs in the short term, although limited fertility data are available following this intervention [25, 29, 44].

12.4.3.2 Uterine Rupture during Pregnancy

Operations on the uterus that affect the wall structure may lead to a uterine rupture during a later pregnancy. This has been known for operations such as caesarean section, myoma enucleation, metroplasties or cone excision from the uterine wall in case of tubal pregnancy. In some cases, there have been reports of uterine ruptures after hysteroscopic operations as well. This concerns mostly operative hysteroscopies, where an intraoperative uterine perforation has occurred. Furthermore, there have been reports of uterine ruptures in rare cases after hysteroscopic septum division, especially when laser systems were used. In these cases, the pathomechanism may possibly be seen in a coagulation necrosis of the uterine wall without perforation up to the serosa.

In case of a uterine perforation during an operative hysteroscopy, the patient should be advised as to the higher risk in a later pregnancy. This risk should also be taken into consideration during the care of delivery. In case of obvious uterine lesions and the wish for later pregnancy, prophylactic suture care may be considered, even if there is no necessity with respect to bleeding.

12.4.3.3 Placenta Accreta

Operations connected with local endometrium denudation may lead to the formation of a placenta accreta or increta in pregnancy. After hysteroscopic septum dissection, a higher rate of this condition has been seen. The same may be possible for hysteroscopic myoma enucleation. A prophylaxis is not known. The risk should be known to the physician taking care of the delivery [45, 46].

12.5 Conclusion

Hysteroscopic myomectomy is a first-line treatment for intrauterine myomas which are the cause of abnormal uterine bleeding and infertility problems.

Limitations for the hysteroscopic approach are size and location of the pathology, but the recent evolution in technique and instrumentation provides the opportunity to deal with most of the symptomatic myomas in a patient-friendly, safe and efficient way.

References

1. Brölmann H, Tanos V, Grimbizis G, et al. On behalf of the European Society of Gynaecological Endoscopy (ESGE) steering committee on fibroid morcellation. Options on fibroid morcellation: a literature review. *Gynecol Surg* 2015;**12**:3–15.

2. Paul PG, Rengaraj V, Das T, et al. Uterine sarcomas in patients undergoing surgery for presumed leiomyomas: 10 years' experience. *J Minim Invasive Gynecol* 2016 Mar–Apr;**23** (3):384–9.

3. Dueholm M, Lundorf E, Sørensen JS, et al. Reproducibility of evaluation of the uterus by transvaginal sonography, hysterosonographic examination, hysteroscopy and magnetic resonance imaging. *Hum Reprod* 2002;**17**(1):195–200.

4. Neuwirth RS, Amin HK. Excision of submucus fibroids with hysteroscopic control. *Am J Obstet Gynecol* 1976;**126**:95–99.

5. Munro MG, Critchley HO, Broder MS, Fraser IS. FIGO classification system (PALM-COEIN) for causes of abnormal uterine bleeding in non-gravid women of reproductive age. *Int J Gynaecol Obstet* 2011;**113**:3–13.

6. Wamsteker K, Emanuel MH, de Kruif JH. Transcervical hysteroscopic resection of submucous fibroids for abnormal uterine bleeding: results regarding the degree of intramural extension. *Obstet Gynecol* 1993;**82**:736–40.

7. Molinas CR, Campo R. Office hysteroscopy and adenomyosis. *Best Pract Res Clin Obstet Gynaecol* 2006;**20**: 557–67.

8. Campo R, Meier R, Dhont N, Mestdagh G, Ombelet W. Implementation of hysteroscopy in an infertility clinic: The one-stop uterine diagnosis and treatment. *Facts Views Vis Obgyn* 2014;**6**(4):235–9.

9. Campo R, Van Belle Y, Rombauts L, et al. Office minihysteroscopy. *Hum Reprod Update* 1999;**5**(1) 73–81.

10. Campo R, Molinas CR, Rombauts L, et al. Prospective multicentre randomized controlled trial to evaluate factors influencing the success rate of office diagnostic hysteroscopy. *Hum Reprod* 2005;**20**:258–63.

11. El-Toukhy T, Campo R, Khalaf Y, et al. Hysteroscopy in recurrent in-vitro fertilisation failure (TROPHY): a multicentre, randomised controlled trial. *Lancet* 2016;387(10038): 2614–21.

12. Li J-J, Chung JPW, Wang S, Li T-C, Duan H. The investigation and management of adenomyosis in women who wish to improve or preserve fertility. *Biomed Res International* 2018;art ID 6832685:12 pages.

13. Gordts S, Grimbizis G, Campo R. Symptoms and classifications of uterine adenomyosis, including the place of hysteroscopy in diagnosis. *Fertil Steril* 2018;109:380–8.

14. Rotenberg L, Verhille R, Schulz-Wendtland R, et al. Multicenter clinical experience with large core soft tissue biopsy without vacuum assistance. *Eur J Cancer Prev* 2004 Dec;13(6): 491–8.

15. Janssens JP, Rotenberg L, Sentis M, Motmans K, Schulz-Wendtland R. Caution with microbiopsies of the breast: displaced cancer cells and ballistics. *Eur J Cancer Prev* 2006 Dec;15(6):471–3.

16. Emanuel MH, Hart A, Wamsteker K, Lammes F. An analysis of fluid loss during transcervical resection of submucous myomas. *Fertil Steril* 1997 Nov;68 (5):881–6.

17. Muzji L, Boni T, Bellati F, et al. GnRH analogue treatment before hysteroscopic resection of submucous myomas: a prospective, randomized, multicenter study. *Fertil Steril* 2010 Sep;94(4):1496–9.

18. Zayed M, Fouda UM, Zayed SM, Elsetohy KA, Hashem AT. Hysteroscopic myomectomy of large submucous myomas in a 1-step procedure using multiple slicing sessions technique. *J Minim Invasive Gynecol* 2015 Nov–Dec;22 (7):1196–202.

19. Ferrero S, Racca A, Tafi E, et al. Ulipristal acetate before high complexity hysteroscopic

myomectomy: a retrospective comparative study. *J Minim Invasive Gynecol* 2016 Mar–Apr;23(3):390–5.

20. Bigatti G. The shaver technique for operative hysteroscopy. In: Tinelli A, Alonso Pacheco L, Haimovich S, editors. *Hysteroscopy.* Cham: Springer; 2018: 635–648.

21. Sancho JM, Delgado VS, Valero MJ, et al. Hysteroscopic myomectomy outcomes after 3-month treatment with either Ulipristal Acetate or GnRH analogues: a retrospective comparative study. *Eur J Obstet Gynecol Reprod Biol* 2016 Mar;198:127–30.

22. Rakotomahenina H, Rajaonarison J, Wong L, Brun JL. Myomectomy: technique and current indications. *Minerva Ginecol* 2017 Aug;69 (4):357–69. doi: 10.23736/S0026-4784.17.04073-4. Epub 26 Apr 2017.

23. Mazzon I, Bettocchi S, Fascilla F, et al. Resectoscopic myomectomy. *Minerva Ginecol* 2016 Jun;68 (3):334–44.

24. Mazzon I, Favilli A, Grasso M, et al. Predicting success of single step hysteroscopic myomectomy: a single centre large cohort study of single myomas *Int J Surg* 2015 Oct;22:10–14.

25. AAGL. Practice report: practical guidelines for the management of hysteroscopic distension media. *J Minim Invasive Gynecol* 2013;20:137–48.

26. Istre O. Managing bleeding, fluid absorption and uterine perforation at hysteroscopy. *Best Pract Res Clin Obstet Gynaecol* 2009;23(5):619–29.

27. Umranikar S, Clark TJ, Saridogan E, et al. BSGE/ESGE guideline on management of fluid distension media in operative hysteroscopy. *Gynecol Surg* 2016;13(4):289–303.

28. Litta P, Leggieri C, Conte L, et al. Monopolar versus bipolar device:

safety, feasibility, limits and perioperative complications in performing hysteroscopic myomectomy. *Clin Exp Obstet Gynecol* 2014;41(3):335–8.

29. Mazzon I, Favilli A. Does cold loop hysteroscopic myomectomuy reduce intrauterine adhesions? a retrospective study. *Fertil Steril* 2014;101:294–8.

30. Di Spiezio Sardo A, Calagna G, Di Carlo C, et al. Cold loops applied to bipolar resectoscope: a safe "one-step" myomectomy for treatment of submucosal myomas with intramural development. *J Obstet Gynaecol Res* 2015 Dec;41 (12):1935–41.

31. Mazzon I, Favilli A, Grasso M, et al. Is cold loop hysteroscopic myomectomy a safe and effective technique for the treatment of submucous myomas with intramural development? a series of 1434 surgical procedures. *J Minim Invasive Gynecol* 2015 Jul–Aug;22(5):792–8.

32. Korkmazer E, Tekin B, Solak N. Ultrasound guidance during hysteroscopic myomectomy in G1 and G2 Submucous Myomas: for a safer one step surgery. *Eur J Obstet Gynecol Reprod Biol* 2016 Aug;203:108–11. doi: 10.1016/j.ejogrb.2016.03.043. Epub 17 May 2016.

33. Wortman M. Sonographically guided hysteroscopic myomectomy (SGHM): minimizing the risks and maximizing efficiency. *Surg Technol Int* 2013 Sep;23: 181–9.

34. Ludwin A, Ludwin I, Pityński K, et al. Transrectal ultrasound-guided hysteroscopic myomectomy of submucosal myomas with a varying degree of myometrial penetration. *J Minim Invasive Gynecol* 2013 Sep–Oct;20 (5):672–85.

35. Bigatti G. BS® Integrated Bigatti Shaver, an alternative approach to operative hysteroscopy.

Gynecol Surg 2011 May;8 (2):187–91.

36. Bigatti G, Ferrario C, Rosales M, Baglioni A, Bianchi S. A 4-cm G2 cervical submucosal myoma removed with the IBS® Integrated Bigatti Shaver. *Gynecol Surg* 2012 Nov;9(4):453–6. Epub 3 Mar 2012.

37. Bigatti G, Franchetti S, Rosales M, Baglioni A, Bianchi S. Hysteroscopic myomectomy with the IBS® Integrated Bigatti Shaver versus conventional bipolar resectoscope: a retrospective comparative study. *Gynecol Surg* 2014 Feb; 11(1):9–18.

38. Vitale SG, Sapia F, Rapisarda AMC, et al. Hysteroscopic morcellation of submucous myomas: a systematic review. *Biomed Res Int* 2017;2017:6848250. Published online 29 Aug 2017.

39. Cohen S, Greenberg JA. Hysteroscopic morcellation for treating intrauterine pathology. *Rev Obstet Gynecol* 2011 Summer;4(2):73–80.

40. Cicinelli E, Mitsopoulos V, Fascilla FD, Sioutis D, Bettocchi S. The OPPIuM technique: office hysteroscopic technique for the preparation of partially intramural leiomyomas. *Minerva Ginecol* 2016 Jun;68 (3):328–33.

41. Haimovich S, Mancebo G, Alameda F, et al. Feasibility of a new two-step procedure for office hysteroscopic resection of submucous myomas: results of a pilot study. *Eur J Obstet Gynecol Reprod Biol* 2013 Jun;168 (2):191–4.

42. Grove JJ, Shinaman RC, Drover DR. Noncardiogenic pulmonary edema and venous air embolus as complications of operative hysteroscopy. *J Clin Anesth* 2004 Feb;16(1):48–50.

43. Van Kruchten PM, Vermelis JM, Herold I, Van Zundert AA. Hypotonic and isotonic fluid overload as a complication of

hysteroscopic procedures: two case reports. *Minerva Anestesiol* 2010 May;76(5): 373–7.

44. Wheeler JM, Taskin O. Second-look office hysteroscopy following resectoscopy: the frequency and

management of intrauterine adhesions. *Fertil Steril* 1993;60:150–6.

45. Tanaka M, Matsuzaki S, Matsuzaki S, et al. Placenta accreta following hysteroscopic

myomectomy. *Clin Case Rep* 2016 Apr 20;4(6):541–4.

46. Mathiesen E, Hohenwalter M, Basir Z, Peterson E. Placenta increta after hysteroscopic myomectomy. *Obstet Gynecol* 2013 Aug;122(2 Pt 2):478–81.

Chapter 13

Modern Management of Intramural Myomas

Dan Yu, Tin-Chiu Li and Enlan Xia

13.1 Intramural Myomas and Fertility

Intramural myomas, the most common type of uterine leiomyoma, develop within the uterine wall and expand either inwards or outwards. According to the FIGO [1] leiomyoma classification system, fibroid types range from 0 to 8. Types 0, 1 and 2 are submucosal myomas, and subserosal myomas refer to type 5 to 7. Both type 3 and type 4 myomas are known as intramural myomas with no involvement of the endometrial cavity (Figure 13.1). The type 3 myomas, which are in the uterine wall but in contact with the endometrium, are more likely to distort the cavity under certain stimulations. Type 4 myomas stay entirely within the myometrium, which does not expand to either the endometrium or the serosa.

It is generally accepted that intramural myomas may be associated with reproductive disorders such as infertility, miscarriage and other adverse pregnancy outcomes. Large intramural myomas (i.e. >5 cm) or intramural myomas distorting the uterine cavity appear to have more adverse impact on fertility. Oliveira et al. [2] evaluated 245 IVF-ICSI patients with uterine myomas and found that patients with intramural myomas more than 4 cm had lower pregnancy

rates than those with smaller myomas. In two other studies, it was found that larger myomas (i.e. >5 cm) had a greater impact on the risk of pregnancy loss as compared to smaller myomas [3, 4]. Furthermore, Sudik et al. [5] noted that women who have myomas of more than 8 cm are more likely to conceive after myomectomy than those with smaller ones. A recent review article concluded that deeply infiltrating intramural myomas which distorted the endometrial cavity negatively affected fertility and so should be removed [6].

However, the impact of smaller intramural myomas on fertility, especially those without endometrial cavity distortion, is still a subject of controversy. There were many observational studies involving assisted conception cycles in which the outcomes in women with myomas were compared to those without (controls). Among published meta-analyses of these studies, three failed to confirm significant adverse impact of intramural myomas on IVF outcome, whereas five concluded significant negative impact [7–14].

The possible mechanisms whereby intramural myomas produce adverse effects on reproduction include cornual occlusion if the intramural myoma is adjacent to the intramural tubal segment [15], altered myometrial contractility, disruption of normal blood supply [16], endometrial inflammation, thinning and atrophy [17], alterations in gene expression [18], as well as adverse effects on gamete migration [19, 20].

13.2 Management of Intramural Myomas

The indication for myomectomy is different for submucosal and intramural myomas. However, the distinction between these two types of myoma is not always so clear-cut. From time to time, ultrasonography or office hysteroscopy may show non-distortion

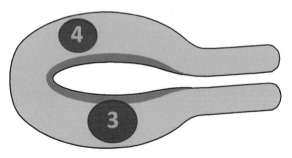

Figure 13.1 Types of intramural myomas according to FIGO classification of uterine myomas published by Munro et al. [1]. Type 3 – the intramural myoma in contact with the endometrium; type 4 – the intramural myoma without the involvement of either the endometrium or the serosa.

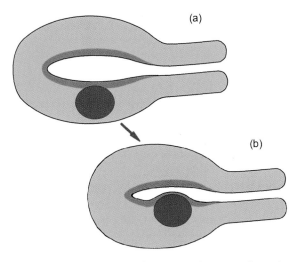

Figure 13.2 The relationship of an intramural myoma to the uterine cavity may change when the uterus contracts, possibly leading to the distortion of the uterine cavity. (a) An intramural myoma stays completely within the myometrial layer, not distorting the uterine cavity; (b) the same intramural myoma protrudes into the cavity when the uterus contracts.

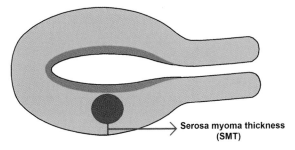

Figure 13.3 Serosa myoma thickness (SMT) – the minimal thickness between the outer margin of the myoma and the serosa.

of the uterine cavity by a myoma in the dormant state, but when the uterus contracts, a type 3 intramural myoma may protrude into and distort the endometrial cavity (Figure 13.2). In this case, the intramural myoma should also be treated as a submucosal myoma and be removed, especially if it is associated with unexplained infertility, recurrent pregnancy loss, mid-trimester loss or other obstetric complications which could be attributed to the myoma.

It is accepted that hysteroscopic surgery is suitable for removal of submucosal myomas including types 0, 1 and 2. As the technique of operative hysteroscopy becomes more advanced, intramural myomas which do not reach and distort the uterine cavity may also be suitable for hysteroscopic myomectomy with a shorter healing time compared with laparoscopic myomectomy. Shen et al. [21] used Doppler ultrasonography to observe the healing of the myometrium after myomectomy and found that the hysteroscopic group had a significantly higher proportion with complete healing at 1, 3 and 6 months post-operation. They found that 88.4% (160/181) of women in the hysteroscopic group achieved complete muscular healing 3 months after the operation, and all cases in the hysteroscopic group achieved complete healing in 6 months; whereas in the laparoscopic group, only 95.2% (320/336) achieved complete healing at 6 months.

In our centre, hysteroscopic myomectomy is considered for intramural myoma if the distance between the endometrium and the myoma is less than 5 mm and the myoma is less than 4 cm in diameter.

In hysteroscopic resection of an intramural myoma (or submucosal myoma with significant intramural involvement), it is useful to determine the 'serosa myoma thickness' (SMT) or 'myometrial free margin', which is measured by ultrasonography and represents the minimal thickness between the outer margin of the myoma and the serosa (Figure 13.3). A minimum thickness of 5 mm is advisable to reduce the risk of uterine perforation during hysteroscopic myomectomy. However, some studies suggested that, during hysteroscopic resection of an intramural myoma, the SMT often increased progressively during the procedure, thereby increasing the safety margin of the resection [22–24]. In the prospective observational study by Casadio et al. [22], the median myometrial free margin increased from 3.9 mm at the beginning of the hysteroscopic surgery to 12.7 mm after the removal of the myoma.

In our centre [25], we have performed 18 cases of hysteroscopic resection of intramural myomas with SMT less than 5 mm under ultrasonographic guidance along with the use of several manoeuvres to promote uterine contractions, including 'water massage', mechanical stimulation with either the cutting loop or the tip of the scope, vacuum aspiration and intravenous oxytocin injection. The mean SMT was 3 mm at the beginning of the operation, which increased to 9 mm at the end of the operation. There was only one incidence of uterine perforation.

Shen et al. [21] carried out a retrospective study to compare the outcome of hysteroscopic myomectomy with laparoscopic myomectomy in women with intramural myoma. Pregnancy occurred significantly earlier in the hysteroscopic group compared with the laparoscopic group; in addition, miscarriage rate in the hysteroscopic group was significantly less than that in the laparoscopic group.

However, hysteroscopic resection of an intramural myoma remains a challenge. We describe below our experience at the Fuxing Hospital of the preoperative protocol, intraoperative techniques and post-operative management of hysteroscopic resection of intramural myomas [26].

13.2.1 Preoperative Assessment and Medication

13.2.1.1 Preoperative Assessment

Pelvic ultrasonography is an essential investigation prior to hysteroscopic resection of intramural fibroids. If the uterus is less than 12 weeks gestational size, transvaginal ultrasonography is preferred to transabdominal ultrasonography. If the uterus is more than 12 weeks gestational size, transabdominal ultrasonography may be more appropriate, but in the presence of significant uterine enlargement, hysteroscopic surgery may not be feasible. Three-dimensional ultrasonography, especially when combined with saline infusion sonography (SIS), is particularly useful to map out the exact location, size and number of the myomas. Not every intramural myoma needs to be removed. In the presence of multiple intramural myomas, the decision regarding which one should be removed or which one to leave undisturbed should be made prior to the operation based on detailed myoma mapping and informed discussion. Magnetic resonance imaging (MRI) may occasionally be required in situations when the margin of the myoma is not so well defined, raising the possibility of an alternative diagnosis such as adenomyoma. In any case, the two most important pieces of information are the minimal thickness between the endometrium and the myoma, and the serosa myoma thickness (SMT).

13.2.1.2 Preoperative Medication

Routine GnRH analogue (GnRHa) treatment is not necessary but it should be considered if the intramural myoma is more than 3 cm in diameter. A 3-month course of treatment may produce a number of advantages. Firstly, the treatment produces shrinkage in size of the myoma, thereby shortening the resection procedure. Secondly, the reduction in vascularity may help to reduce bleeding during operation. Thirdly, it may sometimes lead to the protrusion of the intramural myoma into the uterine cavity because the reduction of uterine volume may be greater than that of the myoma. In addition, the amenorrhoea induced by GnRHa may also help to improve the anaemia.

13.2.2 Operative Techniques

13.2.2.1 Locating the Myoma

By definition, the intramural fibroid to be resected does not normally protrude into the uterine cavity, and so it must be precisely located before the operation. Overdistension of the uterine cavity makes it more difficult to identify the location of the myoma and so should be avoided. Whilst the usual perfusing pressure for hysteroscopic surgery is set at 90–100 mmHg, it may be helpful in the beginning to use a lower pressure, say 40 mmHg, to facilitate the protrusion of the myoma into the cavity and identification under lower pressure.

13.2.2.2 Inducing Uterine Contractions

A number of strategies may be employed to stimulate uterine muscles to contract, which would help not only to reduce intraoperative bleeding but also the extrusion of the myoma into the uterine cavity. Several pharmacological agents such as misoprostol, oxytocin or vasopressin may be administered during the operation. Vasopressin, a potent vasoconstrictor, is particularly effective; it can be injected into the fundus of the uterus under direct vision at the beginning of the hysteroscopic procedure by using an oocyte retrieval needle. Uterine contractions may also be induced with a number of mechanical means including the application of vacuum aspiration, hydraulic uterine massage by rapidly alternating the intrauterine pressure, manual uterine massage and repeatedly stoking the uterine wall with the cutting loop or the beak of the scope. Repeated mechanical pushes on the myoma tissue with the cutting loop may also help to separate the myoma away from the myometrial tissue (Figure 13.4).

13.2.2.3 Ultrasound Guidance

Ultrasound guidance is essential in hysteroscopic resection of intramural myomas. It provides information on the proximity of the intramural myoma to both the endometrium and the serosa (Figure 13.5). Moreover, during the procedure, the changes in

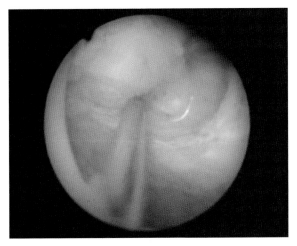

Figure 13.4 After the myometrium covering the intramural myoma was incised, the myoma was seen being pushed mechanically away from the myometrium with the use of the cutting loop.

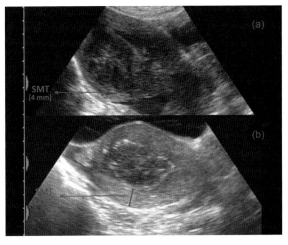

Figure 13.6 Changes of SMT as measured by ultrasonography as the operation proceeded. (a) SMT was 4 mm before the operation; (b) SMT had increased to 12 mm in the middle of the operation.

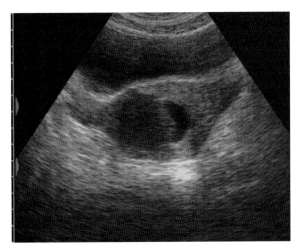

Figure 13.5 A transverse ultrasonographic view of the uterus after fluid medium was introduced into the uterine cavity at the beginning of the hysteroscopic operation. A myoma in the right uterine wall was seen protruding into the cavity.

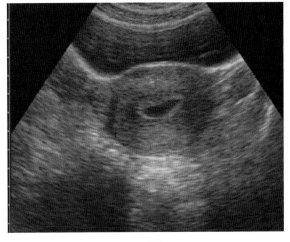

Figure 13.7 At the end of hysteroscopic myomectomy, ultrasonography showed normal appearance of the endometrial cavity.

myometrial thickness between the myoma and the serosa (SMT), which may become thicker when the uterus contracts, can be serially measured (Figure 13.6). At the end of the operation, the shape of the endometrial cavity and the integrity of the uterine wall can be determined (Figure 13.7).

13.2.2.4 Laparoscopic Guidance

Nowadays, ultrasound guidance has largely replaced laparoscopic guidance during hysteroscopic resection of intramural myomas, as the former method is more informative and more effective in preventing perforation.

13.2.3 Surgical Steps

In the Hysteroscopy Centre of Fuxing Hospital, we advocate the use of the following steps in sequence for the removal of myomas, namely: locating the myoma, opening the window, cutting, clamping, twisting, pulling and extraction. Cutting is the first step of the procedure.

The exact location is best ascertained by a combination of ultrasonographic examination and inspection of the uterine cavity with the resectoscope, which may sometimes reveal important clues such as a different degree of vascularization pattern of the endometrium beneath the myoma. If the location is not immediately apparent, a number of manoeuvres may be used, including decreasing the intrauterine perfusing pressure, scrapping the endometrium or applying vacuum aspiration which can stimulate the uterus to contract, making the myoma more easily identified (Figures 13.8 and 13.9) The latter manoeuvre is particularly useful if the endometrium is thickened.

Once the exact location of the myoma is ascertained, a longitudinal incision of endometrium and myometrium above the myoma is made with a hysteroscopic cutting loop or cutting needle. The incision can be repeated until the myoma is visible via the hysteroscope (Figures 13.10 and 13.11). This step is called 'opening the window'.

At this stage, vasoconstrictors such as vasopressin can be administered into the uterus via an oocyte retrieval needle, which will cause the uterus to contract, pushing the myoma via the window already created. The protrusion process may be facilitated

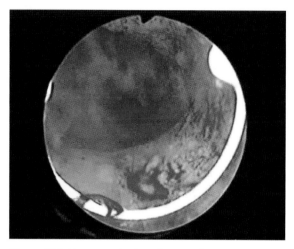

Figure 13.8 Hysteroscopic view of a normal cavity in a woman with an intramural myoma in the posterior wall.

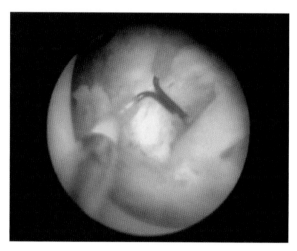

Figure 13.10 The myometrium covering a left posterior wall intramural myoma was being incised by a cutting needle.

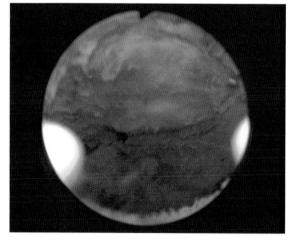

Figure 13.9 Hysteroscopic view of the uterine cavity after vacuum aspiration. An anterior wall intramural myoma was seen protruding into the cavity.

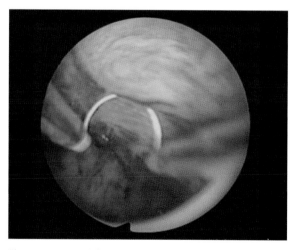

Figure 13.11 A left anterior intramural myoma is visualized after the myometrium covering it was incised by a cutting loop.

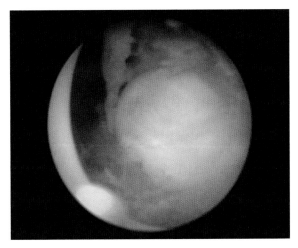

Figure 13.12 After the myometrium covering the myoma had been incised by a cutting needle, the intramural myoma in the left posterior wall could now be seen protruding into the cavity.

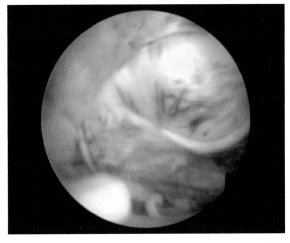

Figure 13.13 After a small submucosal myoma (not shown) had been resected, the underneath intramural myoma was seen protruding into the cavity.

by maintaining a low fluid perfusing pressure at this stage (Figure 13.12).

As the intramural myoma begins to protrude into the cavity, the intracavity component of the myoma should be resected. Meanwhile, the capsule of the fibroid should be identified to avoid resecting into the myometrial tissue. As the resection progresses, frequent mechanical pushes of the myoma or repeated withdrawal and reinsertion of the scope will continue to stimulate the uterus to contract, helping to push the myoma further into the cavity.

Sometimes, it may be possible to deliberately resect only the sidewalls of the myoma, while preserving the central portion, with the aim of converting the spherical myoma into a mushroom-shaped structure with a thick central stalk. In this way, it is possible to speed up the complete removal of the entire myoma by applying a pair of curved grasping forceps to grasp firmly on the thick stalk, followed by twisting either clockwise or anticlockwise, whilst applying a pulling force to loosen and detach the myoma from the surrounding myometrium tissue. With a combination of these manoeuvres, the myoma will descend gradually and be extracted out through the cervix. The steps could be applied repeatedly so that a large myoma can be removed in stages.

From time to time, in women with multiple myomas, following the removal of a submucosal myoma, the intramural myoma underneath it will be exposed to the cavity, leading to intracavity protrusion, especially if the uterus is stimulated to contract. In such a case, the hitherto intramural myoma should be removed (Figure 13.13).

In certain circumstances, the deeply situated intramural myoma which is close to the serosal margin does not protrude towards the cavity or change its location after various manoeuvres to stimulate the uterus. Complete removal of this type of intramural myoma may not be safely performed without a significant risk of perforation. Therefore, partial removal of this type of intramural myoma or just resecting the myometrium covering the myoma (opening the window) should be conducted. Three different outcomes of hysteroscopic resection of intramural myomas are illustrated in Figure 13.14.

At the end of the operation, both the uterine wall and uterus should be checked carefully by combined hysteroscopy and ultrasonography. The endometrial cavity should be normal in shape, and the outer uterine wall should remain intact. Sometimes, a hollow at the original site of the myoma in the uterine wall may be visible (Figure 13.15), but the size should decrease if the perfusing pressure is reduced. Any active bleeding observed should be stopped. If necessary, a Foley balloon catheter can be inserted into the cavity with the balloon inflated for several hours.

13.2.4 Postoperative Management

In all cases, a pelvic ultrasonography should be performed 4–6 weeks after the operation to ascertain if there is any residual fibroid left. It is not necessary to

Type 3 intramural myoma **Type 4 intramural myoma**

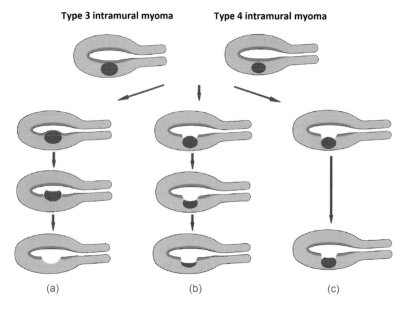

(a)   (b)   (c)

Figure 13.14 An illustration of the three different outcomes of hysteroscopic resection of intramural myomas. (a) Complete removal of an intramural myoma (possible because of myoma protrusion into the uterine cavity in response to uterine contractions); (b) partial removal of an intramural myoma with a remnant in the uterine wall; (c) after resecting the myometrium covering the myoma (opening the window), the myoma stays deep in the uterine wall, making it difficult to proceed with resection.

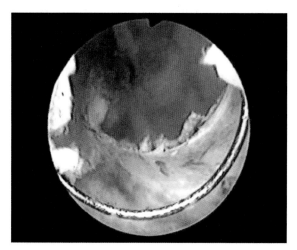

Figure 13.15 After complete removal of an intramural myoma, a hollow appeared over the previous site of the myoma, in the left posterior wall. The space would shrink once the perfusing pressure was reduced.

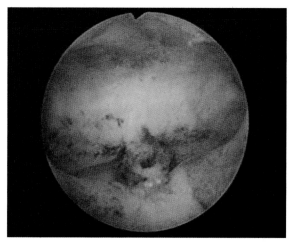

Figure 13.16 A second-look hysteroscopy 4 weeks after hysteroscopic removal of a 4 cm intramural myoma in the posterior wall revealed a normal cavity with a small amount of necrotic and healing tissue on the posterior wall.

do the assessment any earlier because any residual lesion left in the cavity could be extruded out of the cavity, or any residual lesion attached to the bottom of the myometrial wall may be pushed inwards by ongoing uterine contractions.

Routine second-look hysteroscopy (Figure 13.16) may not be necessary but ought to be considered 6–8 weeks after the operation in women (1) with multiple myoma; (2) with possibility of residual lesion; or (3) in whom postoperative ultrasonography showed irregular endometrial echo, raising the possibility of intrauterine adhesions.

For women with the remnants of the myoma left in the uterine wall, postoperative GnRHa therapy should be considered if it has not already been given in the preoperative period.

Infection is more likely to occur in the postoperative period if there are any myoma remnants, which may undergo necrosis and become infected. Women should be advised to report earlier if there are features of infection in order that broad-spectrum antibiotic therapy can be initiated without delay.

13.3 Summary

Intramural myomas may contribute to various forms of reproductive failure. Hysteroscopic resection of intramural myomas without protrusion into the uterine cavity is a challenging operation. The procedure should always be conducted under ultrasonographic guidance. Special preoperative, intraoperative and postoperative measures are required to ensure complete and yet safe removal of the myoma.

References

1. Munro MG, Critchley HO, Fraser IS; FIGO Menstrual Disorders Working Group. The FIGO classification of causes of abnormal uterine bleeding in the reproductive years. *Fertil Steril* 2011;**95**(7):2204–8.

2. Oliveira FG, Abdelmassih VG, Diamond MP, et al. Impact of subserosal and intramural uterine fibroids that do not distort the endometrial cavity on the outcome of in vitro fertilization-intracytoplasmic sperm injection. *Fertil Steril* 2004;**81**(3):582–7.

3. Matsunaga E, Shiota K. Ectopic pregnancy and myoma uteri: teratogenic effects and maternal characteristics. *Teratology* 1980;**21**(1):61–9.

4. Rosati P, Bellati U, Exacoustos C, Angelozzi P, Mancuso S. Uterine myoma pregnancy: ultrasound study. *Int J Gynecol Obstet* 1989;**28**(2):109–17.

5. Sudik R, Husch K, Steller J, Daume E. Fertility and pregnancy outcome after myomectomy in sterility patients. *Eur J Obstet Gynecol Reprod Biol* 1996;**65**(2):209–14.

6. Brady PC, Stanic AK, Styer AK. Uterine fibroids and subfertility: an update on the role of myomectomy. *Curr Opin Obstet Gynecol* 2013;**25**(3):255–9.

7. Pritts EA. Fibroids and infertility: a systematic review of the evidence. *Obstet Gynecol Surv* 2001;**56**(8):483–91.

8. Donnez J, Jadoul P. What are the implications of myomas on fertility? A need for a debate? *Hum Reprod* 2002;**17**(6):1424–30.

9. Benecke C, Kruger TF, Siebert TI, Van der Merwe JP, Steyn DW. Effect of fibroids on fertility in patients undergoing assisted reproduction. A structured literature review. *Gynecol Obstet Invest* 2005;**59**(4):225–30.

10. Somigliana E, Vercellini P, Daguati R, et al. Fibroids and female reproduction: a critical analysis of the evidence. *Hum Reprod Update* 2007;**13**(5):465–76.

11. Pritts EA, Parker WH, Olive DL. Fibroids and infertility: an updated systematic review of the evidence. *Fertil Steril* 2009;**91**(4):1215–23.

12. Sunkara SK, Khairy M, El-Toukhy T, Khalaf Y, Coomarasamy A. The effect of intramural fibroids without uterine cavity involvement on the outcome of IVF treatment: a systematic review and meta-analysis. *Hum Reprod* 2010;**25**(2):418–29.

13. Metwally M, Farquhar CM, Li T-C. Is another meta-analysis on the effects of intramural fibroids on reproductive outcomes needed? *Reprod Biomed Online* 2011;**23**(1):2–14.

14. Guven S, Kart C, Unsal MA, Odaci E. Intramural leiomyoma without endometrial cavity distortion may negatively affect the ICSI–ET outcome. *Reprod Biol Endocrinol* 2013;**11**:102–8.

15. Ingersoll FM. Fertility following myomectomy. *Fertil Steril* 1963;**14**:596–602.

16. Ng EH, Chan CC, Tang OS, Yeung WS, Ho PC. Endometrial and subendometrial blood flow measured by three-dimensional power Doppler ultrasound in patients with small intramural uterine fibroids during IVF treatment. *Hum Reprod* 2005;**20**(2):501–6.

17. Verkauf BS. Myomectomy for fertility enhancement and preservation. *Fertil Steril* 1992;**58**(1):1–15.

18. Arslan AA, Gold LI, Mittal K, et al. Gene expression studies provide clues to the pathogenesis of uterine leiomyoma: new evidence and a systematic review. *Hum Reprod* 2005;**20**(4):852–63.

19. Donnez J, Pirard C, Smets M, et al. Unusual growth of a myoma during pregnancy. *Fertil Steril* 2002;**78**(3):632–3.

20. Nishino M, Togashi K, Nakai A, et al. Uterine contractions evaluated on cine MR imaging in patients with uterine leiomyomata. *Eur J Radiol* 2005;**53**(1):142–6.

21. Shen A-r, Shun-hong Z. The comparative study between transcervical resection of myoma and laparoscopic myomectomy of intramural uterine myoma. *J Int Obstet Gynecol* 2014;**41**(5):522–5 (in Chinese).

22. Casadio P, Youssef AM, Spagnolo E, et al. Should the myometrial free margin still be considered a limiting factor for hysteroscopic resection of submucous fibroids? A possible answer to an old question. *Fertil Steril* 2011;**95**(5):1764–8.

23. Yang JH, Lin BL. Changes in myometrial thickness during

hysteroscopic resection of deeply invasive submucous myomas. *J Am Assoc Gynecol Laparosc* 2001;**8**(4):501–5.

24. Di Spiezio Sardo A, Mazzon I, Bramante S, et al. Hysteroscopic myomectomy: a comprehensive review of surgical techniques.

Hum Reprod Update 2008;**14** (2):101–19.

25. Song WP, Xia EL. Study on feasibility of transcervical resection near serosa myoma combined with B ultrasound monitoring. *The 16th Beijing-International Symposium of*

Gynecological Endoscopy; 2008 (in Chinese).

26. Xia EL, Duan H, Huang XW, Zheng J, Yu D. Transcervical resection of myoma in treatment of hysteromyoma: experience in 962 cases. *Natl Med J China* 2005;**85**(3):173–7 (in Chinese).

14

Outpatient Myomectomy

Mary E. Connor

14.1 Introduction

Uterine fibroids are common. They arise from the myometrium and occur in approximately 20–25% of women aged 35 years or more [1]. They may be found at any position within the myometrium from the serosal surface to lying completely within the uterine cavity in 5–10% [2].

Submucosal fibroids are found close to the inner myometrium and may protrude into the endometrial cavity to a greater or lesser extent; they have been classified according to their position (see Figure 14.1) [3]. Fibroids that are completely within the uterine cavity are classified as type 0 and are sometimes pedunculated with a narrow stalk; type 1 are those having some intramural component, but more than 50% is within the cavity; type 2 are those with less than 50% in the cavity (see Figure 14.2a and b). Pedunculated fibroids may prolapse through the cervical os, having been expelled from the uterine cavity or cervical canal (see Figure 14.2c).

Outpatient or office myomectomy is appropriate for the removal of small and accessible submucosal fibroids, generally those that are less than 2.5 cm diameter and of type 0 or type 1 where most, if not all of the fibroid, is within the uterine cavity. Indications for their removal in an outpatient setting are discussed, and the devices that are available and suitable for use in

these circumstances. Additional equipment is considered too, including systems for fluid management. Appropriate analgesia and anaesthesia is reviewed, as it is important to ensure that the procedure is made tolerable and acceptable for the patient. Potential complications that may occur in this context are discussed. The clinical environment that is required is reviewed and consideration is given to the training necessary to perform such procedures in the outpatient setting.

14.2 Indications for Fibroid Removal

Submucosal fibroids are regarded as an important source of symptoms, such as heavy menstrual bleeding (HMB) and increased menstrual-related pain, possibly due to the uterus trying to expel an intracavitary fibroid [2]. There is an association with increased reproductive failure too, with failed implantation and increased spontaneous miscarriage, though the precise mechanism remains uncertain [1]. Indman argues that given the current evidence it is reasonable to offer hysteroscopic resection of submucosal fibroids to women who desire pregnancy [4]. Pritts has shown in a systematic review that in infertile women with fibroids both pregnancy and delivery rates are increased with removal of submucosal fibroids and become comparable to those of infertile women without fibroids (RR for pregnancy after treatment 1.72 [95%CI 1.13–2.58]; delivery rates 0.98 [95% CI 0.45–2.41]) [5]. However, it has been found that the best improvement in fertility follows removal of the larger submucosal fibroids, with a cumulative pregnancy rate of 25% for fibroids less than 20 mm, but 75% when larger than 30 mm [1]. It is proposed that the best prognostic factors in this context are age less than 35 years, a larger fibroid of at least 50 mm and absence of other infertility factors [6]. By contrast, the best resolution of HMB is seen following removal of the smaller submucosal fibroids ($\leq$30 mm), those which are mainly intracavitary, and

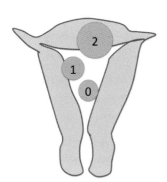

Figure 14.1 The three types of submucosal fibroids: type 0 is entirely within the uterine cavity; type 1 is more than 50% within the cavity and is distinguished by the sharp angle adjacent to the endometrium; type 2 is more than 50% in the myometrium with a wide angle next to the endometrium [4].

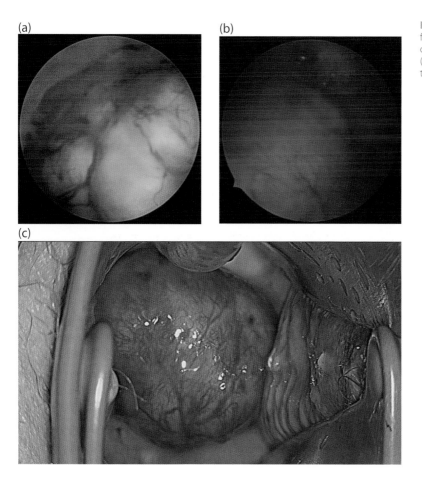

Figure 14.2 (a) Type 0 submucosal fibroid, (b) type 2 submucosal fibroid covered by a layer of endometrium and (c) prolapsed fibroid protruding through the cervical os into the vagina.

with a uterus size of less than or equal to a 6-week gestation [4].

Other circumstances when submucosal fibroids may cause symptoms include postmenopausal bleeding (PMB) arising from the surface of an intracavitary fibroid that has rubbed against the opposing atrophic endometrial surface. Also, intermenstrual (IMB) or irregular bleeding may occur in premenopausal women with the vaginal blood loss made heavier, even if not initiated, by the fibroid. Intracavitary fibroids that have been expelled from the uterine cavity through the cervical os, though relatively uncommon, are another important source of heavy vaginal bleeding.

14.3 Fibroid Removal in an Outpatient Setting: Size and Position

It is apparent that resolution of HMB, PMB, IMB and some fertility problems may arise following removal of submucosal fibroids. The important considerations for removal in an outpatient or office setting are the fibroid size, its position within the uterine cavity and relation to the endometrium and therefore its accessibility, and the patient's willingness to opt for treatment in this context.

The advantages of outpatient treatment and why it is worth considering are similar to those for outpatient endometrial polypectomy and are namely the avoidance of a general anaesthetic with prompter recovery; fewer hospital visits with no requirement for preoperative assessment; shorter stay in hospital, with reduction in associated risks such as hospital-related infections; and quicker return to normal activities including return to work [7]. Patients can be offered a see-and-treat service with a single, short hospital or clinic visit, which may be particularly appreciated by patients awaiting fertility treatment. In addition, in the outpatient setting, the number of clinical staff is lower, with the potential for cost savings; often only the hysteroscopist and usually two nursing and one support staff are required [8]. In the absence of a general anaesthetic or conscious sedation there is no requirement for an anaesthetist or associated support staff.

As for diagnostic hysteroscopy, with an outpatient treatment service it is important to pay attention to minimizing patient anxiety. This is helped by the provision in advance of clearly written information about the procedure, avoiding keeping patients waiting excessively and providing a nurse to support the patient during the procedure [8]. This person, sometimes referred to as the 'local vocal', will act as the patient's advocate and ensure that the clinician is made aware if the patient is distressed and wants the procedure to cease. Some patients wish to have a clear and detailed account of what is going to happen and watch the procedure throughout on the monitor; others ask to be told the minimum without even a glance at the monitor; a few prefer silence and keep their eyes closed. It is important to be responsive to the patient and her wishes.

There are disadvantages too that must be considered: the procedure may be painful during dilatation of the cervix, with distension of the uterine cavity or with activation of some of the hysteroscopic treatment devices, particularly when electrosurgery is involved. It may not be possible to remove all of the fibroid in one session, especially when there is a myometrial component or a larger fibroid. The procedure may take longer than expected, stretching the tolerance of the patient beyond her capacity. An investigation of outpatient endometrial polypectomy found that procedures of up to 15 minutes were well tolerated [9], with a similar finding reported for outpatient fibroid removal [10].

There are, however, important differences between removal of a submucosal fibroid and an endometrial polyp; the latter are softer and so generally easier and quicker to remove [11]. Experience with outpatient see-and-treat hysteroscopic procedures found that polypectomy was successful in 67% compared with only 16% for small submucosal fibroids, though the size and position of the fibroids in this study is not described [12]. The time taken to remove a fibroid is related to its size, as elegantly demonstrated by Emanuel (see Figure 14.3) [13]. The volume of a sphere is determined by the equation $4/3\pi r^3$, and this can be

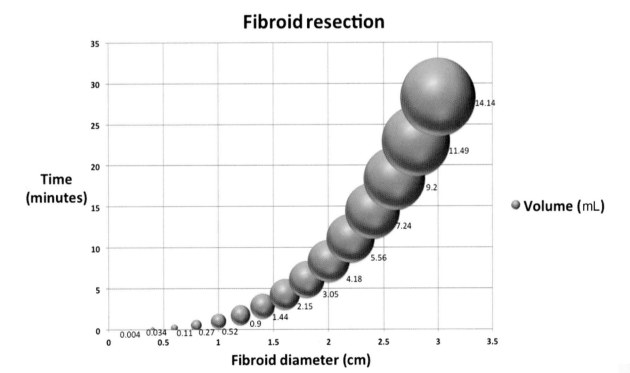

Fibroid resection

Figure 14.3 Estimated fibroid diameter and volume, with resection time as determined by fibroid removal rate of 0.5 mL/minute [13]. Courtesy of Elsevier.

used to approximate the volume of a fibroid. The time taken to resect a fibroid has been calculated as 0.5 mL/minute, so that a fibroid with a diameter of 1 cm (volume 0.52 mL) can be expected to be resected in just over 1 minute, and if 2 cm diameter (volume 4.18 mL) it would take 8.36 minutes, but a 3 cm diameter (volume 14.14 mL) would take 28.28 minutes. If the treatment time is confined to a maximum of 20 minutes, and allows for non-continuous resection, then it is necessary to limit the fibroid size to a diameter of less than 2.5 cm. Larger fibroids are therefore likely to require a second procedure, and this should be negotiated with the patient at the outset, as she may prefer to opt for an inpatient setting with the greater potential for a single treatment.

As previously stated, the position of the fibroid within the uterine cavity is important. Lasmar et al. proposed the STEPW classification of submucosal fibroids that provided a score for complexity of removal [14]. Fibroids that were in the lower third of the cavity were noted to be the easiest to remove, with ones at the fundus or arising from the lateral wall the most difficult.

Access to the intramural portion of a fibroid need not be impossible in an outpatient setting, but requires preparation. As with inpatient fibroid resection, shaving of the intracavity portion allows the intramural component to move into the uterine cavity due to contraction of the surrounding myometrium, allowing for a planned two-stage procedure [15]. Another approach is to make a circular incision with a bipolar needle into the fibroid capsule at the level of the endometrium, several weeks prior to subsequent resection. Bettocchi et al. reported the successful transition of partially intramural fibroids into totally or predominantly intracavitary ones in 55/59 (93%) cases [16]. The mean diameter of the fibroids was 2.9 ± 0.8 cm, all procedures were undertaken in an outpatient setting, and intraoperative pain scores were acceptable and reported as 35.2 ± 12.7 mm on a 100 mm visual analogue score (VAS). However, all subsequent fibroid resections were undertaken as inpatient procedures. Using this preparatory technique, Haimovich et al. adapted the procedure and were able to perform both stages of treatment in an outpatient setting in 34/43 (79%) of patients [17]. They were successful with all fibroids less than 18 mm in diameter and in 85% with 19–30 mm diameter; access was easier for fibroids located in the anterior and posterior walls compared with those in either the fundal or lateral walls.

The removal of a prolapsed cervical fibroid in the outpatient setting is worth considering provided that there is sufficient space in the vagina for insertion of a speculum and manipulation of instruments, such as a monopolar diathermy loop as used in colposcopy (see below).

14.4 Operating Devices and Instruments

14.4.1 Hysteroscopic 5 French Bipolar Needle Electrodes

Small (<15 mm) submucosal fibroids can be resected or vaporized using bipolar needle electrodes passed down the 5 Fr. gauge operating channel found on many diagnostic hysteroscopes. There are several makes of bipolar needles available. The Twizzle and Spring Versapoint™ electrodes are disposable and single-use and must be accompanied by the Gynecare Versapoint™ bipolar generator; they fit down any standard rigid hysteroscope with a 5 Fr. operating channel. They were originally designed to accompany the disposable Versapoint™ sheath and reusable Alphascope™. In the outpatient setting, reduction of the power to its lowest setting (from VC1 to VC3) minimizes myometrial stimulation and pain associated with activation of the device [11]. Reusable bipolar needle electrodes are available from Karl Storz and Richard Wolf (BipoTrode) (see Figure 14.4a and b); these are compatible with most electrosurgical generators, including ones often used in a colposcopy setting.

The difficulties associated with removing solid fibroid fragments larger than the cervical os can be avoided by slicing the fibroid into smaller portions [11]. Otherwise, it may be necessary to dilate the cervix to enable blind removal of the tissue fragments with forceps, though this can cause pain and increases the risk of uterine perforation. A combination of vaporizing and slicing may be used to reduce the fibroid in size before removal; sometimes it can be removed and attached to the tip of the bipolar needle.

14.4.2 TruClear™ Tissue Removal System

The development of mechanical hysteroscopic tissue removal systems has made the resection of intrauterine pathologies significantly easier. The first system,

(a)

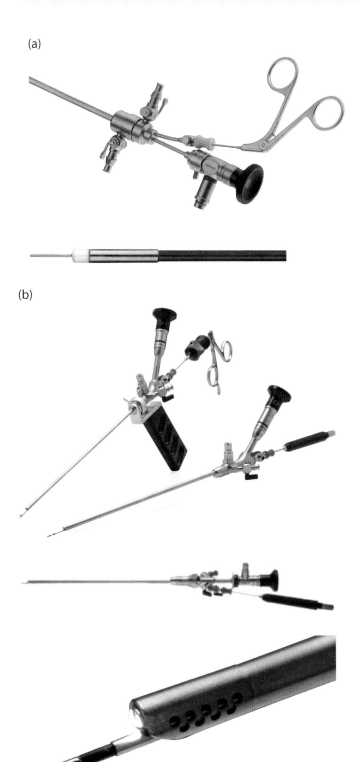

Figure 14.4 Bipolar 'needlepoint' electrodes, all 5 Fr. gauge: (a) bipolar needle electrode with Bettocchi hysteroscope. © KARL STORZ – Endoskope, Germany; (b) BipoTrode bipolar needle with Compact hysteroscopes. Courtesy of Richard Wolf GmbH.

(b)

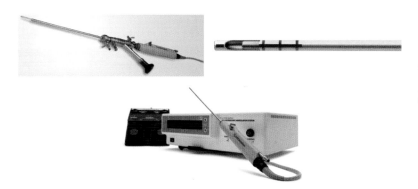

based upon an arthroscope, enables tissue to be excised under direct vision with a moving mechanical device; the tissue is then immediately extracted by suction, so no fragments impede the view [18]. Tissue removal devices are passed down the central core of a rigid hysteroscope with an offset eyepiece; they are attached to a hand piece and activated by a foot-operated control unit.

The larger of the TruClear™ systems has an outer sheath diameter of 7.25 mm (TruClear™ Elite Plus) and so is less amenable for use in an outpatient setting, though this may be possible with a local anaesthetic cervical block. However, since the introduction of the smaller Dense Tissue Shaver Mini for tougher tissue, fibroid removal using the 5 mm hysteroscope (TC5) has become possible (see Figure 14.5) [19]. Cervical dilatation may not be necessary with the TC5. The larger TruClear™ Elite Plus hysteroscope when used with the Dense Tissue Shaver Plus has the advantage over the smaller TC5 hysteroscope of more rapid tissue removal.

The technique for fibroid removal with this system differs from the removal of softer endometrial tissue and polyps. Efficient removal of the firmer fibroid tissue is achieved by pressing the device against the fibroid so that the open jaw is buried (see Video 14.1). Intracavitary tissue is generally readily accessible; any myometrial portion may be made more available by reducing the intrauterine pressure of the irrigating fluid thus allowing the deeper fibroid to become more exposed. The smaller Dense Tissue Shaver Mini, when not activated, may also be used to prise the fibroid away from the surrounding capsule and so push it into the cavity for ease of subsequent resection.

There is evidence that mechanical removal with the TruClear™ 5C system for endometrial polyps is quicker and more effective than electrosurgical resection with Versapoint electrodes [20, 21], and may be less painful [20]; it is not known whether this also applies to the removal of small submucosal fibroids.

14.4.3 MyoSure® Tissue Removal System

The MyoSure® tissue removal system is another hysteroscopic device that combines mechanical excision of intrauterine tissue with immediate extraction by suction. There are two sizes of hysteroscope; the smaller has an outer diameter of 6.25 mm and the larger XL® of 7.25 mm. There are three blades available: (1) the Lite® can be used with either hysteroscope and is best suited for endometrial polyp removal; (2) the newer Reach® blade replaces the previous classic blade and has a shorter tip to improve fundal access and is sufficiently robust to remove small fibroids; it can also be used with both hysteroscopes (see Figure 14.6); and (3) the XL® blade, as its name suggests, is for exclusive use with the larger XL hysteroscope and is suitable for fibroid removal [22]. Cervical dilatation is generally necessary when using either hysteroscope. Recently, Hologic introduced a set of smaller hysteroscopes, the Omni™ set. This consists of a single 0° hysteroscope that may be used with a diagnostic sheath (3.7 mm), or a 5.5 mm operating sheath with either the Lite® or Reach® shaver, or a 6.25 mm operating sheath with the XL® blade.

As with the previous system, the morcellating blade is passed down the central section of the hysteroscope and operated from a control unit by a foot pedal; tissue fragments are again immediately removed by suction. The most efficient method of removing fibroid tissue is also achieved by pressing the blade against the fibroid with the open jaw buried in the tissue and also allowing any deeper tissue to be exposed by reducing the intrauterine pressure (see Video 14.2).

 Video 14.1 Resection of fundal submucosal fibroid: TruClear™ Tissue Removal System using the Dense Tissue Shaver Mini.

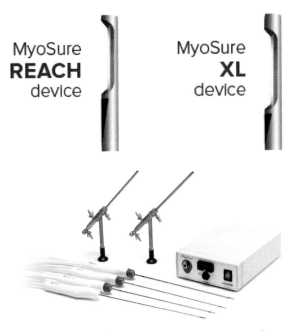

Figure 14.6 MyoSure® tissue removal system with Reach® and XL® blades; both are suitable for removal of small submucosal fibroids in an outpatient setting. The Reach device can be used with either the smaller 6.25 mm, the larger XL (7.25 mm) hysteroscope, or the recently introduced Omni 5.5 mm and 6 mm hysteroscope sheaths. The XL device may be used with the XL scope or the Omni 6 mm. Courtesy of HOLOGIC, Inc. and affiliates.

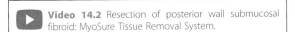

Video 14.2 Resection of posterior wall submucosal fibroid: MyoSure Tissue Removal System.

14.4.4 Resectoscopes

There may be initial scepticism about the use of a resectoscope in the outpatient setting, but the SHINE project in Cardiff established that it was effective and acceptable to patients for a 10 mm resectoscope to be inserted into the uterine cavity for removal of intra-uterine polyps and fibroids following a local anaesthetic cervical block [23]. A monopolar resectoscope was used with glycine for irrigation. The overall pain score for the first 66 patients who responded was an average of 3.3 (SD ± 2.6) on a 0–10 Visual Analogue pain scale, where 0 was no pain and 10 pain as bad as possible. The length of the procedure for 79 patients, from start to finish of treatment, was an average of 30.7 minutes (SD ± 10.4). Patients were asked which anaesthetic they would prefer should they require the procedure again, and 88.6% of 79 women would opt for a repeat local anaesthetic while only 8.9% would want a general anaesthetic.

Successful outpatient resection of fibroids was reported by Papalampros et al., using a narrow 5.3 mm (16 Fr. gauge) diameter prototype monopolar resectoscope [10]. Fibroids of 2–3 cm diameter were removed from four women; the other patients underwent endometrial polypectomy. Importantly, all procedures were completed within 15 minutes and without complication. In total, 16 procedures were accomplished without anaesthesia, and in 14 after an intracervical block with local anaesthetic, as cervical dilatation was required. Patient tolerance was reported as good, with no patients reporting more than slight discomfort.

Resectoscopes currently in use now often use bipolar electrodes, for which an ionic fluid for irrigation is required, such as isotonic normal (0.9%) saline, rather than the non-isotonic glycine or sorbitol.

Standard-sized 9 or 10 mm bipolar resectoscopes are available from several companies, including Karl Storz, Richard Wolf and Olympus, who produce the SurgMaster (Figure 14.7c). There are also now available narrower resectoscopes particularly suitable for outpatient use, with the 15 Fr. (5 mm) bipolar resectoscope from Karl Storz (Figure 14.7a) and the 7 mm resectoscope from Richard Wolf that can be used with the suction device (Chip E-vac™) for removal of resected tissue (see Figure 14.7b). Tissue fragments otherwise need to be removed under direct vision with the resecting loop electrode or blindly with polyp forceps with the risk of uterine perforation.

Techniques for excising fibroid tissue with a resectoscope are the same for outpatient as for inpatient procedures. The resectoscope electrode loop is passed beyond the fibroid and, after activation, the direction of cutting is always towards the cervix. For small fibroids, resection of the full diameter of the fibroid may be achieved by moving just the electrode; for larger fibroids, a combination of withdrawing the resectoscope through the cervix with the electrode extended, then finishing with retraction of the electrode is preferable. The cut strip of fibroid is either immediately removed from the cavity with the loop or placed at the fundus for subsequent removal while other strips of fibroid are resected. For efficient resection, the aim is to remove all of the fibroid with as few strips as possible.

14.4.5 Monopolar Diathermy Loops for Prolapsed Cervical Fibroids

Colposcopy clinics are generally furnished with equipment for taking large cervical biopsies using

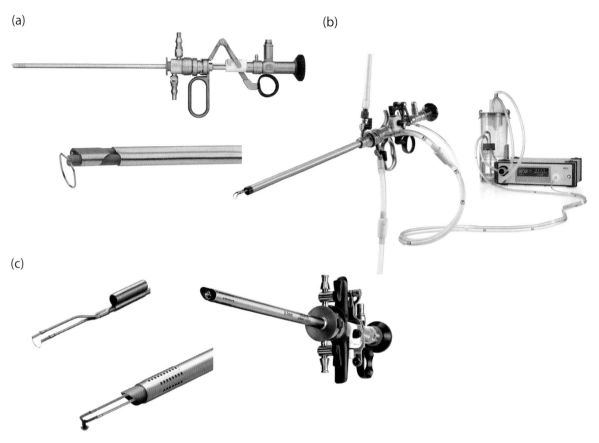

(a)

(b)

(c)

Figure 14.7 Bipolar resectoscopes: (a) bipolar 15 Fr. (5 mm diameter) resectoscope © KARL STORZ – Endoskope, Germany; (b) the 7 mm Princess resectoscope with the Chip E-vac™ suction system. Courtesy of Richard Wolf GmbH; (c) the Olympus SurgMaster resectoscope with 8.5 mm outer sheath for transcervical procedures in saline, with loop electrode for resection and Plasma button for vaporizing tissue. Courtesy of Olympus GmbH.

monopolar diathermy loops, plus an electrosurgery generator, a smoke extractor and insulated speculums, and these can be used for excision of prolapsed cervical fibroids. Infiltration of the fibroid neck with local anaesthetic containing a vasoconstrictor provides analgesia and reduced blood flow. The fibroid can be resected with a hand-held loop electrode, taking care to avoid inadvertent contact with the vaginal wall. If the fibroid stalk is inaccessible within the cervical canal or uterine cavity, it may be resected with one of the hysteroscopic tissue removal systems; dilatation of the cervix is often not required in these circumstances as the cervix will already be open. The limiting factor is the size of the fibroid in relation to the capacity of the vagina, as there needs to be sufficient space to insert the speculum and allow manipulation of the fibroid away from the vaginal

wall. The patient also needs to be willing, though from the author's own experience some are keen to avoid a general anaesthetic, if at all possible.

14.5 Fluid Management

Diagnostic hysteroscopy procedures and removal of endometrial polyps can be readily accomplished with less than a single litre of normal saline (0.9%) and a simple gravity feed or a pressure bag. However, the more solid fibroids, apart from the tiniest ones, take longer to remove and are therefore likely to require more fluid. Maintaining a consistent pressure using a 3 L bag of saline is more difficult and is best established with a fluid management system which also tracks accurately the amount of fluid used and any deficit. A constant pressure ensures a good hysteroscopic view and is more comfortable for the patient than when it waxes and wanes with a pressure cuff (unpublished data, Mary E. Connor). Serious fluid deficit is less likely than during an inpatient procedure as the treatment is likely to be of shorter duration with a smaller fibroid that is superficial and not near to the large blood vessels deep within the myometrium.

14.6 Analgesia and Anaesthesia

14.6.1 Preprocedure Analgesia

The RCOG and BSGE Green-top Guideline for Best Practice in Outpatient Hysteroscopy recommends that patients for whom it is not contraindicated should be advised to take a standard dose of a non-steroidal anti-inflammatory drug (NSAID) around 1 hour before their outpatient procedure [8]. There is limited evidence for its effectiveness, but in a small study, mefenamic acid significantly reduced post-procedural pain at 30 and 60 minutes [24]. However, a Cochrane review found insufficient evidence for either NSAIDs or opioids over placebo for providing pain relief 30 minutes after diagnostic hysteroscopy [25]. Parenteral administration of tramadol an hour before diagnostic hysteroscopy was found to reduce procedural pain [26, 27], but this may be difficult to integrate into an outpatient setting.

Debate continues as to whether cervical softening agents are beneficial for easing cervical dilatation and reducing related pain [8]. The side effects can be troublesome, with misoprostol, causing stomach cramps, nausea and sometimes diarrhoea. Other authors use preprocedure laminaria tents to gently open the cervical canal [4]. However, when compared with self-administered misoprostol laminaria tents, though equally effective, were less favoured by patients and doctors, as an additional hospital visit was required for their insertion [28].

Some particularly anxious patients may benefit from a sedative such as a small dose (2–5 mg) of oral diazepam taken beforehand; this would need to be prescribed in advance and may be provided by the patient's general practitioner.

14.6.2 Cervical Anaesthesia

Cervical anaesthesia is pertinent for patients in this context as relatively large diameter hysteroscopes may be used; at least a 5 mm or so dilatation is often

required. There is evidence that intracervical and paracervical blocks are beneficial at reducing pain associated with hysteroscopy [8]. There is insufficient evidence for recommendation of any particular local anaesthetic preparation; the addition of a vasoconstrictive substance is little needed for hysteroscopic procedures, though the duration of action is increased. Care needs to be taken when using local anaesthetics because of the potential for toxicity, with central nervous and cardiac signs and symptoms. In addition, vasoconstrictive substances may also cause cardiac symptoms; these can be avoided by using felypressin-containing preparations rather than adrenaline.

Convenient preparations for intracervical blocks are those commonly used by dentists, and they can be administered with a dental needle (27 gauge) and syringe. Local anaesthetic is inserted initially to the anterior lip of the cervix if it is to be grasped, and then at four points around the cervical os. Inserting the needle up to the hilt (3–4 cm) is recommended, so that the level of the internal cervical os is reached [29]; a long dental syringe can be useful to enable access whilst maintaining a view of the cervix. A single-toothed tenaculum placed on the anterior lip of the cervix can help provide stability during insertion of the needle so that it can be placed slowly and without bending.

Evidence for the optimum time to wait before proceeding with cervical dilatation is limited; the onset of action of mepivicaine without a vasoconstrictor is 3–5 minutes, with 45–90 minutes duration of action [30].

14.6.3 Inhaled Nitrous Oxide

A number of hysteroscopy clinics have patient-controlled nitrous oxide inhalation readily available for use during both diagnostic and operative hysteroscopy. It can be beneficial at any stage of the procedure, including during insertion of local anaesthesia to the cervix, which can hurt, as well as during the actual hysteroscopic treatment, particularly if uterine distension is painful. There is some evidence for its use in this context [31], and its use is well established on most labour wards, and for endoscopic procedures [32]. Besides providing useful pain relief, it reduces anxiety, it is safe and with few associated complications, and recovery from its use is rapid [33].

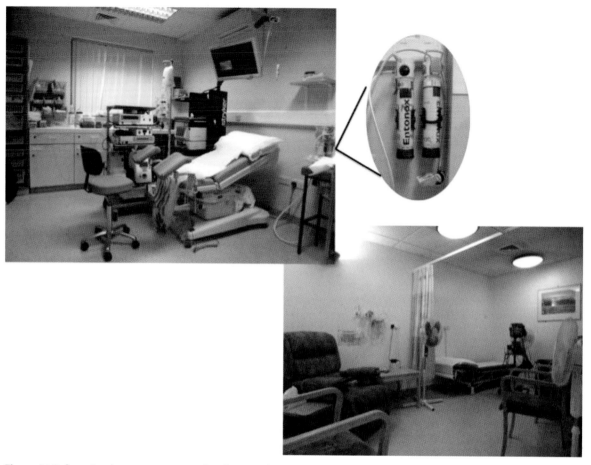

Figure 14.8 Outpatient hysteroscopy room with wall-mounted nitrous oxide (inset), and nearby recovery room.

14.7 Complications of Outpatient Myomectomy

The complications that may occur with inpatient myomectomy may also occur with an outpatient procedure. Incomplete fibroid removal may arise because of poor access to the base of the fibroid due to its position within the uterine cavity or myometrium, poor patient tolerance of the procedure or calcification of the fibroid tissue preventing its resection. The consequence of incomplete removal varies; further treatment may not be necessary if the patient becomes asymptomatic [34].

Uterine perforation may happen during fibroid resection, with a risk of 0.75% [35], though this is unlikely in outpatients when removing small,

superficial fibroids. Also, the patient will complain of increased pain with myometrial penetration before full perforation occurs. Even so, sudden loss of uterine distension or a direct view of peritoneal contents should be taken very seriously, especially if this occurs during activation of a resection device, with the assumption of possible bowel damage and appropriate action taken.

Postoperative endometritis or other infections are uncommon, the incidence varying with how the condition is defined, but can be expected to occur in 0.001–1.6% [36, 37]. Patients need to be warned about what symptoms to expect and where to seek help if concerned. A Cochrane review does not advocate the routine use of prophylactic antibiotics, but patients with a history of pelvic inflammatory disease are at increased risk and so more likely to benefit [38]. Hysteroscopic procedures should not be performed if there is active infection present.

Severe pain sufficient to curtail the procedure may occur, though patients who have tolerated a previous diagnostic hysteroscopy are unlikely to find removal of an intrauterine lesion more painful, provided the myometrium is not stimulated [11].

Vasovagal reactions should be anticipated and managed appropriately; reported incidences vary depending upon the definition used. Van Kerkvoorde et al. reported that 10/1,028 (<1%) patients undergoing office hysteroscopy experienced a vasovagal episode, but with a further five reporting nausea [37]. This symptom could be considered as part of a vagal response, which if combined together would still only give an incidence of 1.5%. In a systematic review of local anaesthesia in outpatient hysteroscopy an incidence for vasovagal episodes of 7.6% was identified. Of note, the use of local anaesthetic did not make a difference; neither did how the response was defined [39].

Fluid overload is of importance particularly when resecting large, deep submucosal fibroids. Whilst this particular complication should not be ignored, the

likelihood of it occurring when removing small, shallow fibroids with a procedure of short duration is small. However, the same guidelines as for inpatient procedures apply, with a maximum deficit of 2.5 L of saline [40].

14.8 Outpatient Facilities

The facilities for outpatient hysteroscopy should be conducive to enabling the patient to feel relaxed. Attention should be paid to maintaining the patient's privacy and dignity by providing changing facilities adjacent to, but separate from the treatment room, and ideally including a toilet [8, 41, 42].

The treatment room should be fully equipped with a couch suitable for hysteroscopy (see Figure 14.8); it may be dedicated to hysteroscopy or a shared

(a)

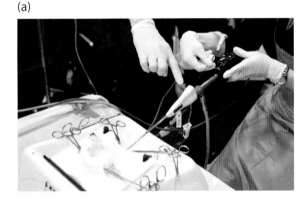

(b)

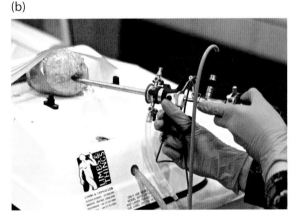

Figure 14.10 Animal and vegetable models used for operative hysteroscopy training: (a) simulated resection of intrauterine tissue with a bipolar needle electrode using a pig's bladder with sewn in 'polyps' and (b) simulated intrauterine resection using a prepared potato. Reproduced with the permission of Royal College of Obstetricians and Gynaecologists.

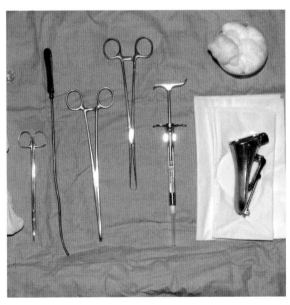

Figure 14.9 Additional equipment required for outpatient hysteroscopy: gloves, long-handled scissors, uterine sound, sponge forceps, single-toothed tenaculum, dental syringe with needle and local anaesthetic ampoule, speculum and cotton swabs.

multi-purpose room. Space is required for the camera stack, resection and fluid-delivery equipment and a trolley with additional equipment laid out ready for use (Figure 14.9).

The recovery room should be separate from the waiting room and furnished with reclining chairs; a bed for lying down may be useful for patients following a vasovagal episode. Adequate resuscitation facilities are essential with readily available oxygen and monitoring equipment; the requirements are the same as for colposcopy and contraceptive coil fitting.

14.9 Training

Resecting submucosal fibroids with an awake and alert patient requires all of the hysteroscopy team to be very familiar with the equipment. Experience can be gained in the inpatient setting, but consideration should be given to the use of simulation models or computer simulators. These can provide the opportunity for training on a variety of

different resection devices and so enable their effective use; models also enable repeated practice (Figure 14.10). There is evidence to suggest that learning to resect tissue with a hysteroscopic tissue morcellator is easier compared with a conventional resectoscope [43].

14.10 Conclusion

Resection of small, shallow submucosal fibroids in an outpatient setting enables patients to undergo prompt, efficient and effective treatment, sometimes as a see-and-treat event. A variety of suitable hysteroscopic devices are available that provide fibroid resection in this setting and causing little more pain than experienced during diagnostic hysteroscopy. The facilities required do not differ from those needed for outpatient hysteroscopic removal of endometrial polyps, though as fibroids are tougher, their removal is more often difficult and will take longer. Additional training to ensure skilful use of the equipment for fibroid removal is required.

References

1. Fernandez H, Sefrioui O, Virelizier C, et al. Hysteroscopic resection of submucosal fibroids in patients with infertility. *Hum Reprod* 2001;**16**:1489–92.

2. Ubaldi F, Tournaye H, Camus M, et al. Fertility after hysteroscopic myomectomy. *Hum Reprod Update* 1995;**1**:81–90.

3. Wamsteker K, Emanuel MH, de Kruif JH. Transcervical hysteroscopic resection of submucous fibroids for abnormal uterine bleeding: results regarding the degree of intramural extension. *Obstet Gynecol* 1993;**82**:736–40.

4. Indman PD. Hysteroscopic treatment of submucous fibroids. *Clin Obstet Gynecol* 2006;**49**:811–20.

5. Pritts EA. Fibroids and infertility: a systematic review of the evidence. *Obstet Gynecol Surv* 2001;**56**:483–91.

6. Varasteh NN, Neuwirth RS, Levin B, Keltz MD. Pregnancy rates after hysteroscopic polypectomy and myomectomy in infertile women. *Obstet Gynecol* 1999;**94**:168–71.

7. Marsh FA, Rogerson LJ, Duffy SR. A randomised controlled trial comparing outpatient versus daycase endometrial polypectomy. *BJOG* 2006;**113**(8):896–901.

8. Best Practice in Outpatient Hysteroscopy. *Green Top Guideline No. 59.* London: RCOG; 2011.

9. Litta P, Cosmi E, Saccardi C, et al. Outpatient operative polypectomy using a 5 mm-hysteroscope without anaesthesia and/or analgesia: advantages and limits. *Eur J Obstet Gynecol Reprod Biol* 2008;**139**:210–14.

10. Papalampros P, Gambadauro P, Papadopoulos N, et al. The mini-resectoscope: a new instrument for office hysteroscopic surgery. *Acta Obstet Gynecol Scand* 2009;**88**(2):227–30.

11. Bettocchi S, Ceci O, Di Venere R, et al. Advanced operative office hysteroscopy without anaesthesia: analysis of 501 cases treated with a 5 Fr. bipolar electrode. *Hum Reprod* 2002;**17**(9):2435–8.

12. Gulumser C, Narvekar N, Pathak M, et al. See-and-treat outpatient hysteroscopy: an analysis of 1109 examinations. *Reprod Biomed Online* 2010;**20**(3):423–9.

13. Emanuel MH. Hysteroscopy and the treatment of uterine fibroids. *Best Pract Res Clin Obstet Gynaecol* 2015;**29**:920–9.

14. Lasmar RB, Barrozo PR, Dias R, Oliveira MA. Submucous fibroids: a new presurgical classification evaluate the viability of hysteroscopic surgical treatment – preliminary report. *J Minim Invasive Gynecol* 2005;**12**:308–11.

15. Di Spiezio Sardo A, Mazzon I, Bramante S, et al. Hysteroscopic myomectomy: a comprehensive review of surgical techniques. *Hum Reprod Update* 2008;**14**:101–19.

16. Bettocchi S, Di Spiezio SA, Ceci O, et al. A new hysteroscopic technique for the preparation of partially intramural myomas in office setting (OPPIuM technique): a pilot study. *J Minim Invasive Gynecol* 2009;**16**(6):748–54.

17. Haimovich S, Mancebo G, Alameda F, et al. Feasibility of a new two-step procedure for office hysteroscopic resection of submucous myomas: results of a pilot study. *Eur J Obstet Gynecol Reprod Biol* 2013;**168**(2):191–4.

18. Emanuel MH, Wamsteker K. The Intra Uterine Morcellator: a new hysteroscopic operating technique to remove intrauterine polyps and myomas. *J Minim Invasive Gynecol* 2005 Jan–Feb;**12**(1):62–6.

19. Truclear System Operating Instructions. www.medtronic .com/content/dam/covidien/ library/us/en/product/ gynecology-products/truclear-system-comprehensive-brochure .pdf (Accessed 19 Sept 2017).

20. Smith PP, Middleton LJ, Connor ME, Clark TJ. Hysteroscopic morcellation compared with electrical resection of endometrial polyps. *Obstet Gynecol* 2014;**123**(4):745–51.

21. Pampalona JR, Bastos MD, Moreno GM, et al. A comparison of hysteroscopic mechanical tissue removal with bipolar electrical resection for the management of endometrial polyps in an ambulatory care setting: preliminary results. *J Minim Invasive Gynecol* 2015;**22**:439–45.

22. Myosure Tissue Removal System Physician Brochure. www.hologic .com/sites/default/files/white-papers/PB-00280-001%20Rev.% 20001_MyoSure_Physician_ Brchr_LowRes.pdf (Accessed 19 Sept 2017).

23. Penketh RJ, Bruen EM, White J, et al. Feasibility of resectoscopic operative hysteroscopy in a UK outpatient clinic using local anesthetic and traditional reusable equipment, with patient experiences and comparative cost analysis. *J Minim Invasive Gynecol* 2014;**21**(5):830–6.

24. Nagele F, Lockwood G, Magos AL. Randomised placebo controlled trial of mefenamic acid for premedication at outpatient hysteroscopy: a pilot study. *BJOG* 1997;**104**(7):842–4.

25. Ahmad G, O'Flynn H, Attarbashi S, Duffy JM, Watson A. Pain relief for outpatient hysteroscopy. *Cochrane Database Syst Rev* 2010;(11). Art. No.: CD007710. DOI: 10.1002/14651858. CD007710.pub2 (Accessed December 2017).

26. Bellati U, Bonaventura A, Costanza L, Zulli S, Gentile C. Tramadol hydrochloride versus mepivacaine hydrochloride: comparison between two analgesic procedures in hysteroscopy. *Giornale Italiano di Ostetricia e Ginecologia* 1998;**20**(10):469–72.

27. Floris S, Piras B, Orru M, et al. Efficacy of intravenous tramadol treatment for reducing pain during office diagnostic hysteroscopy. *Fertil Steril* 2007;**87**(1):147–51.

28. Darwish AM, Ahmad AM, Mohammad AM. Cervical priming prior to operative hysteroscopy: a randomized comparison of laminaria versus misoprostol. *Hum Reprod* 2004;**19**:2391–4.

29. Clark TJ, Gupta JK. *Handbook of Outpatient Hysteroscopy. A Complete Guide to Diagnosis and Therapy.* 1st ed. London: Hodder Education; 2005.

30. Chandrakantan A, Schraga ED, Chang AK, Press CD. Infiltrative Infiltrative Administration of Local Anesthetic Agents. https:// emedicine.medscape.com/article/ 149178-overview#a2. 2018 (Accessed December 2019).

31. del Valle RC, Solano C, Miguel M, et al. Inhalation analgesia with nitrous oxide versus other analgesic techniques in hysteroscopic polypectomy: a pilot study. *J Minim Invasive Gynecol* 2015 May–Jun;**22**(4):595–60.

32. Welchman S, Cochrane S, Minto G, Lewis S. Systematic review: the use of nitrous oxide gas for lower gastrointestinal endoscopy. *Aliment Pharmacol Ther* 2010;**32**:324–33.

33. Maslekar S, Gardiner A, Hughes M, Culbert B, Duthie GS. Randomized clinical trial of Entonox versus midazolam-fentanyl sedation for colonoscopy. *Br J Surg* 2009;**96**:361–8.

34. Van Dongen H, Emanuel MH, Smeets MJ, Trimbos B, Jansen FW. Follow-up after incomplete hysteroscopic removal of uterine fibroids. *Acta Obstet Gynecol Scand* 2006;**85**(12):1463–7.

35. Jansen FW, Vredevoogd CB, van Ulzen K, et al. Complications of hysteroscopy: a prospective, multicenter study. *Obstet Gynecol* 2000;**96**:266–70.

36. Bradley LD. Complications in hysteroscopy: prevention, treatment and legal risk. *Curr Opin Obstet Gynecol* 2002;**14**:409–15.

37. Van Kerkvoorde TC, Veersema S, Timmermans S. Long-term complications of office hysteroscopy: analysis of 1028 cases. *J Minim Invasive Gynecol* 2012;**19**:494–7.

38. Thinkhamrop J, Laopaiboon M, Lumbiganon P. Prophylactic antibiotics for transcervical intrauterine procedures. *Cochrane Database Syst Rev* 2007;**3**: CD005637.

39. Cooper NA, Khan KS, Clark TJ. Local anaesthesia for pain control during outpatient hysteroscopy: systematic review and meta-analysis. *BMJ* 2010; **340**:c1130.

40. Umranikar S, Clark TJ, Saridogan E, et al. BSGE/ESGE guideline on management of fluid distension media in operative hysteroscopy. *Gynecol Surg* 2016 Nov 1; **13**(4):289–303.

41. Standards for Gynaecology. *Report of a Working Party.* London: RCOG; 2008. www.rcog .org.uk/globalassets/documents/ guidelines/wprgynstandards2008. (Accessed 16 July 2017)

42. Providing Quality Care for Women. *Standards for Gynaecology Care.* London: RCOG; 2016. www.rcog.org.uk/ globalassets/documents/ guidelines/working-party-reports/ gynaestandards.pdf (Accessed 16 July 2017).

43. Van Dongen H, Emanuel MH, Wolterbeek R, Trimbos J, Jansen FW. Hysteroscopic morcellator for removal of intrauterine polyps and myomas: a randomized controlled pilot study among residents in training. *J Minim Invasive Gynecol* 2008;**15**:466–71.

Chapter 15

Vaginal Hysterectomy with Fibroids

Swati Jha

15.1 Introduction

Vaginal hysterectomy is the surgical removal of the uterus through the vagina. The first reported vaginal hysterectomy, performed by Themison of Athens, dates back to 50 BC, and the procedure is also known to have been performed by Soranus of Greece in AD 120 [1]. There are also sporadic reports dating to the sixteenth century but with questionable outcomes. In 1670, Percival Willoughby, a male midwife, reported a case of a 46-year-old peasant, Faith Haworth, who was carrying a heavy load when her uterus prolapsed completely and, agitated by this, she pulled it out as far as possible and cut it off using a knife. The bleeding apparently settled soon after and she lived to old age albeit with a fistula [2]. The first detailed reports of planned vaginal hysterectomy were for carcinoma, performed by Langenbeck in 1813. After reporting the operation, he was disbelieved by his peers, and it was only when the patient died of old age 26 years later that she was subjected to a post-mortem, and it was confirmed that the uterus had been removed in its entirety. Sauter described a vaginal hysterectomy for cervical cancer in 1822. This is detailed in a commentary on the history of the procedure by Senn [3]. The early mortality from the procedure was very high, with a figure of 75% quoted by Senn. With developments in anaesthesia, instrumentation and antisepsis, this gradually decreased from 15% in 1886 to 2.5% in 1910 [2], and numbers were significantly lower than the figures for abdominal hysterectomy. In 1934, Noble Sproat Heaney of Chicago reported 627 vaginal hysterectomies resulting in only three deaths [4].

In current practice, the vaginal route is the preferred route of hysterectomy and has several advantages. The Cochrane review comparing routes of hysterectomy for benign gynaecological conditions [5] found that vaginal hysterectomy was superior to abdominal and laparoscopic hysterectomy, with a faster return to normal activities and fewer febrile episodes postoperatively. Where a vaginal hysterectomy is not feasible, other routes are recommended, with the laparoscopic route having advantages over the abdominal, but this is somewhat offset by longer operating time. There are, however, no advantages of the laparoscopic route to the vaginal route.

15.2 Indications

The vaginal hysterectomy is usually performed for benign conditions and is almost never performed in an emergency. It is usually carried out when conservative options have failed, depending on the underlying indication for the procedure. Common indications are similar to those for hysterectomy by other routes with the exception of pelvic organ prolapse and include:

Pelvic organ prolapse: Pelvic organ prolapse is caused by stretching and weakening of the ligamentous supports of the pelvic organs. This can affect the different compartments of the vagina involving the bladder, rectum or uterus. When the apical compartment is prolapsed, a vaginal hysterectomy remains the procedure of choice amongst most urogynaecologists, with 75% performing a vaginal hysterectomy and repair for a uterine prolapse [6].

Abnormal uterine bleeding: Menorrhagia, i.e. heavy uterine bleeding, is a common cause for a hysterectomy.

Fibroids: The symptoms caused by fibroids have been discussed in other chapters of this book. When conservative treatments fail, a woman may opt for a hysterectomy, and where appropriate, and depending on the size and location of the fibroids as well as uterine mobility, this can be done vaginally.

Cervical abnormalities: Pre-cancer abnormalities of the cervix that fail to resolve or recur after treatment can be an indication for a vaginal hysterectomy.

Endometrial hyperplasia: Endometrial hyperplasia is a precursor of endometrial cancer, and if it fails to respond to more conservative treatments, then it can be treated by a vaginal hysterectomy provided invasive cancer can be ruled out.

Chronic pelvic pain: When pain is due to adenomyosis, a vaginal hysterectomy may be indicated.

15.3 Preoperative Assessment

The indication for the hysterectomy should be evaluated preoperatively to determine if a vaginal hysterectomy is the best approach. Preoperatively, an assessment of the patient should take place to assess the menopausal status, size of the uterus, degree of mobility, adnexal pathology, obesity and degree of prolapse if this is present. Other factors such as the patient's cardiac status and the ability to tolerate anaesthesia must be taken into consideration.

A discussion regarding the pros and cons of removal of the tubes and ovaries should also take place. It is not routine practice to remove the ovaries during a vaginal hysterectomy, and elective removal is associated with pros and cons [7]. Alternatively, the tubes can be removed with conservation of the ovaries.

The presence of fibroids is not an automatic exclusion for a vaginal hysterectomy, and in the presence of prolapse this would still be the preferred route as better vaginal support can be achieved. Most clinicians would use a uterine size equivalent to a 16-week gravid uterus as the upper limit for attempting a vaginal hysterectomy, and beyond this size would revert to an abdominal approach. The location of the fibroids is an important determinant of whether the procedure will be feasible vaginally. A cervical fibroid can make a colpotomy difficult, and likewise large lateral fibroids can obstruct access to the uterine cornua and hamper the ability to safely secure the uterine vasculature.

An important assessment to be made prior to a vaginal hysterectomy, therefore, is the degree of pelvic support and uterine mobility. A vaginal approach is feasible if the uterus is mobile, and this can be assessed in the office setting with a Valsalva manoeuvre. In the presence of prolapse, a formal classification of the prolapse using the POP-Q [8] or its alternatives should be undertaken.

Vaginal access should be assessed based on the angle of the pubic arch. An assessment of the bony pelvis provides a guide to the degree of technical difficulty of the procedure. A gynaecoid pelvis usually has an adequate vaginal canal and a deep and wide posterior fornix, which improves surgical access to the uterus and placement of instruments, facilitating the vaginal approach.

Lastly, the breadth of the vaginal apex identifies if there is adequate access for a vaginal hysterectomy. If the apex is greater than 3 cm, access is usually adequate. This assessment is made by performing a bimanual examination and placing two fingers in the posterior fornix. A wider apex provides sufficient space for anterior and posterior entry and allows visualization of the vasculature.

Laboratory tests including haemoglobin, pregnancy test in the premenopausal patient and urinalysis to rule out underlying urinary tract infection should be undertaken. Previous smears should have been negative. Further tests may be required depending on underlying comorbidities. In patients with a large prolapse, an intravenous pyelogram is helpful to rule out hydronephrosis and assess ureteral function [9, 10] but does not change management.

15.4 Procedure

When a vaginal hysterectomy is performed, either there can be a coincidental finding of fibroids during surgery for prolapse or this may be known in advance due to prior investigations such as ultrasound scan. Irrespective of this, the technique of vaginal hysterectomy remains broadly the same as it would in the absence of fibroids. When fibroids are present, special manoeuvres may be required to facilitate removal. If it is known in advance that fibroids are present and these are likely to obstruct surgery, it is sensible to reduce their size either with the use of GnRH analogues or with medications such as uliprystal acetate. GnRH analogues can reduce the size of the uterus by 25–50%. In addition, fibroids can make patients anaemic, so it is beneficial to shrink the fibroids to improve haemoglobin levels before surgery. If there is a coincidental finding of fibroids during surgery and the uterus is too big, it may not be possible to remove it vaginally and an abdominal route will be required.

The decision to perform a vaginal hysterectomy when fibroids are present is usually because there is an element of prolapse and better support of the vaginal vault can be achieved vaginally than abdominally to prevent prolapse recurrence immediately after surgery, which is the main concern if an abdominal approach is used.

Increased uterine size per se is not a contraindication for performing a vaginal hysterectomy [11]. However, as they tend to be technically more difficult, surgeons undertaking these procedures should be adequately trained. There are several case series reported of vaginal hysterectomy in the presence of fibroids which show good outcomes [11–13].

The following steps describe the author's technique of performing a vaginal hysterectomy:

1. Once anaesthetized and in the dorsal lithotomy position, the patient is prepared and draped. An examination is performed to assess the degree of prolapse and defects of other compartments, the size of the uterus and its mobility, and whether or not the procedure is feasible vaginally or better performed abdominally. Most clinicians would use a 16-week-sized uterus as a cut-off for vaginal removal.

2. The cervix is grasped on both the anterior and posterior lip, using a vulsellum forceps. By gentle traction and massaging the uterosacrals, the descent of the uterus can be maximized.

3. Paracervical injection of 20 mL of Marcaine (0.5%) is useful for delineating the surgical planes, and reducing postoperative pain. The author's preference is to inject exclusively paracervically, but it is routine to inject around the uterosacrals, cardinal ligaments and the bladder pillars. Using infiltration with 1:200,000 adrenaline has the advantage of reduced blood loss during surgery but the disadvantage is that the spasm of the vessels caused by vasoconstrictors may mask bleeding from small vessels until the medication wears off and presents as postoperative haemorrhage.

4. With traction on the cervical lips, a circumferential incision is made extending this posteriorly to reach the pouch of Douglas (PoD). The author's preference is to use diathermy for this but a knife can be used. Anteriorly at the cervicovaginal junction, the full thickness of the mucosa is opened and posteriorly vaginal mucosa opened to reach the PoD. Counter-traction provided by the assistant using a lateral vaginal wall retractor is helpful in this dissection. It is important to avoid dissection too low on the cervix or too deep into the cervix anteriorly and posteriorly as this can cause more bleeding and make dissection difficult.

5. Once the circumferential incision is made, sharp dissection is used to dissect the underlying tissue to reach the cul-de-sac anteriorly and posteriorly.

6. The posterior peritoneum is identified and is held with forceps, and the PoD is opened by sharp dissection using scissors, ensuring there are no loops of bowel in it. A speculum can be inserted into the opened posterior cul-de-sac.

7. It is the author's preference to open the anterior cul-de-sac before application of clamps on the uterosacral. This ensures that the ureters are moved out of the operative field by dissecting the bladder up. Access to the peritoneal reflection may require blunt dissection to move the bladder out of the way. Through use of a retractor, the bladder is pushed upwards to identify the peritoneal reflection, and this is then opened to enter the vesicovaginal space. Opening the vesicovaginal fold of peritoneum requires sharp dissection using a scissors with the tips pointing towards the uterus. The peritoneal contents are identified and a retractor is left in place anteriorly once the fold of peritoneum is opened to avoid damage to the bladder till the anterior repair is scheduled to be performed or, when this is not planned, till the vault is due to be closed.

   Where access is not possible due to a failure to identify the peritoneal reflection, entry is delayed till the uterosacral has been clamped, cut and ligated.

8. Once both cul-de-sacs are opened, and whilst applying traction on the cervix, the clamps (the author's preferred is Zeppelins) are placed on the uterosacral, perpendicular to the uterine axis. The pedicle is cut and ligated. During ligation, this pedicle is transfixed to avoid slippage when applying traction for vault support at the end of the procedure. Once tied, the two ends of the ligature on the uterosacral are left long enough to attach to the vaginal mucosa and across the midline at the end of the operation. This reduces the incidence of vaginal vault prolapse [14].

9. The next pedicle is the uterine. Where the vesicouterine fold of peritoneum has not already been opened, it should be done at this point and prior to clamping of the uterine vessels.

Contralateral and downward traction is applied on the cervix, and, by incorporating the anterior and posterior reflections of the peritoneum, the clamp is applied over the uterine vessels. These are then cut and ligated. It is not usual to transfix this as it is a vascular pedicle. It is the author's practice to tie the uterine pedicle incorporating the uterosacral pedicle to secure any bleeders between the two pedicles, and also to ensure that the uterine does not slip.

10. The next pedicle in a normal-sized uterus is the tubo-ovarian pedicle. When the uterus is big, particularly with fibroids, it may be necessary to take one to two more pedicles before the tubo-ovarian can be clamped. If additional pedicles are required, they are clamped cut and ligated in the usual way until the tubo-ovarian pedicle can be reached. The tubo-ovarian pedicle is then clamped cut and ligated. This will usually include the round ligaments as well. It is the author's practice to transfix and double ligate this pedicle as it is usually quite big.

    The ovaries and tubes are inspected to rule out adnexal pathology at this point.

11. In the presence of fibroids and where access to the tubo-ovarian pedicles is obstructed by fibroids, it may be possible to shell these out at this point to reduce the size of the uterus. This may be required for multiple fibroids to allow access. Where it is not possible to shell them out but access to the tubo-ovarian pedicle is restricted, the alternative is to bisect the uterus (Figure 15.1).

    When the fibroids are fundal, enucleation is usually not required but the uterus may need more than the usual three pedicles for removal.

12. Once the uterus has been detached from all its attachments, it can be removed either by delivering the cervix first or by delivering the fundus posteriorly.

13. If adnexal removal is planned as part of the surgery, the round ligaments will need to be clamped cut and ligated separately. The peritoneum between the round ligament and the fallopian tube is excised, and by applying traction on the tubo-ovarian pedicle and drawing it into the operative field using atraumatic forceps, this manoeuvre will allow the infundibulopelvic ligament to be clamped, cut and tied, followed by delivery of the adnexa.

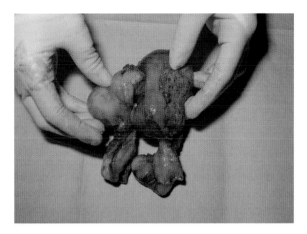

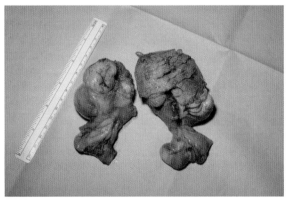

Figure 15.1 Fibroid uterus bisected to reduce uterine size.

14. Closure of the vault can be achieved in several ways. Some surgeons prefer to peritonize the anterior and posterior layers, incorporating the posterior layer as high as possible to close the enterocele sac. This is followed by separate closure of the vaginal mucosa either vertically or horizontally.

15. The author's preference is to start closure posteriorly in the midline at the 6 o'clock position, incorporating both the vaginal mucosa and peritoneum, with closure of the transverse opening of the vaginal vault vertically using a continuous locking stitch. This closes the enterocele sac while closing the posterior cul-de-sac. The last stitch at the 3 and 9 o'clock positions is used to incorporate the uterosacrals on both sides, thereby accomplishing a McCall's culdoplasty for further vault support.

16. Where there has been difficulty with access and bleeding in excess of the usual, as well as in

premenopausal women or women with fibroids, the author inserts a drain (using either a large-bore Foley catheter or a Robinson drain for this purpose) into the vaginal vault. The use of drains in routine vaginal hysterectomy has failed to show a benefit [15], but in well-selected cases this reduces postoperative pyrexia and vaginal vault haematoma formation.

17. When a vaginal wall repair is required for concurrent cystocele, this is completed before closure of the anterior vaginal wall.

18. The author's preference is to insert a pack in the vagina overnight and to leave the catheter in overnight when only a hysterectomy is done, but it may be required for longer when an anterior repair has also been done.

19. Postoperative analgesia and fluid management is necessary. Even with minimal bowel manipulation, the bowel tends to be sluggish and there can be nausea and loss of appetite. Early commencement of oral fluids and diet when the patient is able to tolerate this allows for intravenous fluid administration to be limited to the first operative day.

It is unusual to require a patient-controlled analgesia pump (PCA) following a vaginal hysterectomy and usually oral analgesia is sufficient.

15.5 Complications

The commonest complication of a vaginal hysterectomy is postoperative bleeding. This can present vaginally or with deteriorating vital signs manifesting as low blood pressure, rapid pulse and a falling urinary output. Vaginal bleeding usually represents bleeding from the vaginal cuff or vascular pedicles. When there is no obvious bleeding, the bleeding may be intra-abdominal or retroperitoneal. Abdominal bleeding may present with abdominal distension and retroperitoneal bleed with flank tenderness. In any case, attention to assessing the amount of bleeding, replacing lost blood volume, stabilizing the patient and controlling ongoing bleeding may require a return to operating theatres.

When bleeding is from the vagina, the cuff can be assessed and haemostasis can be achieved by a few stitches, which may be achieved without anaesthetic. If, however, the bleeding is coming from above the cuff, a CT scan helps delineate the location of the

haematoma. A retroperitoneal bleed can be managed conservatively and will usually tamponade, forming a haematoma which will eventually be resorbed. The risk with a haematoma is the development of an infection which will necessitate further surgery. Where there is brisk bleeding, it may be possible to perform selective angiographic embolization.

When there is intraperitoneal bleeding, general anaesthetic may be required for vaginal examination and/or an exploratory laparotomy. If bleeding sites are identified vaginally, these can be ligated; however, if it is not possible to identify the source of bleeding, an abdominal approach will be required. The abdominal exploration should be performed when the patient is stable, and though there is the added morbidity of further anaesthetic and an abdominal incision, it avoids further deterioration and formation of a pelvic abscess later. Once sufficient exposure is obtained, the clots should be evacuated and the pelvis examined systematically to identify the bleeding vessels, which can then be ligated. Where it is difficult to localize bleeding to a specific bleeding point, ligation of the hypogastric arteries may be required. Once haemostasis is achieved, the pelvis should be drained using a closed system.

Postoperative infection is a common complication following a vaginal hysterectomy and varying rates are reported. Infection can be due to pelvic cellulitis, pelvic abscess, infected haematoma or vaginal cuff cellulitis. When there are signs of infection, other causes should be ruled out and examination of the urine, lungs and pelvis should be performed. The diagnosis of pelvic infection is usually one of exclusion. This can be associated with a rise in temperature with or without physical findings. When there is a rise in temperature, parenteral antibiotics may be required. When this fails to address the elevated temperature, the possibility of a pelvic abscess must be considered. This may need drainage.

Other complications that can arise during a vaginal hysterectomy include visceral injury either to the urinary tract or to the bowel. If identified at the time of surgery, this can be adequately repaired; however, when missed, this can cause fistulation and the need for further surgery.

15.6 Conclusion

The modern gynaecologist has so many possible routes of performing a hysterectomy that the art of performing a vaginal hysterectomy is gradually being lost. The vaginal hysterectomy is the oldest route of hysterectomy and should be the default setting for benign disease. Ideally, the gynaecologist should be able to undertake any of the routes and patient selection will be based on a range of factors. Adequate patient selection and good caseload determines the success of the individual approaches.

References

1. Sutton C. Past, present, and future of hysterectomy. *J Minim Invasive Gynecol* 2010 Jul;**17**(4):421–35.

2. Sutton C. Hysterectomy: a historical perspective. *Baillieres Clin Obstet Gynaecol* 1997 Mar;**11**(1):1–22.

3. Senn N. The early history of vaginal hysterectomy. *J Am Med Assoc* 1895 Sep.

4. Baskett TF. Hysterectomy: evolution and trends. *Best Pract Res Clin Obstet Gynaecol* 2005 Jun;**19**(3):295–305.

5. Aarts JW, Nieboer TE, Johnson N et al. Surgical approach to hysterectomy for benign gynaecological disease. *Cochrane Database Syst Rev* 2015 Aug 12;(8):CD003677.

6. Jha S, Cutner A, Moran P. The UK national prolapse survey: 10 years on. *Int Urogynecol J* 2018;29:795–801 Sep 15.

7. Erekson EA, Martin DK, Ratner ES. Oophorectomy: the debate between ovarian conservation and elective oophorectomy. *Menopause* 2013 Jan;**20**(1):110–14.

8. Bump RC, Mattiasson A, Bo K et al. The standardization of terminology of female pelvic organ prolapse and pelvic floor dysfunction. *Am J Obstet Gynecol* 1996 Jul;**175**(1):10–17.

9. Cruikshank SH, Pixley RL. Methods of vaginal cuff closure and preservation of vaginal depth during transvaginal hysterectomy. *Obstet Gynecol* 1987 Jul;**70**(1):61–3.

10. Cruikshank SH, Kovac SR. Role of the uterosacral-cardinal ligament complex in protecting the ureter during vaginal hysterectomy. *Int J Gynaecol Obstet* 1993 Feb;**40**(2):141–4.

11. Quinlan D, Quinlan DK. Vaginal hysterectomy for the enlarged fibroid uterus: a report of 85 cases. *J Obstet Gynaecol Can* 2010 Oct;**32**(10):980–3.

12. Magos A, Bournas N, Sinha R, Richardson RE, O'Connor H. Vaginal hysterectomy for the large uterus. *Br J Obstet Gynaecol* 1996 Mar;**103**(3):246–51.

13. Sahin Y. Vaginal hysterectomy and oophorectomy in women with 12–20 weeks' size uterus. *Acta Obstet Gynecol Scand* 2007;**86**(11):1359–69.

14. Cruikshank SH. Preventing posthysterectomy vaginal vault prolapse and enterocele during vaginal hysterectomy. *Am J Obstet Gynecol* 1987 Jun;**156**(6):1433–40.

15. Dua A, Galimberti A, Subramaniam M, Popli G, Radley S. The effects of vault drainage on postoperative morbidity after vaginal hysterectomy for benign gynaecological disease: a randomised controlled trial. *BJOG* 2012 Feb;**119**(3):348–53.

Chapter 16

Leiomyosarcoma
Implications for the Treatment of Fibroids

Elizabeth A. Pritts

16.1 Introduction

The risk of finding an occult leiomyosarcoma (LMS) at surgery for presumed leiomyomas and subsequent outcomes for patients who have these tumours morcellated is a subject of conflict in gynaecology today. This dispute arose in 2013 from a single case in which a physician underwent surgery for fibroids and power morcellation was utilized. This physician ultimately was diagnosed with an LMS and she and her family began a media campaign and created a public forum to effect a ban on power morcellation. They argued that prevalence of these occult tumours was much higher than originally believed, and the use of power morcellation worsened outcomes. Originally, a friend of the physician performed a cursory meta-analysis using incomplete data suggesting that the rate of uterine sarcoma in women having surgery for presumed fibroids was 1 in 323. The US Food and Drug Administration (FDA) used similar but slightly different methodology and found a prevalence of 1 in 352 for uterine sarcoma, and 1 in 498 for leiomyosarcoma [1]. Neither analysis has been published in a peer-reviewed journal, and both represent incomplete and biased attempts at establishing a prevalence rate.

The FDA also performed a systematic review of the literature addressing outcomes after morcellation of these occult tumours. They found worse outcomes for women after 'power' morcellation compared to intact removal. In the majority of the cases they reported upon, the tumours were morcellated by 'scalpel' or by 'hand'. Nevertheless, their numbers are repeatedly cited and are used as the argument against the use of *power* morcellation.

Two more groups then undertook meta-analyses and systematic reviews to address prevalence and outcomes. Both of these groups found very different prevalence rates and outcome data after morcellation compared with the FDA [2, 3].

What follows is a historical perspective and review of some fundamentals of evidence in medicine. The morcellation controversy will then be addressed and the best available evidence will be provided regarding true prevalence and outcomes after morcellation. This will be followed by a closer look at the reasons for disparities in the findings of the studies.

16.2 The History of Evidence-Based Medicine and Gynaecology

Obstetrics and gynaecology has long been viewed as the specialty that utilizes the lowest-quality research in formulating treatments for patients. In 1979, Archie Cochrane (of the Cochrane Library), awarded obstetrics and gynaecology the 'wooden spoon' for being the least evidence-based medical specialty. The origins of this prize stem from a tradition upheld at Cambridge University until the early twentieth century: an actual 'wooden spoon' was presented each year to the student with the lowest score on the mathematics examination. The implication was that the student was better equipped to become a cook than a scholar. Since this time, our specialty has not only produced better-quality research, but has begun to embrace evidence-based medicine. However, there are still examples of 'junk science' or 'emotional science' being utilized to influence the medical care of women.

Prior to 1980, Bendectin, an antiemetic made of vitamin B6 and an antihistamine, was used in early pregnancy for hyperemesis gravidarum. In 1975, a child was born to a woman that had used many medications, including Bendectin, in her pregnancy. The child had multiple anomalies, and she placed the blame on Bendectin.

This initially resulted in what can be called a legal blitzkrieg with thousands of plaintiffs claiming fetal anomalies due to this drug. This was rapidly followed by a large number of epidemiologic publications of poor quality. The initial reports supported the initial complaint, and due to the publicity of the cases and the cost of litigation, Bendectin was removed from the market. Gradually, however, better data, not influenced by special interests, began to surface. When the dust eventually settled, in fact, there was no convincing evidence that Bendectin was responsible for any type of birth defect. Bendectin has now resurfaced as a category B drug under the name Diclegis. It has been studied more thoroughly than any other drug for pregnant women, and has substantially decreased the suffering of women with hyperemesis gravidarum.

A second glaring example occurred less than 10 years later: the silicone breast implant controversy. Several women that had placement of silicone implants blamed them for autoimmune diseases they acquired. The FDA reviewed the available data and found no evidence to support the claim. However, as with Bendectin, a flurry of poor-quality studies and case reports surfaced, as well as a plethora of 'expert' clinical opinion, supporting the finding of harm with the use of these implants. In 2000, a report was published by the Institute of Medicine with conclusions drawn from high-quality evidence, showing no association between the implantations and autoimmune disease (or any other disease for that matter). However, the court of public opinion had already convened. As researchers that championed evidence-based medicine began speaking out against the claims of harm, they were harassed and threatened with lawsuits. Ultimately, Dow Corning, the makers of the implant, filed bankruptcy, and silicone-based medical technology and research came to a standstill.

16.3 The Current Controversy

Prior to April 2014, there were case reports of occult LMS and single-institution retrospective chart reviews as well as expert opinion regarding the true prevalence of these disorders, but no published meta-analysis or prospective database existed. In April 2014, the FDA issued a warning regarding the use of power morcellation during surgeries for presumed uterine fibroids. They presented an internal meta-analysis and systematic review of the literature. They claimed much higher prevalence rates of occult LMSs than previously presumed and worse outcomes for women when morcellation was utilized during surgery [1].

Since that time, two groups have performed and published meta-analyses addressing the prevalence of these occult tumours and systematic reviews exploring outcomes after unintentional morcellation [2, 3]. Both analyses used more accurate analytic methodology than that of the FDA, and results from these studies were similar to one another, but very different than those claimed by the FDA.

16.4 The Basics of Evidence-Based Medicine

Historically, we have relied less upon science and more upon opinion to formulate treatment plans. Until the early 1990s, clinicians solved clinical problems by considering their own experiences in treating the disease, by considering the underlying physiology and by referring to a textbook or local expert. This meant relying on our veteran physicians; their expert opinion ruled all. An older physician always had the last word when novice physicians were attempting to treat patients. However, attempts to validate this model failed repeatedly. Beginning in the 1970s, there was awareness of the value of answers generated via clinical research rather than mere expert opinion. This was further bolstered by a more thorough understanding of the different types of clinical trials and the relative value of each in determining optimal clinical pathways. It became widely recognized that randomized trials are the gold standard for evaluating clinical issues. Cohort studies are of secondary importance, with prospective data collection deemed more valuable than retrospective review. The hierarchical system of study value gradually became a central tenet of evidence-based medicine. It was clearly successful in that relying on our physiologic rationale continually failed to predict the results of randomized trials. This led to criticism of the practice of evidence-based medicine from those in the position of the authority (more accepted by younger, inexperienced physicians; helping them to have some credibility in their newfound field). Although it is hard for practitioners to admit, we are the largest source of bias in forming treatment plans for our patients [4].

As stated above, retrospective cohort studies are relatively low in the hierarchy of trusted outcomes. They are generally used as a step in the creation of scientifically valid patient treatment regimens. Retrospective cohort studies have numerous inherent biases and unmeasured confounders which serve to reduce their reliability.

An example of a bias at work is in the collection of prevalence rates, affecting the results in either direction. For example, someone with an occult LMS may have her chart sent directly to the hospital risk management department, rendering it inaccessible to the researchers. This could falsely lower prevalence rates. Conversely, retrospective studies can be initiated due to an index case. When the index case is included in the prevalence calculations, the resulting bias potentially can overestimate the rate of prevalence. By restricting or extending the range of years included in the chart mining, the numerator (or overall population count) could easily be manipulated. This was actually the case in several studies that have been included in several recent meta-analyses. The most significant came from a referral centre that identified an occult LMS during a surgery for presumed fibroids. The index case was included in the study, but the retrospective chart review went back only 2 years [5]. The prevalence rate for this particular study was disparate to other studies that included longer study periods and larger populations.

The origin of retrospective datasets may also confound results. Referral centres are different from the average medical centre in that patients are often much sicker or suffer from unusual maladies. Thus, clinical studies performed in such centres often draw from patient populations radically different from the general populations seen in community hospitals. When dealing with prevalence rates, relatively rare diagnoses are overrepresented, as is disease severity.

The best available evidence comes from studies in which the data are prospectively collected. It includes randomized trials and/or prospective cohort data. In comparing retrospective versus prospectively collected data, retrospective data collection is measurably less accurate than prospective collection. In some instances, more than 50% of the data is unavailable if collected in a retrospective fashion [6].

In prospective investigations, the data collection is begun at a predefined time point, consecutive cases are included and the data are uniformly collected on all patients until the study is completed. This lessens the confounding factors such as selection bias, patient exclusion and referral bias.

16.5 The Utility of the Meta-Analysis

Rigorously conducted systematic reviews and meta-analyses are widely recognized as among the highest standards of evidence for informed medical decision making [7]. This technique involves combining results of multiple studies in an attempt to discern a single best pathway or rate. With rare events, this may be the only reliable and accessible approach to formulate sound medical treatments.

Some have argued that prevalence rates for occult LMSs can be calculated from the current literature using the crude method of summing number of reported cases of disease, and dividing this by the total number of surgeries performed. However, the combination of data from multiple populations is not the same as data from a single large population undergoing sampling. The heterogeneity among studies for inclusion and exclusion, confounders, and even definitions of risk factors and outcomes leads to tremendous bias in calculating a crude prevalence [8, 9] Crude calculations are only appropriate if (1) each study was an independent and identically distributed measure of the overall population and (2) the variance of each study's estimate is known. These conditions are rarely if ever met.

Heterogeneity among studies in a meta-analysis also dictates the type of analysis performed. When studies investigate the same population with the same research questions and structure, a fixed effects model can be used. The clear majority of most studies in meta-analyses are not designed to estimate similar populations and with the same questions, so some degree of statistical heterogeneity is likely. A random effects meta-analysis corrects for design differences.

There are also several random effects models from which to choose. Many choose the classical model, but this model does not correct for variation in study size. The FDA in their meta-analysis chose to use this model. Bayesian random effects meta-analysis has been used extensively for clinical decision making and policy analysis. This type of analysis is much more robust and automatically corrects for variation in study size. It has proven to be the method of choice for combining multiple studies to determine rates of rarely occurring diseases.

16.5.1 Prevalence: The Data

The meta-analysis presented by the FDA was executed by the Senior Advisor in the Office of Planning and Policy and has yet to be formally published. The FDA initially identified 41 studies, but only 9 met inclusion/exclusion criteria. Eight of the studies were retrospective; only one included prospectively collected data. Nineteen occult leiomyosarcomas were identified from their dataset comprised of 9,160 uterine fibroid surgeries, and the FDA utilized the classical meta-analytic model. The estimated prevalence rate of occult leiomyosarcoma was 2.01/1,000 or 1 occult leiomyosarcoma for every 498 surgeries for presumed fibroids [1].

The next meta-analysis was completed by our group, utilizing comparable study dates, from 1980 to early 2014. We included data from studies where pathology was confirmed for every study participant. Our database, however, was stratified based upon the quality of evidence. Sensitivity analyses confirming the validity and robustness of our calculations were also performed. We initially identified 4,864 candidate studies; excluding 3,844 after abstract review. The remaining 1,020 manuscripts were reviewed in their entirety. One hundred thirty-three publications fit the inclusion/exclusion criteria and comprised our evidence base. We identified 32 total occult leiomyosarcomas in 30,193 surgeries.

We initially analysed the information using only the prospectively collected data. These data were extracted from 64 published prospective analyses: 38 as prospective cohorts and 26 as part of randomized clinical trials. The women were undergoing a combination of hysterectomy and myomectomy. These analyses encompassed 5,223 women, with 3 leiomyosarcomas identified postsurgically. The prevalence of occult leiomyosarcoma using only data derived from prospective studies was 0.12 per 1,000 surgeries. Stated alternatively, surgeons can expect to find one occult leiomyosarcoma per each 8,300 surgeries for presumed benign uterine fibroids, with a 97.5% probability of being less than 0.75 per 1,000 surgeries.

Seventy published analyses with retrospective cohorts also qualified for our analysis, encompassing a total of 24,970 patients. There was a mix of patients undergoing myomectomy and hysterectomy. Of these, 29 were noted to have leiomyosarcomas postsurgically. The prevalence of occult leiomyosarcoma using all of the data derived from both prospective and retrospective databases was 0.51/1,000 surgeries. When including all the data, we confirmed that surgeons could expect to find one occult leiomyosarcoma per each 2,000 surgeries performed for fibroids, with a 97.5% probability of being less than 0.98 per 1,000 surgeries [2]. These data were reported to the FDA during the medical device special meeting in July of 2014, and subsequently published in peer-reviewed journals. If only hysterectomies and no myomectomies

are included in the analysis, the rate remains similar at 0.55 per 1,000 surgeries (CI 0.06–1.3) or 1 in 1,818 procedures (D. Olive and D. Vanness, personal communication).

The third meta-analysis to estimate prevalence of occult leiomyosarcomas comes from an analysis by the Agency for Healthcare Research and Quality (AHRQ) of the Department of Health and Human Services that was published on 14 December 2017. They confirmed and validated our search analysis then expanded the search to include data published after our cut-off date in 2014. They were able to identify 539 more candidate publications and found another 24 retrospective studies, 2 prospective studies and a single randomized controlled trial that fit exclusion and inclusion criteria. They included studies with women undergoing either myomectomy and/or hysterectomy for presumed benign fibroid tumours where pathology results were available for all women in the publication. An additional 71,153 more retrospective cases were analysed along with the 24,970 cases in our original database. An additional 34,842 prospective cases were added to our original 5,230. Using the Bayesian analytical model, the predicted prevalence rate using only the prospective data was 2.1 per 10,000 surgeries or 1 occult LMS per every 4,761 surgeries and 8.5 per 10,000 surgeries when looking at retrospective data, or 1 occult tumour per 1,176 surgeries. They initially combined both prospective and retrospective datasets, but chose to separate them due to statistical heterogeneity making the approximations markedly different. Sub-analyses were performed using data that excluded hysteroscopy as well as restricting the analyses to prospective data in which they had high confidence of histopathologic evaluation for all subjects. Using all of the above exclusions, a prevalence risk of 0.5 occult LMSs per 10,000 surgeries or 1 occult tumour in each 20,000 surgeries was found [3].

Taken together, the more comprehensive meta-analyses reveal an estimated prevalence of LMSs in surgeries for presumed leiomyomas that is substantially less than that previously estimated by the FDA.

16.6 Exploring the Disparities in the Data

The variation in outcomes between the initial FDA analysis and the ensuing meta-analyses can be ascribed to both the statistical methodology employed and the base of evidence identified.

Classical meta-analytic techniques were utilized by the FDA, while Bayesian techniques were utilized by our group and the AHRQ. This accounted for 8% of the variation between studies.

The remaining 92% of the difference is attributed to the datasets themselves. The search terms used in the two comprehensive meta-analyses included any studies in which surgery was performed for presumed benign fibroids with histopathology explicitly provided for every subject. This strategy yielded 134 studies for our dataset and 160 for the AHRQ dataset. In contrast, to obtain their evidence, the FDA performed a targeted search using the search terms 'uterine cancer' AND 'hysterectomy or myomectomy' AND 'incidental cancer or uterine prolapse, pelvic pain, uterine bleeding, and uterine fibroids'. By using the conjunction 'and' during their search, the term 'uterine cancer' was necessary in the title, abstract, or key words. Those studies not including the search term 'uterine cancer' in title, abstract or listed keywords would be overlooked. Indeed, this was the case: eight of the nine studies found in the FDA database contained at least one LMS; the ninth study used the term malignancy in the abstract.

We note that in the FDA's review of the nine studies referenced, eight were retrospective studies and one was a report from prospectively collected data, while all nine in the unpublished dataset were retrospective. Such a preponderance of retrospective reports raises concerns of significant ascertainment bias in the resulting prevalence rate. The subsequent two analyses contained a sufficient number of both retrospective and prospective studies to allow analyses restricted to each, producing what we believe to be the most appropriate evidence base from which to calculate prevalence.

Another difference lies in the fact that only studies with more than 100 subjects were included in the evidence base compiled by the FDA, while the unpublished work required 50 subjects for inclusion; their reasoning was that this would reduce bias from smaller studies. Recognizing the arbitrary nature of any predefined size threshold, our preferred approach included eligible studies of all sizes, while using a statistical model that allowed weighting of each study according to its size and degree of statistical heterogeneity. This was possible due to the collaboration of both published groups with professors of biostatistics that specialize in analysis of complex clinical research and meta-analyses. The

FDA did not have a statistician collaborate in their endeavours.

Third, the FDA and the unpublished analysis included only studies that exclusively examined procedures performed for presumed leiomyomas; if multiple indications were listed by the author of the study, it was excluded from their evidence base and was unavailable for analysis. However, many publications containing multiple indications for surgery contained unequivocal information about those women with a primary surgical indication of fibroids and the data were easily extractable. They were included in the published evidence bases if the patients undergoing hysterectomy or myomectomy for fibroids were clearly identified, if histopathology was performed on all cases, and if results were explicitly provided.

Fourth, the FDA and non-published group excluded all non-English articles from consideration, a decision that makes reviews much easier to perform but is highly elitist and incomplete. We felt the inclusion of non-English publications made for a more comprehensive review of the subject, and thus included studies regardless of the language of publication. The AHRQ and our group were able to expand our database further by including all languages of publication as long as they were in peer-reviewed journals. This also leads to a more real-world application of the data.

The FDA included one non-peer-reviewed abstract and one letter to the editor in their dataset. We excluded these and other similar data, restricting our analysis to peer-reviewed publications containing five or more applicable subjects. Parenthetically, the letter to the editor included in the FDA evidence base was written in English. The original data were reported in their entirety in a French language publication. We excluded the letter to the editor, but found the original, peer-reviewed publication and included it in our evidence base. There were three LMSs presented in this study.

In examining our own data, we found that seven of the leiomyosarcomas defined were inconsistent with the World Health Organization (WHO) criteria utilized to diagnose a tumour as such. The criteria used for classification are the so-called Stanford criteria [10] published in 1994 and later adopted by the WHO [11]. These criteria indicate that a uterine smooth muscle tumour with coagulative tumour cell necrosis (not hyaline necrosis) is an LMS. If no such necrosis exists, then the diagnosis is made only if the

Table 16.1 Tumours inconsistent with World Health Organization 2003 Leiomyosarcoma Criteria (benign with no metastatic potential) [2]

Author	Leiomyoma subtype	Age (years)	Pathology	Recurrence
Leibsohn [12]	Atypical	36	6 mitoses/10 HPF, 'poorly demarcated', cellular atypia	NED 6 months
	Atypical	48	7 mitoses/10 HPF, cellular atypia	NED 16 months
Parker [13]	Atypical	30	Irregular infiltrative borders, mild nuclear atypia, 5–8 mitoses/10 HPF	NED 'Years'
Seki [14]	Mitotically active	33	6 mitoses/10 HPF, NO cellular atypia	NED 11 months
	Mitotically active	34	5 mitoses/10 HPF, NO cellular atypia	NED 57 months
	Mitotically active	43	8 mitoses/10 HPF, NO cellular atypia	NED 61 months
	Mitotically active	43	9 mitoses/10 HPF, NO cellular atypia	NED 92 months

HPF, high-powered field; NED, no evidence of disease.

mitotic index is ≥10 mitoses per 10 high-power fields and there is diffuse, moderate to severe cytological atypia. As seen in Table 16.1, seven of these did not fit criteria [12–14].

In order to be very conservative in our estimates, we analysed these tumours as LMSs. In the several cases in which no histopathology was specified for the LMSs, we included these as identified by the authors.

Based upon the best available evidence, the prevalence of occult leiomyosarcoma is much less than estimated by the FDA [2].

16.7 Outcomes after Morcellation

Some have argued that even if the prevalence is low, 'power' morcellation of these tumours leads to worse outcomes. In this case, power morcellators should be prohibited.

One author recently suggested that 'it has been established that motorized morcellation of uterine leiomyosarcoma during surgery adversely affects disease-free survival and overall survival' [15]. The warning presented by the FDA also was focused upon the dangers of power morcellation.

The FDA identified 196 studies and found 7 that fit inclusion and exclusion criteria for outcome investigations. Only six studies addressed leiomyosarcoma in particular and five contained comparative data. Outcomes consisted of (1) dissemination, (2) recurrence, and (3) disease-free or overall survival compared with women that had their tumour removed intact.

They identified two studies addressing the risk of dissemination [16, 17]. The first author, Dr George, found that of the seven women that had power morcellation of occult leiomyosarcoma and then completion surgery for staging immediately thereafter, two of the seven (28%) had disseminated peritoneal disease.

For the second author [17], the findings were not as straightforward. Seidman and his group identified 14 cases of atypical smooth muscle tumours in women undergoing surgery for fibroids. Of those 14, 9 (64%) had dissemination if completion surgery was performed. They identified seven cases of leiomyosarcoma, and four of those showed dissemination. They used this number to fuel their argument.

However, upon further evaluation of the publication, this was not the case. Their conclusion was that unexpected diagnoses occurred in 1.2% of cases using power morcellation (12/1,091). These tumours included one cellular leiomyoma, six atypical leiomyomas, three smooth muscle tumours of unknown malignant potential, one endometrial stromal sarcoma and a single LMS. They went on to explain that 'when examining follow-up laparoscopies, from both in-house and consultation cases, disseminated disease occurred in 64% of all tumours … and 4/7 LMS. Only disseminated LMS, however, was associated with mortality.'

However, when looking only at the 1,091 in-house surgeries, there were 12 atypical tumours identified, but only 7 with follow-up surgery, and only 4/7 had dissemination (57%). The single endometrial stromal sarcoma and the single LMS identified in-house did NOT have dissemination and had NO evidence of disease at 34 and 42 months, respectively.

How then, did the authors account for the identification of seven leiomyosarcomas, with four disseminated at the time of completion surgery, and mortality linked only with an LMS diagnosis?

They included six more women that had been referred to the centre and added those to the numerator in their calculation, without including the number of women with LMS *not* referred. Two women with power-morcellated LMS were referred at 13 and 16 months. One of the two women referred at recurrence was deceased by publication. The remaining four women were referred within 1 month post their initial surgeries. Two had dissemination at follow-up surgery, two did not. The mortality rate was 50% for each of these groups.

In this paper, power morcellation of these occult tumours is censured for worse outcomes, particularly for LMS. However, the actual evidence does not support this assertion as only the in-house data can be used for analysis due to the lack of a denominator for referred cases of LMS; that is, while six cases of LMS were referred, we have no idea how many were *not* referred. One woman at their institution had an occult LMS power morcellated and that woman had no evidence of dissemination during follow-up surgery nor disease at 42 months. It is not possible to make any assertions regarding dissemination of tumours based upon this evidence.

Next the FDA looked at recurrence data following both power and non-power morcellation of LMS. They gleaned data from George et al. [16] with 58 patients, Park et al. [18] with 56 patients, and Morice et al. [19] with 53 patients. Park and George had statistically significant odds for local recurrence at 9.4 (CI 2.6–33.7), and 5.3 (CI 1.4–19.7), but Morice did not. In his study, he compared recurrence rates for LMS at 3 and 6 months. None of the 17 women with or the 36 women without morcellation had recurrence at 3 months, and 1/15 with and 5/36 without morcellation had recurrence at 6 months (non-significant [NS]).

Only George and Park provided data regarding disease-free survival or overall survival. Both authors found lower disease-free states following morcellation with odds at 0.3 (0.1–0.7) and 0.4 (0.2–1.0), respectively. Overall survival rates, however, were significantly lower only for Park, with odds of 0.3 (0.1–0.95).

Our group also looked at the data in a systematic review and identified 4,864 papers, and excluded 4,804 through evaluation of the title or abstract [20]. Sixty papers were evaluated in full, and 16 with outcomes data were included. They were categorized as to whether and how they addressed the principal question of the outcomes after inadvertent morcellation compared with women with tumour removed intact.

During evaluation of the data, it became clear that 3 of the 16 authors published data on overlapping patient cohorts. The studies covered equivalent dates, and came from the same institutions. Since we had no means to differentiate the patient populations, we suspect that we do not have unique patient data. Nonetheless, all datasets were analysed as if they were exclusive. See Table 16.2 [15–17].

We identified six studies in which comparison data were available, three already identified by the FDA and three additional investigations. All but one were retrospective. Due to the small numbers of patients and the heterogeneity of studies, no pooled analyses could be performed. Some studies did

Table 16.2 Authors with overlapping patient cohorts

Author, Morcellation type	Study dates	Institutions	'All' patients treated at their institution	Outcome
George [16] Power/Hand	2007–12	Brigham & Women's, Mass General, Dana Farber	Yes	Total population recurrence and survival
Oduyebo [15] Power/Hand	2005–12	Brigham & Women's, Mass General, Dana Farber	Yes	Individual patient upstaging and survival
Seidman [17] Power	2005–10	Brigham & Women's		Individual patient upstaging

Table 16.3 Confirmed power morcellation cases

Author	Power	Non-power or unknown	En bloc
Einstein et al. [21]	2	1 (abdominal fragmentation)	2
George et al. [16]	?	19 (scalpel or power morcellation hysterectomy)	39
Leibsohn et al. [12]	0	1 (abdominal myomectomy)	4
Morice et al. [19]	?	17 (biopsy, hysteroscopy, myomectomy, hysterectomy)	36
Park et al. [18]	1	24 (18 laparoscopic assisted vaginal hysterectomy, 1 vaginal hysterectomy, 5 mini-laparotomy myomectomies)	31
Perri et al. [22]	0	16 (2 laparoscopic hysterectomies, 4 hysteroscopies, 2 'injury', 4 myomectomies)	21

3/81 with confirmed power morcellation.
42/81 with confirmed non-power morcellation
36/81 with unknown type or mixed type of morcellation.

confirm that en bloc uterine removal conferred better outcomes for women compared with morcellation. However, that conclusion was 'tenuous and difficult to quantify'.

When further evaluating the study by George et al., it appears that the morcellation was performed with a 'spinning blade or a scalpel', without delineation of exact numbers. The results are relevant in regards to morcellation in general, not for any specific method of morcellation.

When addressing the data reported by Dr Park, he arguably had the best-quality data as it came from a cancer registry where prospective entry of much information is likely. The data come from a referral centre, however, with many women referred at an unknown time from original surgery, and only one of the 25 underwent power morcellation.

Morice, on the other hand, made no mention of type of morcellation, and only had a follow-up of 6 months, again without much meaningful information.

The additional studies we found included work from Einstein et al. [21], Leibsohn et al. [12], and Perri et al. [22]. Einstein published results of five women who were referred for treatment of leiomyosarcoma to their centre after power morcellation, tumour fragmentation, or en bloc removal of the specimen by hysterectomy. The outcomes were comparable between the groups.

Leibsohn reported on five patients with unsuspected leiomyosarcoma – four had hysterectomies, and one had an abdominal myomectomy. Of the four patients with en bloc removal, three were deceased at 6, 8 and 12 months. The patient with removal of her leiomyosarcoma via abdominal myomectomy was alive with disease at an unspecified time.

Lastly, Perri compared 21 women who underwent abdominal hysterectomy with 16 women in whom the LMS was disrupted: the overall survival was better with en bloc uterine removal (OR 2.8; 95% CI 1.02–7.67). The women undergoing morcellation had a variety of techniques used, but none were via power morcellation.

A recurring theme noted in our evaluation of the data was the lack of power morcellation cases. Only three cases of the 81 included in our analysis confirmed utilization of power morcellation. A full 42 women underwent morcellation with sharp instrumentation or fragmentation, and the remaining 36 cases included mixed groups without identification of type. This implies that any form of occult tumour morcellation may be injurious. See Table 16.3 [12, 16, 18, 19, 21, 22].

16.8 Outcomes after Power or Scalpel Morcellation

Our group, as well as the AHRQ, were obliged to ask the next question: Is there a variation in outcomes between simple sharp morcellation or fragmentation of tissue compared with power morcellation?

The only study we found comparing morcellation types was by Oduyebo and colleagues [15], who examined 15 patients with occult LMS that underwent morcellation, 10 by electromechanical means and 5 by hand or scalpel. Due to limited numbers and heterogeneity of stages and treatment approaches, no assessment could be made.

As an alternative, we collected data from publications that included type of morcellation and length of survival. Thirty-two such cases were found in various studies, small series and case reports. Of these, 24 surgeries employed power morcellation, and 8 hand or scalpel. Nine of 24 were deceased after power morcellation (follow-up 3–61 months) and 2 of 8 deceased after hand morcellation (length of follow-up 1–72 months). Life table analysis comparing these two datasets showed no significant difference in the two, no great surprise given the paucity of data [20].

We then identified 25 cases in which upstaging data were available. We identified 27 women that had staging surgery completed, with 11 upstaged between 2 and 36 months after original surgery. Upstaging rates were not significantly different regardless of the type of morcellation. See Figure 16.1.

Subsequent to our systematic review, the AHRQ identified a total of 16 studies with evaluable data for survival after power morcellation, hand morcellation or en bloc removal of these tumours. They also identified 16 studies with data regarding disease progression.

The AHRQ addressed outcomes after power versus non-power morcellation, but were able to add newer data from women who had intact removal of these tumours as well. Based upon outcome data from 384 women, they found that survival rates at 5 years were 30% for women undergoing power morcellation, 59% for women undergoing scalpel morcellation, and 60% for women with no use of morcellation. However, the uncertainty within these estimates was so high that they did not reach statistical significance [4].

At this point, it is unclear that power morcellation causes worse outcomes compared with scalpel morcellation or intact removal.

16.9 Conclusion

There has been much debate, of late, regarding surgical removal of occult uterine tumours. If we utilize the best available evidence and fully evaluate the data, it appears that the prevalence of occult leiomyosarcoma in hysterectomy and myomectomy for presumed leiomyomas is far lower than previously estimated, with the best estimate from the most recent prospective data being at approximately 1 in 4,700. We believe that further efforts to refine these data via large prospective registries are warranted.

The data point to no differences in outcomes when looking at power versus non-power morcellation, and no statistical difference in 5-year survival when comparing any type of morcellation or intact removal. Even though the point estimates differ, with worse outcomes after power morcellation, this is a non-significant finding. Neither the creation of new standards of care nor the establishment of public policy is warranted at this time. Unfortunately, both of these were constructed when the FDA gave their initial warning and their recent reaffirmation. Gynaecological patients and the federal regulating communities have been focusing energy and resources on castigation of gynaecologists and instrumentation companies, blaming them for 'thousands of unnecessary deaths'. This effort is erroneous. Neither prevalence nor outcomes after morcellation is the key determinant if we wish to improve health care for women. Preoperative diagnosis of these aggressive tumours would mitigate any putative risks of morcellation. This could also lead to earlier diagnosis and

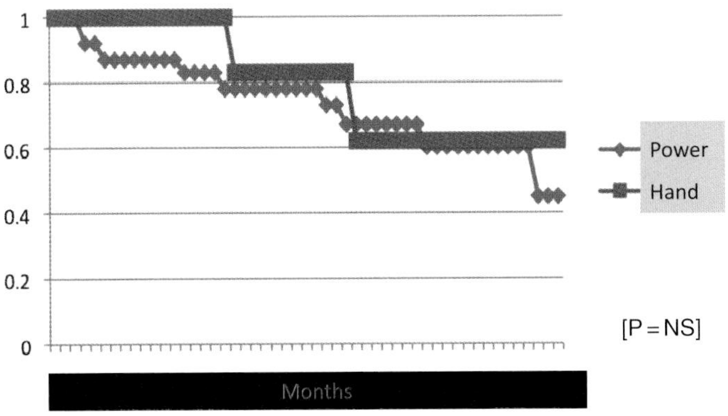

Figure 16.1 Life table survival analysis and upstaging outcomes comparing power versus non-power morcellation [20].

treatment, certainly improving survival rates. It is our hope that in the future, more and better data will be available to further refine answers to these important issues. We also hope that in the future, evidence-based medicine rather than emotion-based medicine is used for medical and public health decision making.

References

1. FDA. Quantitative assessment of the prevalence of unsuspected uterine sarcoma in women undergoing treatment of uterine fibroids: summary and key findings, April 17, 2014. www.fda.gov/media/88703/download. Accessed April 2020.

2. Pritts EA, Vanness DJ, Berek JS, et al. The prevalence of occult leiomyosarcoma at surgery for presumed uterine fibroids: a meta-analysis. *Gynecol Surg* 2015;**12**:165–77.

3. Hartmann KE, Fonnesbeck C, Surawicz T, et al. Management of uterine fibroids. Comparative effectiveness review no. 195 (Prepared by the Vanderbilt Evidence-based Practice Center under Contract No. 290-2015-00003-I.) AHRQ Publication No. 17(18)-EHC028-EF. Rockville, MD: Agency for Healthcare Research and Quality; 2017. https://effectivehealthcare.ahrq.gov/sites/default/files/pdf/cer-195-uterine-fibroids-final-revision.pdf. Accessed April 2020.

4. Olive DL. The dangers of junk science in obstetrics and gynecology: lessons from the power morcellation controversy. *Curr Opin Obstet Gynecol* 2015;**27**:249–52.

5. Mettler L, Alvarez-Rodas E, Semm K. Hormonal treatment and pelviscopic myomectomy. *Diagn Ther Endosc* 1995;**1**:217–21.

6. Nagurney JT, Brown DF, Sane S, et al. The accuracy and completeness of data collected by prospective and retrospective methods. *Acad Emerg Med* 2005 Sept;**12**(9):884–95.

7. Harbour R, Miller J. A new system for grading recommendations in evidence-based guidelines. *Br Med J* 2001;**323**:334–6.

8. Bradburn MJ, Deeks JJ, Berlin JA, et al. Much ado about nothing: a comparison of the performance of meta-analytical methods with rare events. *Stat Med* 2007;**26**:53–77.

9. Altman DG, Deeks JJ. Meta-analysis, Simpson's paradox, and the number needed to treat. *BMC Med Res Methodol* 2002;**26**:53–77.

10. Bell SW, Kempson RL, Hendrickson MR. Problematic uterine smooth muscle neoplasms. A clinicopathologic study of 213 cases. *Am J Surg Pathol* 1994 Jun;**18**(6):535–58.

11. WHO Classification of Tumours. In: Tavassoli FA, Devilee P, editors. *Pathology and Genetics of Tumours of the Breast and Female Genital Organs*. Lyon: IARC Press; 2003:233–8.

12. Leibsohn S, d'Ablaing G, Mishell D, et al. Leiomyosarcoma in a series of hysterectomies performed for presumed uterine leiomyomas. *Am J Obstet Gynecol* 1990;**162**:968–76.

13. Parker WH, Fu YS, Berek JS. Uterine sarcoma in patients operated on for presumed leiomyoma and rapidly growing leiomyoma. *Obstet Gynecol* 1994;**83**:414–18.

14. Seki K, Hoshihara T, Nagata I. Leiomyosarcoma of the uterus: ultrasonography and serum lactate dehydrogenase level. *Gynecol Obstet Investig* 1992;**33**:114–18.

15. Oduyebo T, Rauh-Hain AJ, Meserve EE, et al. The value of re-exploration in patients with inadvertently morcellated uterine sarcoma. *Gynecol Oncol* 2014 Feb; **132**(2):360–5. doi: 10.1016/j.ygyno.2013.11.024.

16. George S, Varysauskas C, Serrano C, et al. Retrospective cohort study evaluating the impact of intraperitoneal morcellation of outcomes of localized uterine leiomyosarcoma. *Cancer* 2014 Oct 15; **120**(20):3154–8. doi: 10.1002/cncr.28844.

17. Seidman MA, Hinchcliff E, George S, et al. *PLoS One.* 2012; 7(11):e50058. doi: 10.1371/journal.pone.0050058.

18. Park JY, Park SK, Kim DY, et al. The impact of tumour morcellation during surgery on the prognosis of patients with apparently early uterine leiomyosarcoma. *Gynecol Oncol* 2011;**122**:255–9.

19. Morice P, Rodriquez A, Rey A, et al. Prognostic value of initial surgical procedure for patient with uterine sarcoma: analysis of 123 patients. *Eur J Gynaecol Oncol* 2003;**24**:237–40.

20. Pritts EA, Parker WH, Brown JB, et al. Outcome of occult uterine leiomyosarcoma after surgery for presumed uterine fibroids: a systematic review. *J Minim Invasive Gynecol* 2015;**22**:26–33.

21. Einstein MH, Barakat RR, Chi DS, et al. Management of uterine malignancy found incidentally after supracervical hysterectomy or uterine morcellation for presumed benign disease. *Int J Gynecol Cancer* 2008;**18**:1065–70.

22. Perri T, Korach J, Sadetzki S, et al. Uterine leiomyosarcoma: does the primary surgical procedure matter? *Int J Gynecol Cancer* 2009;**19**:257–60.

MRI-Guided Ultrasound Lysis of Fibroids

Jessica Gelman and Charles E. Miller

17.1 Introduction

Magnetic-resonance-guided focused ultrasound surgery (MRgFUS) is the only truly non-invasive procedure for the treatment of uterine fibroids. In MRgFUS, high-frequency ultrasound beams target specific tissue, in this case fibroids, causing increased temperatures leading to destruction of the tissue by coagulative necrosis. The resultant fibroid shrinkage occurs under the guidance of real-time magnetic resonance imaging (MRI) for accuracy and preservation of healthy surrounding myometrium [1]. This chapter will begin with an overview of the history of MRgFUS, then examine the technical parameters of the procedure and measurement of success, discuss patient eligibility and selection, preparation for the procedure, recovery, potential complications, and finally, outlooks for fertility and other outcomes.

17.2 History

MRI has the best resolution and sensitivity for fibroids compared to other modalities, such as ultrasound or CT scanning, and allows for real-time three-dimensional thermal mapping [2]. The Food and Drug Administration (FDA) approved MRgFUS for the treatment of fibroids in 2004 [1]. At that time, the treatment could only be used to ablate 33% of a fibroid, as it was yet unclear whether this procedure was safe for the surrounding non-target tissue. In 2006, the FDA approved ablation of 50% of any given fibroid, and by 2009 ablation of 100% of a fibroid was approved, with the caveat that the fibroid had to be more than 10 mm from the serosal surface [3]. Today, the FDA has approved this technique for the ablation of uterine fibroids in pre- or perimenopausal women with symptomatic uterine fibroids desiring a procedure that spares the uterus, and whose uterus size is less than 24 weeks.

The original system that the FDA approved for MRgFUS was the ExAblate 2000 (InSightec, Haifa, Israel). Newer platforms, including the ExAblate 2100 (InSightec, Haifa, Israel) and the Sonalleve MR-HIFU (Philips Healthcare, Vantaa, Finland), offer novel sonication techniques allowing for more efficient fibroid lysis [4].

17.3 How It Works

High-frequency ultrasound beams cause heating between 56°C and 70°C which subsequently leads to protein degradation, cell death, and coagulative necrosis that is eventually absorbed by the body [1, 5]. More specifically, temperatures between 50°C and 52°C for 4–6 minutes cause cellular damage that is irreversible; between 60°C and 100°C they will cause desired protein degradation and coagulative necrosis. Heating past 105°C will cause carbonization and vaporization of tissue, which can worsen ablation potential by impeding US wave transmission [6–9].

17.4 Measuring Treatment Success

The amount of tissue that has been effectively ablated after MRgFUS is termed non-perfused volume (NPV). Studies have shown NPV to be the best predictor of success for this procedure. Increased NPV correlates with better symptom improvement as measured in several studies by the Symptom Severity Score (SSS), which is included within the Uterine Fibroid Symptom and Quality of Life (UFS-QOL) scale, a validated questionnaire. Higher NPV is also associated with increased fibroid shrinkage and decreased rates of reintervention [4–6, 10–12].

17.5 Patient Selection

When MRgFUS was first approved for use on uterine fibroids, it was difficult to find eligible patients. In addition to the ablation percentage restrictions that were initially present as mentioned earlier in this chapter, several other factors were considered contraindications to this procedure. For example,

MRgFUS was previously contraindicated for anyone who had loops of bowel or abdominal scars in the pathway of the US beam. One study showed that bowel interposition affected 60.4% of women, and thus only 38.9% of women were eligible for MRgFUS, while 99.2% were eligible for uterine artery embolization (UAE) [13]. Today's techniques, which circumvent many of these obstacles, have increased the number of eligible patients immensely.

Candidate selection is based upon the likelihood of achieving an acceptable NPV. Part of determining a patient's likelihood of success involves pre-screening all patients with an MRI to assess for certain fibroid features, namely size, number of fibroids, vascularity, accessibility, and texture. Assessing for other uterine or other pelvic disorders is also prudent.

17.5.1 Size Restrictions

A maximum diameter of 10 cm has been suggested for best success of MRgFUS. This number is dependent on the time it takes to ablate a fibroid of such girth. For example, an 8 cm fibroid takes about 3 hours to achieve an ideal NPV. For patient procedure tolerance (as the procedure requires lying still in a confined space, which can be uncomfortable), as well as deep vein thrombosis (DVT) risk, 3–4 hours is the time limit for any given ablation session [6].

In addition to maximum size restrictions, there are also minimum fibroid sizes that are considered safe for MRgFUS. A single focal ablation is about 2.5 cm in length along the anterior–posterior (A-P) direction. Thus, attempting to sonicate a fibroid less than 3 cm in diameter may result in undesired over-ablation of healthy tissue. For this reason, treating fibroids less than 3 cm with MRgFUS should be reserved for those with severe symptoms in whom the benefit of ablating such a fibroid outweighs the risks of injuring healthy intra- or extrauterine tissue [5].

17.5.2 Location

Each ablation system also has a finite range or distance of tissue that it is able to reach. Thus, fibroids that fall outside of this range are unsuitable for treatment with this modality [5].

Fibroids may also be in dangerous proximity to other vital structures that might be at risk of being sonicated. Because high-density tissues absorb ultrasound energy more readily, low doses of energy can significantly heat bone, like the sacrum. Overheating the sacrum can in turn damage nearby nerves, causing pain or damage to that nerve. For this reason, fibroids lying close to the bone and specifically sacrum may not be good candidates for MRgFUS. A distance of at least 4 cm from the spine or nerve roots has been recommended [14]. Other high-density areas, such as abdominal scars, can pose a challenge. Scars often have increased energy absorption and thus are at risk for thermal injury with less than expected energy levels. Alternatively, low-density matter, like air, reflects US rays. Thus, a mass of intestines between the transducer and the fibroid is a relative contraindication to MRgFUS [5].

Some studies argue that limits on proximity to endometrium, such as >1.5 cm away, may be prudent, but this is not standardly recognized or practised as of yet [15].

17.5.3 Vascularity

Fibroids that are very vascular may not reach therapeutic temperatures because the high volume of blood flow carries heat away from the tissue of interest. High vascularity can be detected if the intensity of the fibroids seen on T2W MRI is increased relative to the wall of the uterus [5]. Hyperintense fibroids, which are more common in younger women, are associated with decreased NPV and worse post-treatment SSS [4].

17.5.4 Indications

Anything that distorts the focal point of the beam, such as copious adipose tissue or distorted muscle, may cause suboptimal treatment or pose an additional risk to non-target structures [5].

There are other factors to consider in selecting for optimal patient outcome aside from the likelihood of achieving high NPVs. For one, fibroids that are seemingly optimal for MRgFUS based on size, vascularity, and accessibility may not be appropriate targets if they are not relevant to a patient's symptoms. For example, a woman with abnormal uterine bleeding may not experience relief of symptoms from ablation of a subserosal fibroid. However, ablation of a submucosal fibroid invading the endometrium may very well decrease her bleeding. Alternatively, attempting to ablate a subserosal fibroid in a woman having bowel or bladder symptoms may be appropriate. Furthermore, if a woman's uterus is overrun by numerous small fibroids, it is unlikely that one or a few of these fibroids alone are causing her symptoms. It is thus recommended that treatment is concentrated on the "dominant" fibroid, which is the one most likely associated with the patient's symptoms [5].

While no cases have yet been reported, pedunculated subserosal fibroids have a theoretical risk of amputation, followed by dislodgement into the intraperitoneal cavity [5]. One study retrospectively looked at stalk-sparing MRgFUS treatments in nine women. Results showed that with an average NPV of 67%, mean fibroid volume had decreased by 30% and stalk diameter by 13% at 6-month follow-up. This translated into average baseline SSS of 30 diminishing to 14.6, with no cases of stalk separation or untoward outcomes [4].

African-American women, who are more likely to have symptomatic and early-onset fibroids, are also less likely to be eligible for the MRgFUS procedure, as one study found. These authors noted the most likely reasons for failed eligibility were multiple small fibroids or significant abdominal wall scarring. However, African-American women, when eligible, have equivalent outcomes to others undergoing MRgFUS [16].

There are few absolute contraindications to this procedure, but patients with suspected uterine or gynaecologic malignancy, current pregnancy, and acute inflammatory diseases should not undergo MRgFUS for fibroids. One must recognize the increased risk of leiomyosarcoma in women beginning in their 40s [17]. Any contraindications to having an MRI, such as implantable metal devices (intrauterine devices, cardiac pacemakers, etc.), allergy to contrast agents, or morbid obesity over limits for the MRI machine, are also contraindications to this procedure [18].

17.6 Optimizing Patient Selection

Today, certain methods have been demonstrated to circumvent several of the barriers mentioned above and thus increase patient eligibility for this procedure.

17.6.1 Interposed Bowel

As mentioned previously, the presence of bowel loops in the path of the transducer is a contraindication to MRgFUS because the low-density air can reflect beams; or worse, unpredictable bowel contents can result in thermal damage or even bowel perforation. While this factor is one of the most common barriers,

it is also one of the most modifiable. One way to displace bowel is through bladder filling, whereby a Foley catheter is inserted and the bladder is backfilled with normal saline. The Foley catheter is then clamped. Urine production over the course of the procedure can cause bladder distension and distortion of the mapped area, so small drainages from the catheter should be done frequently with MRI re-verification of the anatomy.

Rectal filling is another method to mechanically shift interposed bowel. Using ultrasound gel transrectally or a rectal balloon can shift the uterus forward. Not only can this displace the anterior bowel loops, but it can also decrease the distance between the anterior abdominal wall and the uterus, and increase the space between the uterus and the spinal nerves and bones. Perhaps most simply, a convex gel pad can be placed on the table directly under the patient's abdomen to apply central pressure and shift the bowel. One study used vaginal pessaries to manipulate bowel. Any combination of these methods can be trialled to optimize patient eligibility [6].

17.6.2 Scars

Abdominal scars are other common barriers to eligibility for this procedure. Scar tissue is often more dense than non-scarred tissue and thus has increased US absorption. Also, scar tissue is often less vascular than other tissue, and thus experiences decreased cooling and risk for underestimation of accumulated heat. Since sensation may be decreased in scarred tissue, patients may not recognize and verbalize that injury is happening as readily as with normal tissue. Plus, once a burn has progressed to second or third degree, even less sensation is appreciable due to thermal nerve damage.

Thus, visualizing scars on MRI is imperative but not always easy. Older scars are much more difficult to visualize, but fortunately more safe to sonicate through. Newer, thick, pronounced scars are often the densest and thus the worst to attempt to treat through. Scars of the epidermis, dermis, and subcutaneous tissue are usually much easier to visualize than scars on muscle or uterus through MR imaging. Special MRI sequences or even MRI paint (like nail varnish or dedicated contrast with paramagnetic iron oxide particles) can help pick up scars on imaging. Reflective acoustic patches, which are visible on MRI, suitable for scars of many shapes, water-resistant, and easily adherent to skin, are another newer and viable option. One clinical study found a small risk of hyperemic changes on skin and muscle but otherwise no major adverse events. These may reflect energy too well, though, and can damage the machine's transducer [19].

Positioning the patient to remove the scar from the field of interest is also possible through tilting or bladder filling [6]. Beam shaping, which is possible with some platforms, can disable one part of the beam to avoid the scarred tissue.

Sonicating through a scar can sometimes be appropriate, and certain patient factors make this process safer. For example, attempting to sonicate a deep fibroid means the focus of energy will be less intense close to the skin, leaving lower risk of overheating a scar. Conversely, fibroids that are very vascular or cellular that will require high energies for ablation are not suitable for treatment if there is an unavoidable scar. If the decision is made to sonicate through a scar, real-time mapping, ample cooling time, and constant patient feedback are crucial.

17.6.3 Pretreatment with GnRH

Pretreatment with GnRH agonists has been shown to shrink fibroids prior to the procedure and improve outcomes of MRgFUS [20–23]. Other studies have shown that GnRH agonists can help reduce fibroid vascularity [24]. While there have been no specific studies to date examining the effect of GnRH and reduced vascularity in relation to MRgFUS outcomes, one can predict that decreased vascularity through GnRH treatment would improve the success rate of MRgFUS since, as mentioned above, MRgFUS is superior for fibroids with lower vascularity [6].

17.6.4 Vascularity

Other methods have been used for optimizing conditions with highly vascular fibroids. Vessel targeting can specifically ablate vessels that are feeding fibroids by taking a non-enhanced MR angiography (MRA) image immediately before the procedure. While this technique has shown extremely promising results, the outermost circumference of the fibroid must still not be treated for the safety of surrounding healthy tissue [19]. Using oxytocin as a pretreatment has also been shown to decrease energy level requirements and sonication time [25]. With extreme caution, some

practitioners have been using higher temperatures than average to effectively treat very vascular fibroids.

17.6.5 MRgFUS Platforms

Certain MRgFUS systems can modify the size, energy level, and transmission of each sonication beam, such as the ExAblate. This can help optimize treatment by tailoring each ablation attempt to the precise tissue of interest. For example, a long area of ablation can be targeted if the energy level is increased parallel to the beam, while increasing the level perpendicular to the beam will create a thicker, deeper spot [5]. The Sonalleve system has the option for volumetric ablation (as opposed to the standard point-by-point method), which is more energy-efficient and thus can sonicate a larger fibroid in a shorter period of time. It does so by ablating in a circular manner, thus pre-heating the next area to be treated and limiting time needed to reach therapeutic temperatures [19].

17.6.6 Large Fibroids

To circumvent the issue of a fibroid being too large, physicians can pre-plan for two separate treatment sessions, one for the superior aspects of the fibroid and one of the inferior aspects, for example. Of note, it may be prudent to avoid sonicating parts of the fibroids that have already been treated, as those now drier areas may absorb too much energy. Sometimes, though, such a procedure may be beneficial and thus intentionally planned. For instance, a fibroid that is too close to the sacrum could have one ablation anteriorly, followed by another session targeting the rest of the fibroid once it has moved further from the bone [5].

17.7 Patient Preparation

All patients should have a screening gadolinium-enhanced MRI. This will assess for eligibility and allow for patient-specific preprocedure planning.

On the day of the procedure, the patient should arrive having fasted for at least 6 hours. Some recommend that bowel cathartics, glucagon, and a low-residue diet prior to fasting may also minimize bowel activity during the procedure [3]. The abdominal wall should be shaved from the umbilicus down to the pubic symphysis. Patients can be asked to do this the night before the procedure. The abdomen should also be free of creams or lotions, as sonicating through these can result in skin burns. An intravenous line will then be placed so conscious sedation can be administered. This helps with patient comfort, decreased anxiety, and minimized movement. The patient should, however, be able to converse with the operators and verbalize if they are feeling burning, pain, or cramping. Some highly compliant and relaxed patients may not require any sedation. A Foley catheter is also placed to keep the bladder empty, unless bladder filling is desired for bowel manipulation as described above, in which case the Foley will be used for filling and then clamped [14, 18, 26].

17.8 Procedure

The MRgFUS system is integrated with a special table that can be docked to a compatible MRI machine. On top of this table is a degassed water tank coupled to a gel pad upon which the patient lies prone. There should be ultrasound gel on both sides of the solid gel pad. The gel and water help to propagate ultrasound waves, as any air between the beam and the patient can cause beam reflection. Then the T2-weighted MRI is used to locate and map fibroids in relation to surrounding structures in three orthogonal planes. After mapping, a low-energy test dose is performed. During the procedure, there is real-time, quantitative temperature mapping that identifies minute temperature changes in non-target tissues before irreversible damage can occur. The full ablation session then ensues with constant MRI monitoring and modified sonication as necessary. Between each sonication, down time is allowed for adequate cooling, as thermal buildup can damage surrounding tissues. The two newest platforms, the ExAblate 2100 and the Sonalleve, automatically pause for cooling. At the end of the procedure, the new area of NPV is measured with gadolinium-enhanced MRI. The results seen immediately post-treatment may be a good indicator of the thermal dose received for a small treatment area; for larger treatment volumes, however, there will likely be a delay in visualizing the full treatment effect. This is thought to be due to vessel occlusion causing a slow downstream effect, or perhaps from underestimation of temperature at the edges of the field that are too distant from the transducer to detect the small changes [4, 14, 26].

17.9 Recovery

There is minimal time needed for immediate postoperative recovery as patients have not been under general anaesthesia and have had an incision-free procedure. Thus, patients usually do not require hospitalization after MRgFUS, can often leave 1 hour after the procedure, and can even return to work within 1–2 days [27]. Most people note symptomatic improvement within 6 months with an average improvement in Symptom Severity Score (SSS) to 50% of pretreatment values [4].

17.10 Complications

Initial studies during clinical phase trials showed no unintended second procedures, no life-threatening events or deaths after MRgFUS [28]. To date, there have been no reports of death or hysterectomy as direct outcomes of this procedure [2]. One of the most serious complications reported is sciatic nerve injury, but this resolved without intervention by 1 year post-procedure [2]. Risks of urinary tract infection and minor skin burns have been reported to be less than 2%, and risk of major skin burn requiring further treatment is less than 0.5% [29]. All reports of major skin burns have been through a previously existing abdominal scar [2]. DVTs are infrequent and bowel perforation is an extremely rare complication of this procedure [18]. More commonly, a patient may experience lower abdominal pain, leg pain, or buttocks pain after the procedure [27].

17.11 Fertility Outlook

MRgFUS is believed to be a suitable option for women with infertility related to intrauterine fibroids, as this procedure is uterus- and endometrium-sparing, non-invasive, and does not use radiation [18].

While there have been no studies on women who have infertility as their main complaint, to date there have been 54 documented pregnancies in 51 women who have previously been treated with MRgFUS for uterine fibroids. Each of these women had reported being family complete, as desiring future fertility was previously a contraindication to having this procedure. The study that describes these cases reports the mean age for the women who became pregnant to be 37.2 years and the miscarriage rate as 26%. The average time between MRgFUS treatment and pregnancy was 8.2 months. At the time of publication, only 42%

of the women had delivered, but 64% of them had normal spontaneous vaginal deliveries with a mean birth weight of 3.3 kg. There were two cases of placenta praevia reported and one serious complication relating to a myomectomy that was done at the time of the caesarean section; however, this woman went on to have a second uncomplicated pregnancy [30]. Other studies have shown that the caesarean section rate after MRgFUS treatment and the rate of low birth weight or stillborn infants (of which there were zero) were lower than after uterine artery embolization [30].

Currently, there is one randomized controlled trial offering MRgFUS treatment to women whose chief complaint is infertility. The first published report coming from this study demonstrated a successful conception 3 months following two sessions of MRgFUS. This patient went on to have an uncomplicated pregnancy and full-term normal spontaneous vaginal delivery [31]. There is also a case report showing the first successful case of in vitro fertilization after MRgFUS for fibroids [32].

At the time of this publication, there is still much to be learned and researched regarding the role of MRgFUS in infertility and pregnancy. Thus, it is important to follow patients closely who become pregnant after MRgFUS treatment. As of yet, there is no evidence of worsening fertility after MRgFUS, but the appropriate period between treatment and conception is still to be determined [18].

17.12 Outcomes

A meta-analysis of 38 studies found that MRgFUS is safe, cost-effective, efficient, and improves quality of life and infertility. When focusing in on quality of life, this analysis notes improvements on the validated Uterine Fibroid Symptoms Quality of Life Questionnaire (UFS-QOL) of between 15 and 44 points at 6 months and between 21 and 47 points at 12 months

post-procedure [33]. One particular study that pretreated with GnRH for 3 months found 28.35 points of improvement at 6 months and 30.3 points at 12 months [34]. Another study of 359 women treated with MRgFUS used the UFS-QOL over time and found improved quality of life scores that persisted for over 2 years [11]. When comparing quality of life scores for MRgFUS to abdominal hysterectomy, one study concluded that while the scores for improvement in quality of life were not significantly different at 6 months post-procedure, MRgFUS had significantly fewer complications [35]. Another study, however, comparing MRgFUS to UAE, found that UAE had superior total health-related quality of life and symptom severity scores [36]. Importantly, 60% of women who were informed about the different treatment modalities for fibroids chose MRgFUS as their top choice [37].

A recent study notes that an NPV greater than 80% is necessary to define clinical success [38]. Alternatively, one study notes that having greater than 45% NPV correlated with a 15% reintervention rate at 2 years, while an NPV between 10% and 20% was associated with a 40% risk of reintervention [39]. Another study looking at 5-year follow-up found that the overall reintervention rate was 58.64%. When stratified for NPV, those with more than 50% NPV postprocedure had a 50% reintervention rate at 5 years [2, 23]. Newer technologies are reporting NPVs at a range of 33–100% [2].

17.13 Conclusion

MRgFUS is a newer, non-invasive technique for ablation of uterine fibroids in symptomatic women. Maximizing patient eligibility using various methods is crucial for the success of this safe and effective treatment. Outcomes of using MRgFUS in women with a chief complaint of infertility are looking positive, though much more research is necessary.

References

1. Carranza-Mamane B, Havelock J, Hemmings R. The management of uterine fibroids in women with otherwise unexplained infertility. *J Obstet Gynaecol Can* 2015;**37**(3): 277–85.

2. Quinn SD, Gedroyc WM. Thermal ablative treatment of uterine fibroids. *Int J Hyperthermia* 2015;**31**(3):272–9.

3. Silberzweig JE, Powell DK, Matsumoto AH, Spies JB. Management of uterine fibroids: a focus on uterine-sparing interventional techniques. *Radiology* 2016;**280**(3): 675–92.

4. Clark NA, Mumford SL, Segars JH. Reproductive impact of MRI-guided focused ultrasound surgery for fibroids: a systematic review of the evidence. *Curr Opin Obstet Gynecol* 2014;**26**(3):151–61.

5. Yoon SW, Lee C, Cha SH, et al. Patient selection guidelines in MR-guided focused ultrasound

surgery of uterine fibroids: a pictorial guide to relevant findings in screening pelvic MRI. *Eur Radiol* 2008;**18**(12):2997–3006.

6. Kim YS, Bae DS, Park MJ, et al. Techniques to expand patient selection for MRI-guided high-intensity focused ultrasound ablation of uterine fibroids. *AJR Am J Roentgenol* 2014;**202**(2):443–51.

7. Goldberg SN, Gazelle GS, Halpern EF, et al. Radiofrequency tissue ablation: importance of local temperature along the electrode tip exposure in determining lesion shape and size. *Acad Radiol* 1996;**3**(3):212–18.

8. Solbiati L, Ierace T, Goldberg SN, et al. Percutaneous US-guided radio-frequency tissue ablation of liver metastases: treatment and follow-up in 16 patients. *Radiology* 1997;**202**(1):195–203.

9. Goldberg SN, Gazelle GS, Mueller PR. Thermal ablation therapy for focal malignancy: a unified approach to underlying principles, techniques, and diagnostic imaging guidance. *AJR Am J Roentgenol* 2000;**174**(2):323–31.

10. Lenard ZM, McDannold NJ, Fennessy FM, et al. Uterine leiomyomas: MR imaging-guided focused ultrasound surgery – imaging predictors of success. *Radiology* 2008;**249**(1):187–94.

11. Stewart EA, Gostout B, Rabinovici J, et al. Sustained relief of leiomyoma symptoms by using focused ultrasound surgery. *Obstet Gynecol* 2007;**110**(2 Pt 1):279–87.

12. LeBlang SD, Hoctor K, Steinberg FL. Leiomyoma shrinkage after MRI-guided focused ultrasound treatment: report of 80 patients. *AJR Am J Roentgenol* 2010;**194**(1):274–80.

13. Froling V, Kröncke TJ, Schreiter NF, et al. Technical eligibility for treatment of magnetic resonance-guided focused ultrasound surgery. *Cardiovasc Intervent Radiol* 2014;**37**(2):445–50.

14. Fennessy FM, Tempany CM. A review of magnetic resonance imaging-guided focused ultrasound surgery of uterine fibroids. *Top Magn Reson Imaging* 2006;**17**(3):173–9.

15. Zhao WP, Chen JY, Zhang L, et al. Feasibility of ultrasound-guided high intensity focused ultrasound ablating uterine fibroids with hyperintense on T2-weighted MR imaging. *Eur J Radiol* 2013;**82**(1):e43–9.

16. Machtinger R, Fennessy FM, Stewart EA, et al. MR-guided focused ultrasound (MRgFUS) is effective for the distinct pattern of uterine fibroids seen in African-American women: data from phase III/IV, non-randomized, multicenter clinical trials. *J Ther Ultrasound* 2013;**1**:23.

17. Howlader N, Noone AM, Yu M, Cronin KA. Use of imputed population-based cancer registry data as a method of accounting for missing information: application to oestrogen receptor status for breast cancer. *Am J Epidemiol* 2012;**176**(4):347–56.

18. Masciocchi C, Arrigoni F, Ferrari F, et al. Uterine fibroid therapy using interventional radiology mini-invasive treatments: current perspective. *Med Oncol* 2017;**34**(4):52.

19. Yoon SW, Seong SJ, Jung SG, et al. Mitigation of abdominal scars during MR-guided focused ultrasound treatment of uterine leiomyomas with the use of an energy-blocking scar patch. *J Vasc Interv Radiol* 2011;**22**(12):1747–50.

20. Fennessy FM, Tempany CM, McDannold NJ, et al. Uterine leiomyomas: MR imaging-guided focused ultrasound surgery – results of different treatment protocols. *Radiology* 2007;**243**(3):885–93.

21. Smart OC, Hindley JT, Regan L, Gedroyc WG. Gonadotrophin-releasing hormone and magnetic-resonance-guided ultrasound surgery for uterine leiomyomata. *Obstet Gynecol* 2006;**108**(1):49–54.

22. Cura M, Cura A, Bugnone A. Role of magnetic resonance imaging in patient selection for uterine artery embolization. *Acta Radiol* 2006;**47**(10):1105–14.

23. Quinn SD, Vedelago J, Gedroyc W, Regan L. Safety and five-year re-intervention following magnetic resonance-guided focused ultrasound (MRgFUS) for uterine fibroids. *Eur J Obstet Gynecol Reprod Biol* 2014;**182**:247–51.

24. Deligdisch L, Hirschmann S, Altchek A. Pathologic changes in gonadotropin releasing hormone agonist analogue treated uterine leiomyomata. *Fertil Steril* 1997;**67**(5):837–41.

25. Huang X, He M, Liu YJ, Zhang L, Wang ZB. [Effect of oxytocin on uterine fibroids treated by ultrasound ablation]. *Zhonghua Fu Chan Ke Za Zhi* 2011;**46**(6):412–15.

26. Fischer K, McDannold NJ, Tempany CM, Jolesz FA, Fennessy FM. Potential of minimally invasive procedures in the treatment of uterine fibroids: a focus on magnetic resonance-guided focused ultrasound therapy. *Int J Womens Health* 2015;**7**:901–12.

27. Pérez-López FR, Ornat L, Ceausu I, et al. EMAS position statement: management of uterine fibroids. *Maturitas* 2014;**79**(1):106–16.

28. Stewart EA, Rabinovici J, Tempany CM, et al. Clinical outcomes of focused ultrasound surgery for the treatment of uterine fibroids. *Fertil Steril* 2006;**85**(1):22–9.

29. Chudnoff SG, Berman JM, Levine DJ, et al. Outpatient procedure for the treatment and relief of

symptomatic uterine myomas. *Obstet Gynecol* 2013;**121**(5):1075–82.

30. Rabinovici J, David M, Fukunishi H, et al. Pregnancy outcome after magnetic resonance-guided focused ultrasound surgery (MRgFUS) for conservative treatment of uterine fibroids. *Fertil Steril* 2010;**93**(1):199–209.

31. Bouwsma EV, Gorny KR, Hesley GK, et al. Magnetic resonance-guided focused ultrasound surgery for leiomyoma-associated infertility. *Fertil Steril* 2011;**96**(1): e9–12.

32. Zaher S, Lyons D, Regan L. Successful in vitro fertilization pregnancy following magnetic resonance-guided focused ultrasound surgery for uterine fibroids. *J Obstet Gynaecol Res* 2011;**37**(4):370–3.

33. Gizzo S, Saccardi C, Patrelli TS, et al. Magnetic resonance-guided

focused ultrasound myomectomy: safety, efficacy, subsequent fertility and quality-of-life improvements, a systematic review. *Reprod Sci* 2014;**21**(4):465–76.

34. Smart OC, Hindley JT, Regan L, Gedroyc WM. Magnetic resonance guided focused ultrasound surgery of uterine fibroids – the tissue effects of GnRH agonist pre-treatment. *Eur J Radiol* 2006;**59**(2):163–7.

35. Taran FA, Tempany CM, Regan L, et al. Magnetic resonance-guided focused ultrasound (MRgFUS) compared with abdominal hysterectomy for treatment of uterine leiomyomas. *Ultrasound Obstet Gynecol* 2009;**34**(5):572–8.

36. Froeling V, Meckelburg K, Schreiter NF, et al. Outcome of uterine artery embolization versus MR-guided high-intensity focused

ultrasound treatment for uterine fibroids: long-term results. *Eur J Radiol* 2013;**82**(12): 2265–9.

37. Borah BJ, Nicholson WK, Bradley L, Stewart EA. The impact of uterine leiomyomas: a national survey of affected women. *Am J Obstet Gynecol* 2013;**209**(4):319 e1–319 e20.

38. Zhao WP, Chen JY, Chen WZ. Dynamic contrast-enhanced MRI serves as a predictor of HIFU treatment outcome for uterine fibroids with hyperintensity in T2-weighted images. *Exp Ther Med* 2016;**11**(1):328–34.

39. Machtinger R, Inbar Y, Cohen-Eylon S, et al. MR-guided focus ultrasound (MRgFUS) for symptomatic uterine fibroids: predictors of treatment success. *Hum Reprod* 2012;**27**(12):3425–31.

Chapter 18

Embolization for the Management of Uterine Fibroids

John Mark Regi, Krit Dwivedi and Trevor J. Cleveland

18.1 Introduction

Uterine fibroids are the most common benign tumour in premenopausal women, with a lifetime prevalence of almost 70% in Caucasian women and more than 80% in women of Afro-Caribbean descent. About half of these women experience symptoms, with the most common being menorrhagia, dysmenorrhoea, pressure symptoms and infertility. Whilst hysterectomy is still the most commonly offered and performed operation to treat uterine fibroids, over the last 20 years minimally invasive therapies have been gaining popularity and uterine fibroid embolization is now a mainstream option for most women who wish to preserve their uterus. Since its introduction, a strong body of evidence has built demonstrating safety and efficacy with low rates of complication. Uterine fibroid embolization (UFE) was first described as a treatment for symptomatic leiomyomas in 1995 by Ravina et al. and has proved so popular that in the last year there were over 25,000 uterine fibroid embolization procedures performed worldwide [1].

18.2 Background/History

UFE was first performed as an adjunct to myomectomy. One of the significant complications of myomectomy was (and remains) bleeding. In a number of areas of the body, embolization was known to be a useful tool for limiting the blood loss at the time of surgery (e.g. nephrectomy and spinal fusion for tumour). In an attempt to reduce the risk of significant intraoperative bleeding, Ravina et al. performed embolization [1]. Subsequently, it was found that a significant proportion of those treated by embolization no longer required the intended myomectomy, and this was notably so in those whose surgery was delayed. On the basis of this observation, the concept of UFE as a standalone treatment was born, trials were performed, and then UFE was introduced to mainstream clinical practice.

18.3 Anatomy and Patient Selection

Almost all patients with uterine fibroids who are suitable for hysterectomy and/or myomectomy are suitable for UFE; in fact there are very few anatomical configurations that are considered unsuitable for fibroid embolization in modern practice. Interventional radiologists are best placed to make the assessment on suitability, but this should not be in isolation and the patients should benefit from a multidisciplinary approach, having already discussed the surgical options with a gynaecologist, preferably in a clinic with the benefit of both specialties. The most common indications for UFE in the United Kingdom are menorrhagia, dysmenorrhoea, pressure-type symptoms and infertility.

An analysis of available practice guidelines [2] states that the absolute contraindications for UFE are consistent across most bodies, and are active pregnancy or active infection. Relative contraindications include endovascular technical considerations such as renal impairment, coagulopathy and contrast allergy. Previous surgery that may lead to altered fibroid blood supply or visible utero-ovarian arterial anastomoses are also quoted as relative contraindications, although in practice these can often be seen and treated at the time of embolization and a safe treatment performed. Razavi et al. describe three types of common anastomoses, and it is important for the operator to recognize these, and to understand the effect that UFE may have on the ovarian artery and that the anastomoses may have with regard to clinical failure of the treatment [3]. Non-visualization of these anastomoses does not exclude small underlying connections and there is very little evidence that they are linked to ovarian failure, with many authors questioning the clinical importance, quoting other factors such as the patient's age as far more likely to contribute to early menopause.

Over time, the indications for UFE have grown to include all fibroid types and characteristics. Some guidelines suggest patients with pedunculated and/or submucosal and/or subserosal fibroids should not be offered embolization, but as experience with the technique has grown, most practitioners will offer UFE to almost all fibroid types, with areas of uncertainty being discussed on an individual basis. The reasoning behind the reticence is the fear that pedunculated subserosal and pedunculated submucosal fibroids may detach into the peritoneum or uterine cavity, respectively, after embolization and cause complications. The Society of Interventional Radiology (SIR) USA guidance (2014) cites evidence that these fibroids cause no more complications than fibroids in other anatomical locations [4]. This area is important, because as part of the consent process, patients who have a pedunculated submucosal fibroid must be aware that there is a risk of vaginal expulsion after embolization, although in practice this is rare. One common misconception is that once they have been embolized, fibroids will be passed PV. This is highly unlikely, unless the previous imaging has indicated a pedunculated submucosal fibroid. Once the patient is fully aware of the relative merits of the treatment options, she can make an informed decision as to whether UFE is the most suitable for her.

The size of the fibroid burden often is included in the decision making. Whilst there are definitive limits to the size of fibroid that can be treated by UFE, common sense would say that the larger the fibroid, the more embolic agent it will require to treat and the longer the procedure, with an increase in the radiation dose. Recently, however, there been a number of reports demonstrating the efficacy and safety of UFE to treat fibroids as large as 10 cm.

18.4 Clinic and Consent

The majority of interventional radiologists (IRs) in the United Kingdom will consult with patients who are considering UFE in clinic prior to intervention. They will assess the patient's symptoms, age, wish for future fertility, previous interventions and understanding of the surgical and conservative options. They will review the risks and benefits of embolization including the risks of the procedure and what happens if the patient opts for no treatment at all. The positive aspects of UFE are its effectiveness in dealing with the symptoms caused by fibroids, its safety profile and minimally invasive nature. The advantages of UFE over surgery are a short hospital stay with a quick return to normal activities (usually 1–2 weeks), fewer major complications and the preservation of the patient's uterus and fertility in most cases. The disadvantages are that these patients, especially if young, may require reintervention at some point, and that the end result is not immediate and it often takes a few months before the symptoms stabilize. Patients are all counselled that whilst the procedure itself is relatively painless, over the first 24–48 hours after the procedure, they can experience some significant discomfort. However, this is usually relatively easily managed.

The patients are warned about the risks of the UFE, which include induction of an early menopause (very uncommon in young women under 40 years), infection, post-embolization syndrome, and the potential need for hysterectomy at some point. The patients are also told about the rare complication of non-target embolization.

The therapeutic effect of UFE peaks at 6 months post treatment, with most exhibiting a significant reduction in fibroid size and related symptoms. However, if the patient wants an immediate and final result then she should be advised towards hysterectomy. If the patient wishes to watch and wait, then she should be informed that the symptoms caused by fibroids are likely to subside after menopause.

Whilst most fibroids involute after menopause, there is a subset of postmenopausal women who continue to suffer with symptoms. Obesity and hormone replacement therapy have been associated with continuing symptoms. UFE for the treatment of pressure or bulk-type fibroid symptoms has been shown to be safe but postmenopausal women presenting with bleeding symptoms need to be thoroughly investigated for malignancy prior to consideration of UFE.

Patients should also be informed that the speed of symptom resolution and efficacy of embolization depend on the symptoms with which they present. It is the authors' experience that women who present with menorrhagia tend to benefit from a relatively quick resolution of symptoms, whereas those presenting with pressure-type symptoms may need to be more patient for the final results as the fibroids take time to shrink.

18.5 Imaging

Most patients will at some point have undergone pelvic ultrasound investigation which confirms the presence of uterine fibroids, but it has become the standard of treatment to perform contrast-enhanced MRI. This has been shown to be more accurate in characterizing lesions as it provides accurate information on fibroid location, fibroid enhancement or blood supply and the presence of other disorders that may mimic the symptoms of fibroids, such as adenomyosis [5]. MRI will also help identify the feared complication of leiomyosarcoma and differentiate between a benign fibroid and malignant lesion. The standard MRI sequences used are fairly universal with non-contrast T1 and T2 imaging to assess characteristics, size and position. This is followed by post-gadolinium T1 imaging to assess the enhancement of the fibroids and blood supply (Figure 18.1). After treatment, most centres will follow these patients with further imaging (Figure 18.2).

Many centres are using magnetic resonance angiography (MRA) time-resolved imaging to assess the enhancement and blood supply of the patient's fibroids. This gives an angiogram type of picture which is also very useful for identifying the presence of ovarian artery supply to the fibroid (Figure 18.3).

18.6 Technique

There are two considerations to plan for prior to intervention. Firstly, it has been traditionally considered a potential risk of postoperative infection if a woman has an intrauterine contraceptive device (IUCD) in situ. Studies have shown the risk of performing UFE with an IUCD in situ is very low (less

than 1 in 1,300) and so it is very much a matter of preference of the operator whether they consider it important to remove any device prior to embolization. The second consideration surrounds those patients on gonadotrophin-releasing hormone (GnRH) agonists for short-term symptomatic relief from menorrhagia. GnRH agonists have been associated with a reduction in the vascularity of uterine fibroids (indeed that is their mode of action) and may reduce the efficacy of UFE. Some units will stop these medications 3 months prior to embolization to ensure that the uterine arteries have returned to normal prior to treatment. Kim et al. reported a study using GnRH agonists to reduce the size of large fibroids prior to embolization showing this was safe and did not compromise the embolization [6].

The standard technique for UFE is relatively uniform across most centres; however, the finer points of the technique can vary widely between operators. The choice of embolic material, for example, depends on operator preference as a rule, with no strong evidence that one embolic material is superior to another.

Prior to the intervention, the patients are given pre-medications, often including antibiotics and anti-inflammatories. Usually a patient-controlled analgesia system is established and the patients familiarized in its use. This allows access to either opiate or opioid medicines in a controlled fashion. During the procedure, the patients are also given intravenous (IV) paracetamol (acetaminophen).

Prior to the procedure starting, some centres use a superior hypogastric nerve block (SHNB) to reduce the ischaemic pain experienced by the patient. This technique is performed under fluoroscopic guidance

(a)

(b)

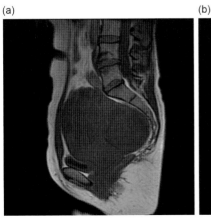 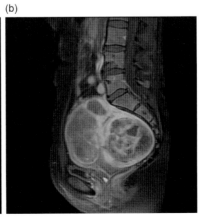

Figure 18.1 T1-weighted MRI images pre- (a) and post-gadolinium (b) contrast showing the enhancing fibroids prior to embolization.

(a)

(b)

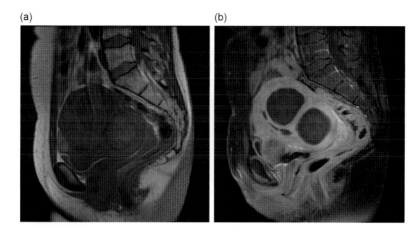

Figure 18.2 Post-embolization. Pre-contrast (a) and post-contrast (b) after embolization T1-weighted images showing that the fibroids are no longer enhancing, and have been successfully treated.

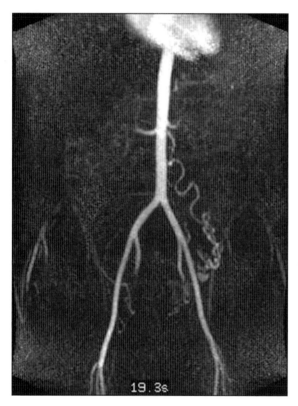

Figure 18.3 A single MRA image from the time-resolved sequences (at 19.3 seconds after contrast injection) showing left ovarian artery supply to a fibroid.

with a long 21 gauge skinny needle, under local anaesthetic and aseptic conditions, placed through the anterior abdominal wall down to the level of the L5 vertebral body [7]. The aortic bifurcation is often marked with an arterial catheter to avoid inadvertent puncture of the aorta or aortic bifurcation. Once the

bone is reached, a small amount of contrast is injected to delineate the nerve sheaths (Figure 18.4). Once in position, 10 mL of bupivacaine is injected. This has been shown to be safe and to decrease the need for opiate analgesia at 4 hours post embolization. Yoon et al. performed a prospective, double-blinded RCT comparing SHNB with a placebo and showed this reduced the opioid analgesia and antiemetic requirements in the immediate post-embolization period but failed to demonstrate a reduction in the hospital inpatient stay [8].

The arterial system is accessed most commonly via the common femoral arteries (CFA) under local anaesthetic using ultrasound guidance with a small arterial sheath (4 or 5 Fr.). Some units will access both CFAs with sheaths as bilateral access allows simultaneous bilateral uterine artery embolization, reducing the radiation burden to the patient. However, arterial bleeding from the puncture sites is probably the most common minor complication of UFE and bilateral punctures increase this risk, and the authors prefer a single-puncture protocol. Some units have adopted unilateral radial artery access as the primary access point as there is growing evidence that this is preferred by patients and leads to quicker recovery time [9, 10]. Most units will give unfractionated heparin depending on weight to prevent peri-catheter thrombus formation.

The fixed image intensifier and imaging equipment are all set to a low-dose protocol with the majority of the imaging performed with digital image grabs rather than the traditional subtraction angiography, which has a much higher radiation dose. Digital zoom rather than image magnification also reduces patient dose. The ALARA (as low as

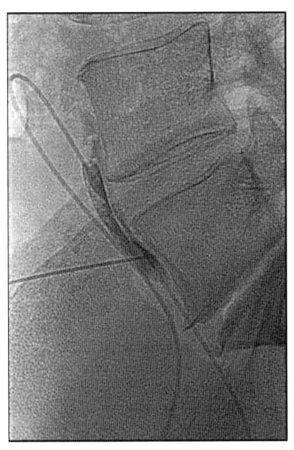

Figure 18.4 Fluoroscopic image taken in the lateral aspect showing the correct needle position in SHNB with injected contrast showing the nerve sheath. There is an angiographic catheter demonstrating the aortic bifurcation.

reasonably achievable) principle is practised with all these young patients to minimize dose.

The uterine arteries are commonly the first branch from the anterior division of the internal iliac artery (IIA). Once identified, the uterine arteries have a characteristic appearance with a vertical segment followed by a horizontal one and then a corkscrew appearance. The uterine arteries are susceptible to spasm, and many units will give medication to treat or prevent this. The uterine arteries can be accessed (sequentially) with a standard imaging catheter (4 or 5 Fr.) of the operator's choice. Some operators choose to use a micro-catheter system to embolize the uterine arteries with the intention of reducing the risk of spasm (Figure 18.5). If the artery does go into spasm, this will reduce the efficacy of the embolization. The catheter or micro-catheter is placed in the horizontal segment of the uterine artery to decrease the risk of reflux of embolic agent into non-target branches of the IIA or the cervicovaginal branches.

The most commonly used embolic agents are calibrated particles, with the accepted method being to start with smaller particles to allow distal embolization followed by gradual upsizing of particle size (typically in the region of 500 μm or larger). All embolic agents are combined with a radio-opaque contrast agent to allow their progress to be tracked. It is important to monitor the progress of the embolic agents carefully to ensure there is no significant shunting through the fibroid into the venous system and to ensure that there is no reflux of embolic agent

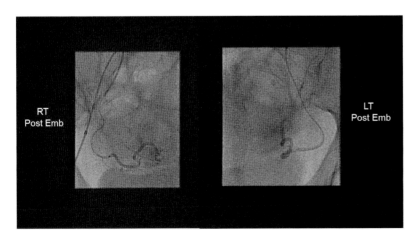

Figure 18.5 Right and left uterine arteries selectively catheterized using a 4f catheter and micro-catheter combination. The tip of the micro-catheter has a radio-opaque marker on it and the tip is located in the horizontal portion of the uterine artery.

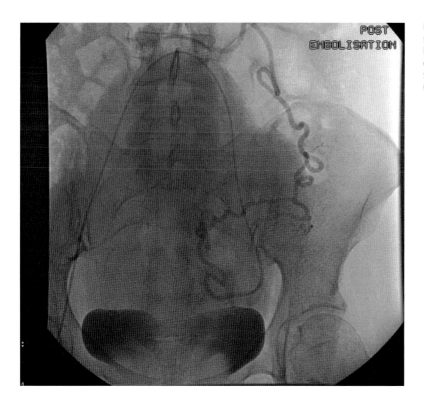

Figure 18.6 Catheter angiogram showing left ovarian artery supply to a large fibroid. Note this is a low-dose digital image acquisition and not standard digital subtraction angiography (DSA).

backwards into any of the other branches of the IIA, or ovarian communications (Figure 18.6).

There is often a misunderstanding by non-interventional radiology medical professionals and patients that the fibroids are selectively embolized. The uterine arteries are embolized to near-stasis, and so the unaffected uterus will receive some embolic agent. The fibroids are preferentially supplied by the uterine arteries, whereas the uterus has a rich collateral supply of other vessels, and as a result uterine necrosis is very rare. As embolization progresses, the fibroids can be seen to enhance as the embolic material preferentially collects within the capillaries of the fibroid. Occasionally, the uterus has a single uterine artery supply, and rarely it is possible to access only one of the uterine arteries due to technical issues. In these cases, there is good evidence that the patients can still derive a good symptomatic improvement from single uterine artery embolization.

If significant fibroid supply is noted from an ovarian artery (OA) source, there is evidence that direct embolization of the OA has very little effect on ovarian function. Hu et al. compared standard UFE with UFE plus OA embolization and found there was no effect on ovarian function or symptoms of menopause. However, most operators will avoid embolization of the ovarian supply if possible [11].

Once the uterine artery has been embolized to near-stasis, which is very sluggish flow in a patent uterine artery, many clinicians will pause and wait a few minutes before checking for further antegrade flow or near-stasis again. A slow infusion of intra-arterial lidocaine, when uterine artery flow is slow, has been used to decrease postoperative pain [12]. Once both arteries have been embolized to stasis, the procedure is complete and the groin puncture is closed with either direct pressure or an arterial closure device. Most patients will remain in hospital overnight and go home the next day if well. The patients are often discharged home on antibiotics, although there is no consensus on a prophylactic regime in the literature or in the guidelines.

Clinical outcomes from UFE have been described in multiple papers – the patients can expect a 50–60% reduction in the size of the fibroids with a similar reduction in uterine size. A 90% reduction in pressure-related symptoms and a greater than 90% reduction in menorrhagia have been reported, with 80–90% of patients being satisfied with the early results [13]. At 3 years, the overall reintervention rate is about 14%, and the number of embolization patients who remain satisfied is approximately the same as among those who underwent surgery.

Follow-up varies between clinicians and units; however, most patients are reviewed in the clinic between 6 weeks and 3 months with the benefit of a repeat MRI to assess reduction in uterine and fibroid size as well as degree of infarction. If there is residual perfusion of fibroids following UFE, there is a higher risk of clinical recurrence in time (depending upon the timing of other factors such as menopause) [13].

18.7 Potential Complications

Major complications from UFE are rare and patient satisfaction rates are high post procedure. Major complications are less common than for the surgical alternatives; however, minor complications are more common than in surgery. The most common complication of UFE is a groin haematoma from the arterial access in the CFA. Active arterial bleeding is very rare. The infection rate post-UFE is around 2%, with 0.5% of patients requiring hysterectomy. Pain post embolization should not be considered as a complication as it is an expected result.

One of the most feared complications is non-target embolization, which occurs either due to an anatomical anastomosis between the uterine arteries and the ovarian arteries across the broad ligament or from a technical complication/failure of the procedure. Shunts through the fibroids into the venous system can sometimes be seen on preoperative MRA imaging and should be suspected during the procedure if there is failure to slow the arterial flow with introduction of the embolic agent. If the embolic agent's progress is not carefully monitored, then it is possible for it to reflux back up the uterine artery into any of the branches of the IIA and into the pelvis or buttock blood supply or the external iliac artery and down the leg. This is a very rare complication, less than 1 in 1,000, particularly with the use of careful technique and high-quality imaging chains.

18.8 College/NICE Guidance

The current guidance and body of literature robustly demonstrates the safety and efficacy of UFE in providing symptomatic relief. Clinical trials have shown UFE patients to have a shorter length of stay and operative blood loss compared to patients after

surgery, and similar quality of life and satisfaction rates. There is paucity of data looking at comparison of outcomes such as complications and cost-effectiveness of UFE versus other surgical procedures, and further large multicentre prospective studies comparing the two are required before more definite recommendations can be made. There is especially very low evidence and a paucity of data looking at conception, fertility and pregnancy post procedure, and caution must be exercised when drawing any conclusions. These outcomes have been recognized by NICE, RCOG, CIRSE and Cochrane.

18.8.1 NICE Guidance (2014)

NICE guidance, last updated in 2014, recognized uterine artery embolization (UAE – which is interchangeable with UFE) as efficacious for symptom relief in the short and long term for a substantial portion of patients [14]. No major safety concerns were noted, and patient selection should be carried out by a multidisciplinary team including both a gynaecologist and an interventional radiologist. In line with the current evidence of time, it suggested that patients be informed that in some cases symptom relief may not be achieved, symptoms may return, and that further procedures, such as a myomectomy or hysterectomy, may therefore be required in the future.

NICE encouraged further research into the effects of UFE compared with other procedures. It identified fertility as a particular region of interest and recommended informing patients who undergo the procedure that its effects of fertility and pregnancy were uncertain.

18.8.2 Royal College of Obstetricians and Gynaecologists (RCOG) (2013)

The latest RCOG guidance (third edition, 2013) recognized UFE as being as effective as surgery for symptom control, and recommended that for women with symptomatic fibroids, UFE should be considered as one of the treatment options alongside other surgical treatments, endometrial ablation, medical management and conservative measures [15]. It highlighted good early- and medium-term results. However, it cautioned that about a third of women would require a second intervention in 5 years.

Like NICE, it highlighted the paucity of evidence for fertility and pregnancy outcomes after UFE and myomectomy. It also noted there is 'no robust evidence' comparing UFE or myomectomy looking specifically at fertility or pregnancy. Therefore, it stated that it was 'impossible to make an evidence-based recommendation about treatment (UFE or myomectomy) for women with fibroids who wish to maintain their fertility'.

18.8.3 Cochrane Guidance (2014)

The most recent Cochrane review [16] included seven studies, with 793 participants. It both looked at UFE as an independent entity and tried to compare outcomes versus other surgical procedures such as hysterectomy or myomectomy. Three studies compared UFE versus hysterectomy, two versus myomectomy and two versus hysterectomy or myomectomy. The quality of evidence was rated 'very low' for fertility, and 'moderate' for satisfaction ratings and most safety outcomes. Evidence on fertility was deemed to be of a 'very low quality', with 'extreme caution' to be applied to any definitive claims.

Findings on patient satisfaction were considered inconclusive, with a large variance in reported outcomes (from 41% lower to 48% higher). UFE was associated with shortened hospital stay and more rapid return to daily activities. Evidence on complications was inconclusive. Overall, there was some evidence to suggest the risk of minor complications was higher with UFE compared to myomectomy and that there was a higher likelihood of the patient needing further intervention. There are now more data from the 10-year EMMY trial regarding this.

18.8.4 Cardiovascular and Interventional Radiological Society of Europe (CIRSE) (2015)

The CIRSE standards of practice (2015) [17] recognized UFE as a true alternative to hysterectomy in women who wanted to preserve their uterus, and recommended that every symptomatic patient be offered it as a choice. It noted the 5-year prevention of hysterectomy post successful UFE to be 75–80%.

18.9 Clinical Trials Overview

18.9.1 Summary of Evidence

Support for UFE as a safe and effective treatment of uterine fibroids has progressed over three decades from small case series to numerous multicenter trials and studies, and a meta-analysis of the literature. UFE had a lower risk of major complications than surgery but an increased risk of minor complications, a shorter hospital inpatient stay and shorter recovery time. Since the first case series by Ravina et al., there have been multiple randomized and single-arm non-randomized trials both looking at UFE itself and comparing it with surgical alternatives. We summarize four major randomized trials of note, and their subsequent outcomes.

18.9.2 FIBROID

The Fibroid Registry for Outcomes Data (FIBROID Registry) was established in 1999 by the Society of Interventional Radiology (SIR) foundation [18]. This enrolled 72 sites across all settings, with 2,000+ patents eligible for long-term follow-up. The aim was to assess outcomes following UFE over 3 years. It included a questionnaire to assess symptom control and quality of life, and data on subsequent interventions. The questionnaire used was termed the Uterine Fibroid Symptom and Quality of Life (UFS-QOL) questionnaire, and results from its analysis showed a significant improvement at both 6 months and 3 years post procedure. The reintervention rates included myomectomy, hysterectomy and repeat UFE at 2.82%, 9.79% and 1.83%, respectively. In all, 28.6% patients were amenorrhoeic 3 years post procedure; however, no causal relationships between UFE and amenorrhoea could be established.

18.9.3 EMMY

The EMMY trial was a multicenter RCT conducted in the Netherlands, comparing 1:1 hysterectomy with UFE. It is the only study with 10 years of long-term follow-up reported outcomes, most recently in December 2016 [19]. After 10 years, 69% of all women undergoing a technically successful UFE avoided a hysterectomy. Recovery time was faster in UFE and there was no significant difference in complication rates.

18.9.4 REST

REST was a UK multicentre RCT study that randomized patients 2:1 UFE with hysterectomy or myomectomy [20]. There was no difference at 1 and 5 years between patient satisfaction scores, and there were similar adverse event rates between surgery and UFE. An important finding was a higher cumulative need for reintervention at 5 years for UFE (32%), compared to surgery (4%). This was commonly due to recurrent or persistent symptoms. REST also conducted economic trial analysis and showed both UFE and surgery to have equal cost-effectiveness. UFE initially showed better cost-effectiveness at 12 months, but this was not the case at 5 years due to the need for reinterventions.

18.9.5 HOPEFUL

HOPEFUL was a large UK retrospective cohort study comparing UFE with hysterectomy, looking at safety, efficacy, cost-effectiveness and patient's perspective on the procedure [21]. Although fewer complications were observed in UFE compared to hysterectomy, the rate of serious complications was similar. The cost-effectiveness analysis favoured UFE, even when reinterventions and complications were included. However, for younger women with recurrent fibroids and additional future procedures, this may not be the case.

18.9.6 FEMME

FEMME is a multicentre trial in the United Kingdom comparing UFE with myomectomy, with results yet to be published [22]. The primary outcome is the quality of life (QoL) score. An important secondary outcome is pregnancy outcomes and measurements of ovarian reserve post procedure. As noted above in all guidelines, this is a clinically important outcome that lacks robust evidence. Other outcomes include adverse events such as complications, reinterventions, major complications, length of stay, time to return to work or usual activity and menstrual blood loss.

In summary, there appear to be both some advantages and disadvantages for UFE when compared to traditional surgical methods, and further evidence is required before definite recommendations can be made favouring one over the other. Therefore, careful counselling of patients and management of expectations is required pre-procedure, and a multidisciplinary approach with both gynaecology and interventional radiology involvement recommended. The informed individual patient should be given the choice as to her preferred treatment option.

18.10 UFE and Conception

Despite the paucity of evidence in this field, it is the authors' experience that most units offering UFE to younger women who want to conceive can point to a handful of successful pregnancies each, and this can give women hope. There are a number of case series describing successful uncomplicated pregnancies and childbirths after UFE [23]. Reproductive outcomes post-UFE have been reported in a number of retrospective reviews. Goldberg et al. looked at 53 pregnancies post-UFE and 139 pregnancies post-laparoscopic myomectomy. They noted that pregnancy post-UFE was associated with a higher rate of preterm labour and malpresentation, although the UFE group were markedly older and possessed larger fibroids [24]. Homer and Saridogan compared pregnancies between UFE patients and pregnant patients with untreated fibroids, and found a higher rate of caesarean section, miscarriage and postpartum haemorrhage. However, there were significant differences between the demographics of the two groups [25]. Pisco et al. reported more positive findings with low overall pregnancy complications in post-UFE patients [26]. Mohan et al. published a thorough review of UFE and fertility quoting preterm delivery rates similar to the general population [27]. Chen and Athreya recently looked at the national and international guidance available for UFE and specifically looked at UFE and conception [2]. They found a number of differing interpretations of the same pool of limited evidence and questioned the objectivity of the current practice guidelines. Given the paucity of good evidence in the area, the SIR in the USA no longer considers the desire to maintain fertility or have children as a relative contraindication to UFE.

Informed consent in clinic is vital in this area, with both young and older women increasingly keen to maintain their fertility after treatment of fibroids. This is a very personal decision, with the clinicians offering the best advice given the available evidence. One of the potential and well-documented risks of UFE is amenorrhoea post treatment, and women should be aware of this prior to any intervention. The rate of affected women is highly age-dependent, and it is uncommon in women under the age of 40, with 3% of those under 40 years of age and 41% aged 50 years and older exhibiting temporary or permanent cessation of menstruation, according to a large Canadian trial [28].

Kitson et al. cite concerns with increased rates of postpartum haemorrhage (PPH) and abnormal placentation, with a slight increase in the c-section rate in these patients, pointing to a case report of a patient in their institution [29]. The other risks appeared to be unchanged from the general population. They recommend myomectomy (from a 2004 paper) in those patients with fibroids wishing to achieve pregnancy. However, the regional placental abnormalities unit for the North of England has not seen or reported a trend in abnormal placentation in UFE patients. The FEMME trial (a larger multicenter RCT) is due to publish its results in the near future and one of the study endpoints is looking at UFE fertility outcomes [22].

18.11 Combined UFE and Surgery

It is technically possible to combine UFE and surgical options. Clearly, there is little to be gained by UFE in a patient in whom hysterectomy is planned, unless there is a need to reduce the size of the fibroids to facilitate the surgery.

A much more likely combination is UFE and myomectomy or hysteroscopic resection. Myomectomy (particularly if considered laparoscopically) is well suited to subserosal and pedunculated subserosal fibroids. Similarly, hysteroscopic fibroid resection for intracavity fibroids is technically well suited. UFE has more potential complications in these circumstances, but is more suited to the intramural fibroids (which are more difficult to resect endoscopically). Therefore, there are some anatomical features where there is a large fibroid load, throughout the uterus, where a combination of techniques may be advantageous. Such circumstances may be considered on an individual patient and multidisciplinary team (MDT) basis.

18.12 Future Developments

UFE is a safe and effective treatment for vascular fibroid disease, but one of its limitations is that the level of postoperative pain that women experience means that the majority of patients require an inpatient hospital stay. Developing techniques to augment traditional UFE such as superior hypogastric nerve block and intra-arterial lidocaine for pain relief and radial artery access for increased patient mobility and decreased bleeding complications may improve patients' experience and recovery time and allow these procedures to be performed routinely as day cases. Further work and additional trials are required to validate the safety and feasibility of performing UFE on an outpatient basis. As already discussed, UFE can be used in combination and just prior to myomectomy to reduce blood loss during surgery. An expansion of this role may benefit patients, potentially reducing operative time and hospital length of stay. Given the limited literature on this topic, additional studies are required before this becomes more common practice.

References

1. Ravina JH, Herbreteau D, Ciraru-Vigneron N, et al. Arterial embolization to treat uterine myomata. *Lancet* 1995;**346**: 671–2.

2. Chen HT, Athreya S. Systematic review of uterine artery embolization practice guidelines: are all the guidelines on the same page? *Clin Radiol* 2018;**73**:507. e9–15.

3. Razavi MK, Wolanske KA, Hwang GL, et al. Angiographic classification of ovarian artery-to-uterine artery anastomoses: initial observations in uterine fibroid embolization. *Radiology* 2002;**224**:707–12.

4. Smeets AJ, Nijenhuis RJ, Boekkooi PF, et al. Safety and effectiveness of uterine artery embolization in patients with pedunculated fibroids. *J Vasc Interv Radiol* 2009;**20**:1172–5.

5. Rajan DK, Margau R, Kroll RR, et al. Clinical utility of ultrasound versus magnetic resonance imaging for deciding to proceed with uterine artery embolization for presumed symptomatic fibroids. *Clin Radiol* 2011;**66**:57–62.

6. Kim MD, Kim YM, Kim HC, et al. Uterine artery embolization for symptomatic adenomyosis: a new technical development of the 1-2-3 protocol and predictive factors of MR imaging affecting outcomes. *J Vasc Interv Radiol* 2011;**22**:497–502.

7. Binkert CA, Hirzel FC, Gutzeit A, Zollikofer CL, Hess T. Superior hypogastric nerve block to reduce pain after uterine artery embolization: advanced technique and comparison to epidural anesthesia. *Cardiovasc Intervent Radiol* 2015;**38**:1157–61.

8. Yoon J, Valenti D, Muchantef K, et al. Superior hypogastric nerve block as post–uterine artery embolization analgesia: a randomized and double-blind clinical trial. *Radiology* 2018. https://doc.org/10.1148/radiol .2018172714

9. Resnick NJ, Kim E, Patel RS, et al. Uterine artery embolization using a transradial approach: initial experience and technique. *J Vasc Interv Radiol*; 2014;**25**:443–7.

10. Posham R, Biederman DM, Patel RS, et al. Transradial approach for noncoronary interventions: a single-center review of safety and feasibility in the first 1,500 cases. *J Vasc Interv Radiol* 2016;**27**:159–66.

11. Hu NN, Kaw D, McCullough MF, Nsouli-Maktabi H, Spies JB. Menopause and menopausal symptoms after ovarian artery embolization: a comparison with uterine artery embolization controls. *J Vasc Interv Radiol* 2011;**22**:710–1.

12. Noel-Lamy M, Tan KT, Simons ME, et al. Intraarterial lidocaine for pain control in uterine artery embolization: a prospective, randomized study. *J Vasc Interv Radiol* 2017;**28**:16–22.

13. Pelage J-P, Guaou NG, Jha RC, Ascher SM, Spies JB. Uterine fibroid tumors: long-term MR imaging outcome after embolization. *Radiology* 2004;**230**:803–9.

14. National Institute for Health and Care Excellence. Uterine artery embolization (Interventional procedures guidance [IPG367]). 2010. Available at www.nice.org.uk/guidance/IPG367. Accessed 22 May 2018.

15. Royal College of Obstetricians and Gynaecologists. Uterine artery embolization in the management of fibroids. 2013. Available at: www.rcog.org.uk/en/guidelines-research-services/guidelines/uterine-artery-embolization-in-the-management-of-fibroids. Accessed 22 May 2018.

16. Gupta JK, Sinha A, Lumsden MA, Hickey M. Uterine artery embolization for symptomatic uterine fibroids. *Cochrane Database Syst Rev* 2014;(12): CD005073.

17. van Overhagen H, Reekers JA. Uterine artery embolization for symptomatic leiomyomata. *Cardiovasc Intervent Radiol* 2015;**38**:536–42.

18. Myers ER, Goodwin S, Landow W, et al. Prospective data collection of a new procedure by a specialty society: the FIBROID registry. *Obstet Gynecol* 2005;**106**:44–51.

19. de Bruijn AM, Ankum WM, Reekers JA, et al. Uterine artery embolization vs hysterectomy in the treatment of symptomatic uterine fibroids: 10-year outcomes from the randomized EMMY trial. *Am J Obstet Gynecol* 2016;**215**:745.e1–12.

20. Moss JG, Cooper KG, Khaund A, et al. Randomised comparison of uterine artery embolization (UAE) with surgical treatment in patients with symptomatic uterine fibroids (REST trial): 5-year results. *BJOG* 2011;**118**:936–44.

21. Dutton S, Hirst A, McPherson K, Nicholson T, Maresh M. A UK multicentre retrospective cohort study comparing hysterectomy and uterine artery embolization for the treatment of symptomatic uterine fibroids (HOPEFUL study): main results on medium-term safety and efficacy. *BJOG* 2007;**114**:1340–51.

22. McPherson K, Manyonda I, Lumsden M-A, et al. A randomised trial of treating fibroids with either embolization or myomectomy to measure the effect on quality of life among women wishing to avoid hysterectomy (the FEMME study): study protocol for a randomised controlled trial. *Trials* 2014;**15**:100–11.

23. Carpenter TT, Walker WJ. Pregnancy following uterine artery embolization for symptomatic fibroids: a series of 26 completed pregnancies. *BJOG* 2005;**112**:321–5.

24. Goldberg J, Pereira L, Berghella V, et al. Pregnancy outcomes after treatment for fibromyomata: uterine artery embolization versus laparoscopic myomectomy. *Am J Obstet Gynecol* 2004;**191**:18–21.

25. Homer H, Saridogan E. Uterine artery embolization for fibroids is associated with an increased risk of miscarriage. *Fertil Steril* 2010;**94**:324–30.

26. Pisco JM, Duarte M, Bilhim T, Cirurgiao F, Oliveira AG. Pregnancy after uterine fibroid embolization. *Fertil Steril* 2011;**95**:1121.e8.

27. Mohan PP, Hamblin MH, Vogelzang RL. Uterine artery embolization and its effect on fertility. *J Vasc Interv Radiol* 2013;**24**:925–30.

28. Pron G, Bennett J, Common A, et al. The Ontario Uterine Fibroid Embolization Trial. Part 2. Uterine fibroid reduction and symptom relief after uterine artery embolization for fibroids. *Fertil Steril* 2003 Jan;**79**(1):120–7.

29. Kitson SJ, Macphail S, Bulmer J. Is pregnancy safe after uterine artery embolization? *BJOG* 2012;**119**:519–21.

Chapter

19

Uterine Fibroids in Postmenopausal Women

Mohamed Ali, Zunir Tayyeb Chaudhry and Ayman Al-Hendy

19.1 Introduction

19.1.1 Uterine Fibroids

Uterine fibroids (UFs), also known as leiomyomas or myomas, are the most common benign gynaecologic neoplasm in premenopausal women worldwide and estimated to occur in 7–8 women out of 10 during their lifetime [1]. The aetiology behind UFs is thought to involve genetic, biologic, and environmental factors [1]. Growth factors have been implicated in certain molecular processes involved in the pathogenesis of UFs which includes inflammation, cell proliferation, fibrosis, and angiogenesis [2]. Numerous studies and clinical observations have shown that growth of UFs is dependent on ovarian steroid hormones. Accordingly, there have been no documented cases of UFs prior to menarche, while its prevalence increases with age and peaks during the fifth decade of life [3]. Consequently, the risk tends to decline after menopause, especially in women over the age of 70 years [4]. About 20% of UF patients present with heavy or abnormal bleeding and pelvic pressure; additionally, UFs can cause infertility or loss of pregnancy [2].

19.1.2 Ovarian Steroid Hormones and Uterine Fibroids

The role of oestrogen and progesterone has been critical in understanding the pathogenesis of UFs and how to manage them accordingly. Fibroids have an increased expression of oestrogen receptors (ERs) and progesterone receptors (PRs) as compared to the adjacent myometrium [5]; moreover, oestrogen recently has been shown to increase the expression of PRs, thus increasing the sensitivity of progesterone-responsive tissue including UFs to its actions [6].

Evidently, fibroid growth has been suppressed when treated with a continuous gonadotrophin-releasing hormone (GnRH) agonist for a period of 3 months, this is due to inhibition of oestrogen and progesterone release in response to GnRH receptor down-regulation at the pituitary gland, thus mimicking a postmenopausal hormonal profile [7]. Combined, these findings implicate the critical role of ovarian steroid hormones, especially progesterone, on fibroid growth [8]. Other clinical observations have noted success in suppressing fibroid growth with therapies targeting oestrogen, progesterone, and their respective receptors [5, 6].

19.2 Menopause and Uterine Fibroids

19.2.1 Menopause

Menopause, the permanent cessation of menstruation, happens due to a decline in ovarian function, while perimenopause is the period prior to complete cessation of menses, and it is marked by fluctuations in ovarian steroid hormones reflecting the woman's transitions from her reproductive years to non-reproductive years. Postmenopause is described as the period following a 12-month history of amenorrhea, signifying unresponsive ovaries and a collapse of the hypothalamic–pituitary–ovarian axis [9, 10]. In the United States, the average age for menopause is between 50 and 52 years. Women will typically present with hot flashes, night sweats, insomnia, vaginal atrophy, dysuria, urinary urgency, and sexual dysfunction [11].

19.2.2 Uterine Fibroids in Postmenopausal Women

Postmenopausal women classically have been found to have smaller, shrinking, and fewer fibroids, most likely due to the decline in ovarian steroid hormones [12]. Early onset of menarche and late onset of menopause act as risk factors for increased incidence of

UFs. Noticeably, by the time women reach the age of 50, it is estimated that over 80% of black women and nearly 70% of white of women will have developed at least one fibroid during their lifetime [1]. Thus, reaching menopause does not totally eliminate the risk of new fibroids being diagnosed and women in the perimenopausal period should be considered to have higher risk of developing UFs. It is also possible that existing fibroids may continue to grow at a higher rate with an increase in patients' age [13].

A large cohort study of teachers from California found that among 1,790 subjects, over 30% of those with newly diagnosed fibroids were between the ages of 45 and 49 years, followed by the second highest incidence in the age group of 50–54 years. The study results also showed that highest prevalence overall was between 45 and 49 years, with 40–44 years as a close second. The study trends also indicated a decline in newly diagnosed fibroids from 50 years old onwards, but it remained above 1% until the age of 80 years [14].

19.2.3 Postmenopausal Fibroids and BMI

The California teachers cohort study reported a statistically positive correlation between high body mass index (BMI) among premenopausal and perimenopausal women and surgical diagnosis of UFs. Such association desisted once women became postmenopausal [14]. Furthermore, a large prospective cohort study exploring the impact of obesity and hormone replacement therapy (HRT) on fibroids in postmenopausal women documented that obesity (defined by the World Health Organization as BMI >30 kg/m^2) doubled the risk of UFs independent of HRT use [15]. The investigators went on to state that the use of HRT increased the risk of fibroids, regardless of BMI.

As uterine fibroids are known to be oestrogen-responsive, the increase in adiposity seen in obese women is likely to create a higher oestrogenic environment from the peripheral conversion favouring oestrogens. The study results signified that postmenopausal women continue to deal with fibroids, and the highest risk of surgically confirmed fibroids was found in obese women who had used HRT [15].

19.2.4 Postmenopausal Fibroids and Aromatase Enzyme Expression

Fibroid cells were shown to express the enzyme aromatase; therefore, they are able to locally synthesize oestrogen from androgenic substances such as androstenedione. This may explain why fibroids sometimes do not consistently regress in postmenopausal women, and this suggests a possible therapeutic role for aromatase inhibitors in the treatment of symptomatic fibroids in premenopausal and menopausal women. Moreover, aromatase is present in subcutaneous fat, so aromatase activity and plasma oestrogen levels correlate with BMI in postmenopausal women. This again supports the possible therapeutic benefit of an aromatase inhibitor in obese postmenopausal women [16–19].

19.2.5 Postmenopausal Fibroids and Bone Health

Postmenopausal loss of oestrogen greatly increases the risk of bone loss and, subsequently, development of osteoporosis [11]. Conversely, hyperoestrogenic states, such as obesity, have been shown to have protective effects on bone mineral density (BMD) even after factoring in mechanical load on bones [20]. Women with UFs are thought to have higher intrinsic oestrogen levels throughout their lifetime, which raises the question of whether the presence of fibroids influences bone health. As such, a prospective study published in 2006 demonstrated lower fracture risk and better bone health in peri- and early postmenopausal women who underwent hysterectomies for symptomatic UFs and never used HRT [20]. The study found a 31% reduction in any type of fracture in postmenopausal women with UFs in comparison to women without fibroids. The assumption is that fibroids causing symptoms severe enough to require hysterectomy are typically large and may have a higher intrinsic oestrogen level than smaller fibroids not requiring hysterectomies [20].

19.2.6 Leiomyosarcoma

Continued growth of any uterine masses and/or bleeding after menopause is worrisome and urgently warrants further evaluation for possible uterine sarcoma. Uterine leiomyosarcoma (uLMS) is the most common type of uterine sarcoma; they are rare but highly aggressive tumours with a poor long-term survival rate and account for an estimated 1% of all uterine malignancies [21]. Most investigators believe that leiomyosarcomas arise de novo from the myometrium and are not a progression from UFs [22].

They typically present with abnormal vaginal bleeding, pelvic pain, and pelvic mass, which all paint a similar clinical picture to UFs, thus making a preoperative diagnosis very difficult [22]. Occasionally, uLMS will have suspicious characteristics on MRI; also elevated serum levels of lactate dehydrogenase (LDH) isozyme 3 have been proposed as a possible biomarker [23]. However, these methods have poor positive predictive value and better uLMS diagnostics are urgently needed. Histologically, uLMSs are usually less well-circumscribed in comparison to fibroids and typically present as a single large myometrial mass [24].

All uLMS should be treated by en-bloc hysterectomy to avoid intraoperative abdominal spread of malignant cells [25]. However, as preoperative discrimination between benign UFs and malignant uLMS is currently difficult, laparoscopic power morcellation of possible uLMS lesions recently became a major surgical controversy [24, 26]. Morcellation uses a rotating blade to slice tissue into smaller pieces for ease of removal when undergoing a laparoscopic procedure [26]. Yet, it is argued that morcellation may lead to cancerous cells being spread throughout the abdominal cavity, thereby increasing the risk of further malignancy and possible worsening of patient prognosis. This is especially worrisome as one study estimates more than half of uLMS are not diagnosed until after surgical removal [26]. On the other hand, the FDA ban on power morcellation in the USA has led to a surge in open gynaecologic surgeries, with the expected increase in morbidity and complications [27].

19.2.7 Rare Cases of Postmenopausal Fibroids

Many case reports of rare, different types of fibroids in postmenopausal women have been published; for example, a severely calcified fibroid of broad ligament was identified in a 49-year-old postmenopausal woman and treated with hysterectomy [28], and another case of a large uterine fibroid with associated secondary polycythaemia was presented in a postmenopausal woman who underwent total abdominal hysterectomy [29]. A rare case of ovarian leiomyoma coexisting with a uterine lipoleiomyoma in a 59-year-old postmenopausal woman can postulate a common pathway as a stimulus for further research [30]. Other cases include a 23 kg giant fibroid removed from a

67-year-old postmenopausal woman that mandated urgent surgery [31], an ovarian leiomyoma [32], and a paraurethral leiomyoma [33].

19.3 Postmenopausal Fibroids and Hormone Replacement Therapy

19.3.1 Hormone Replacement Therapy

Many postmenopausal women opt to use hormone replacement therapy (HRT) due to its effectiveness to ameliorate symptoms associated with menopause as well as slow the progression of osteoporosis [11]. Hormone therapy can also provide cardioprotective effects during the first 10 years of early menopause [34]. As the natural regression of fibroids during menopause is understood to be due to the withdrawal of oestrogen and progesterone, supplementation of ovarian hormones in postmenopausal women has understandably made many clinicians apprehensive, due to the fear that therapy will increase fibroid size or at the very least prevent their regression. The use of HRT, however, can raise concern in women with a history of fibroids, as these hormones play a pivotal role in UF growth [35, 36].

Although HRT in postmenopausal women with fibroids may cause fibroid regrowth, it is not significant enough to contraindicate use, as most women will remain asymptomatic. Research on effects of HRT on fibroids remains inadequate, with conflicting and inconsistent results among many studies [37]. Nevertheless, it is suggested that women opting to use HRT should have ultrasound follow-ups every 3 months, and that therapy should be discontinued if fibroids show an increase in size after starting HRT [37].

19.3.2 Clinical Studies of HRT Effect on Postmenopausal Fibroids

In one trial, postmenopausal women were treated with continuous combined regimens of conjugated equine oestrogen (CEE) 0.625 mg/day along with oral medroxyprogesterone acetate (MPA) at 5 mg/day [38]. This trial showed increased growth of UFs during the first 2 years of therapy in comparison to women not on HRT. However, during the third year of therapy, there was a significant reduction of fibroid volumes, dropping from 13.5% of women experiencing fibroid growth in the first 2 years to 8.1% after the third year [38]. Several prospective studies have affirmed that fibroid growth peaks within the first 2 years of combined hormone therapy [14]. Another study compared 50 µg transdermal oestradiol plus 5 mg oral MPA continuously versus a regimen of 0.625 mg oral CEE plus 2.5 mg oral MPA continuously [36]. The results of this trial showed significant increase in fibroid size in the transdermal oestradiol group with 5 mg MPA after 1 year of therapy and no change in the oral CEE plus 2.5 mg MPA group; it also noted that fibroid size immediately shrunk after discontinuing therapy. These results suggest transdermal oestrogens and the increased dose of MPA may put patients at more risk for increase in fibroid size.

However, clinically, most studies have shown women remain asymptomatic and have low study dropout rates, regardless of whether the women had fibroid growth. Due to the increased risk of endometrial malignancy from unopposed oestrogen therapy, combined regimens are preferred [39]. Consequently, if therapy does include progestin, it is advised to use the lowest efficacious dose to avoid increased risk of fibroid growth [40].

19.3.3 Tibolone

Tibolone, a synthetic steroid with semi-oestrogenic, progestogenic, and androgenic activities, is used to treat menopausal symptoms. It seems to have the least effect on fibroid growth in postmenopausal women and so is preferred over combination therapies. One small study conducted with 56 postmenopausal women evaluated tibolone (2.5 mg) compared to transdermal HRT of oestradiol 0.05 mg for 4 weeks and norethisteron acetate 0.25 mg for 2 weeks [41]. The results showed that neither tibolone nor combined transdermal therapy had statistical significance for fibroid growth. Conversely, another small randomized study showed statistically significant increase in uterine volume, fibroid size and numbers with oestrogen–progestin therapy (transdermal system releasing 0.05 mg/day oestradiol with oral 10 mg/day MPA for 12 days), especially after 6 and 12 months of therapy [42]. One randomized trial indicated postmenopausal women who received tibolone 2.5 mg showed no statistical significance in fibroid volume change after 1 year of treatment [36]. Overall, most studies showed preference for tibolone over combined or transdermal HRT, as it does not increase uterine and fibroid size while still providing relief from menopausal symptoms [36, 42].

19.4 Management of Postmenopausal Women with/at Risk of Uterine Fibroids

As women with symptomatic UFs approach menopause, clinicians may consider a "watch and wait" approach to management with the expectation that small fibroids will shrink or spontaneously resolve on their own [43]. In persistent cases with increasing symptoms, the treatment choice for postmenopausal women is often hysterectomy. Alternative medical treatment options do exist and should also be considered, and hysterectomy should probably be considered as the last resort.

19.4.1 Aromatase Inhibitors

Aromatase inhibitors markedly suppress plasma oestrogen levels in postmenopausal women by inhibiting or inactivating aromatase enzyme. The ability of aromatase inhibitors to suppress endogenous oestrogen levels in postmenopausal women has led to their use as adjuvant therapy in the treatment of breast cancer [16].

Anastrozole, a third-generation non-steroidal aromatase inhibitor, may prove of value in treating fibroid-related uterine bleeding in obese postmenopausal women. Moreover, women taking aromatase inhibitors seem less likely to experience hot flashes than those using tamoxifen.

Use of aromatase inhibitors, in contrast to tamoxifen use, does not increase the risk of endometrial neoplasia or thromboembolism. A study has reported the successful use of an aromatase inhibitor in reducing the dimensions of a fibroid tumour causing urinary retention in a perimenopausal woman [18, 19].

19.4.2 Selective Oestrogen Receptor Modulators (SERMs)

Selective oestrogen receptor modulators (SERMs) elicit tissue-specific actions through a mixed agonistic and antagonistic effect on oestrogen receptors [5]. Two SERMs have been investigated: tamoxifen, which is used in treating breast cancer especially after surgical resection, and raloxifene, which is used in the prevention of osteoporosis. In one study, 17 postmenopausal women with fibroids were given a regimen of tamoxifen 20 mg daily. At the time of follow-up, the study found a significant increase in overall mean fibroid volume and volume of each fibroid on ultrasound scan [36]. However, all women remained asymptomatic and none discontinued therapy. Additionally, Palomba and colleagues evaluated raloxifene in postmenopausal women with fibroids and concluded that it is safe for use after studying its effect on fibroid dimensions, growth, and symptom severity, especially that of abnormal uterine bleeding. Their results suggested raloxifene significantly decreased uterine fibroid size after 6, 9, and 12 cycles of therapy [7, 44]. Studies on the impact of therapy for fibroids should be performed not exclusively with premenopausal women but also with perimenopausal and postmenopausal women, both users and non-users of HRT.

19.4.3 Uterine Artery Embolization

A retrospective study was conducted to explore the efficacy of uterine artery embolization (UAE) for postmenopausal symptomatic fibroid treatment. In all, 88.9% of patients demonstrated resolution of symptoms. UAE therefore could be considered as an alternative treatment to hysterectomy [45].

19.5 Conclusion

Uterine fibroids are very common and their symptoms have a significant impact on women's quality of life. The disease and the symptoms may persist in the peri- and even postmenopausal periods. The postulation that UF cases will resolve with the onset of the menopause is realistic, but it does not necessarily happen in every case. Classically, postmenopausal women had to go for hysterectomy if their UF-related symptoms persist, but alternative medical options now exist. Aromatase inhibitors currently may be effective in treating fibroid-related uterine bleeding or bulk symptoms in postmenopausal women, especially when obesity is involved. The triage of a suspicious uterine mass into benign fibroids versus malignant sarcoma is currently unattainable due to lack of reliable imaging characteristics or biomarkers. There is urgent need in the field to develop better diagnostics for uterine sarcoma in pre- and postmenopausal women.

References

1. Bulun SE. Uterine fibroids. *N Engl J Med* 2013;**369**(14):1344–55.

2. Islam MS, et al. Growth factors and pathogenesis. *Best Pract Res Clin Obstet Gynaecol* 2016;**34**:25–36.

3. Stewart EA, Laughlin-Tommaso SK, Catherino WH, et al. Uterine fibroids. *Nat Rev Dis Primers* 2016;**2**:16043.

4. Stewart EA, Cookson CL, Gandolfo RA, Schulze-Rath R. Epidemiology of uterine fibroids: a systematic review. *BJOG* 2017;**124**(10):1501–12.

5. Borahay MA, Asoglu MR, Mas A, et al. Estrogen receptors and signaling in fibroids: role in pathobiology and therapeutic implications. *Reprod Sci* 2017;**24** (9):1235–44.

6. Reis FM, Bloise E, Ortiga-Carvalho TM. Hormones and pathogenesis of uterine fibroids. *Best Pract Res Clin Obstet Gynaecol* 2016;**34**:13–24.

7. Palomba S, Sena T, Noia R, et al. Transdermal hormone replacement therapy in postmenopausal women with uterine leiomyomas. *Obstet Gynecol* 2001;**98**(6):1053–8.

8. Tan H, Yi L, Rote NS, Hurd WW, Mesiano S. Progesterone receptor-A and -B have opposite effects on proinflammatory gene expression in human myometrial cells: implications for progesterone actions in human pregnancy and parturition. *J Clin Endocrinol Metab* 2012;**97**(5):E719–30.

9. Prior JC. Perimenopause: the complex endocrinology of the menopausal transition. *Endocr Rev* 1998;**19**(4):397–428.

10. Soules MR, Sherman S, Parrott E, et al. Executive summary: Stages of Reproductive Aging Workshop (STRAW). *Fertil Steril* 2001;**76** (5):874–8.

11. Marjoribanks J, Farquhar C, Roberts H, Lethaby A, Lee J. Long-term hormone therapy for perimenopausal and postmenopausal women. *Cochrane Database Syst Rev* 2017;**1**:CD004143.

12. Cramer SF, Patel A. The frequency of uterine leiomyomas. *Am J Clin Pathol* 1990;**94**(4):435–8.

13. Stewart EA. Clinical practice. Uterine fibroids. *N Engl J Med* 2015;**372**(17):1646–55.

14. Templeman C, Marshall SF, Clarke CA, et al. Risk factors for surgically removed fibroids in a large cohort of teachers. *Fertil Steril* 2009;**92**(4):1436–46.

15. Sommer EM, Balkwill A, Reeves G, et al. Effects of obesity and hormone therapy on surgically-confirmed fibroids in postmenopausal women. *Eur J Epidemiol* 2015;**30**(6):493–9.

16. Shozu M, Murakami K, Inoue M. Aromatase and leiomyoma of the uterus. *Semin Reprod Med* 2004;**22**(1):51–60.

17. Smith IE, Dowsett M. Aromatase inhibitors in breast cancer. *N Engl J Med* 2003;**348**(24):2431–42.

18. Kaunitz AM. Aromatase inhibitor therapy for uterine bleeding in a postmenopausal woman with leiomyomata. *Menopause* 2007;**14** (5):941–3.

19. Shozu M, Murakami K, Segawa T, Kasai T, Inoue M. Successful treatment of a symptomatic uterine leiomyoma in a

perimenopausal woman with a nonsteroidal aromatase inhibitor. *Fertil Steril* 2003;**79**(3):628–31.

20. Randell KM, Honkanen RJ, Tuppurainen MT, et al. Fracture risk and bone density of peri- and early postmenopausal women with uterine leiomyomas. *Maturitas* 2006;**53**(3):333–42.

21. Wen KC, Horng HC, Wang PH, et al. Uterine sarcoma Part I – Uterine leiomyosarcoma: the topic advisory group systematic review. *Taiwan J Obstet Gynecol* 2016;**55**(4):463–71.

22. D'Angelo E, Prat J. Uterine sarcomas: a review. *Gynecol Oncol* 2010;**116**(1):131–9.

23. Goto A, Takeuchi S, Sugimura K, Maruo T. Usefulness of Gd-DTPA contrast-enhanced dynamic MRI and serum determination of LDH and its isozymes in the differential diagnosis of leiomyosarcoma from degenerated leiomyoma of the uterus. *Int J Gynecol Cancer* 2002;**12**(4):354–61.

24. Cui RR, Wright JD, Hou JY. Uterine leiomyosarcoma: a review of recent advances in molecular biology, clinical management and outcome. *BJOG* 2017;**124**(7):1028–37.

25. Park JY, Park SK, Kim DY, et al. The impact of tumor morcellation during surgery on the prognosis of patients with apparently early uterine leiomyosarcoma. *Gynecol Oncl* 2011;**122**(2):255–9.

26. Skorstad M, Kent A, Lieng M. Uterine leiomyosarcoma – incidence, treatment, and the impact of morcellation. A nationwide cohort study. *Acta Obstet Gynecol Scand* 2016;**95**(9):984–90.

27. Ebner F, Friedl TW, Scholz C, et al. Is open surgery the solution to avoid morcellation of uterine sarcomas? A systematic literature review on the effect of tumor morcellation and surgical techniques. *Arch Gynecol Obstet* 2015;**292**(3):499–506.

28. Pal S, Mondal S, Mondal PK, et al. Severely calcified leiomyoma of broad ligament in a postmenopausal woman: report of a rare case. *J Midlife Health* 2016;**7**(3):147–9.

29. Abdul Ghaffar NA, Ismail MP, Nik Mahmood NM, Daud K, Abu Dzarr GA. Huge uterine fibroid in a postmenopausal woman associated with polycythaemia: a case report. *Maturitas* 2008;**60**(2):177–9.

30. Kelekci S, Eris S, Demirel E, Aydogmus S, Ekinci N. Lipoleiomyoma of the uterus and primary ovarian leiomyoma in a postmenopausal woman: two rare entities in the same individual. *Case Rep Pathol* 2015;**2015**:564846.

31. Konstantinov S, Slavov S, Chernev A, Slavchev B. [A rare case of giant leiomyoma in postmenopausal woman]. *Akush Ginekol (Sofiia)* 2014;**53**(4):59–61.

32. Sasikala R, Rupavani K, Rekha R, Amel Ivan, E. Postmenopausal huge ovarian leiomyoma: a rare presentation. *J Clin Diagn Res* 2014;**8**(11):OD03–4.

33. Shim S, Borg CS, Majeed HG, Humaidan P. Paraurethral leiomyoma in a postmenopausal woman: first European case. *Case Rep Obstet Gynecol* 2015;**2015**:542963.

34. Kase NG. Impact of hormone therapy for women aged 35 to 65 years, from contraception to hormone replacement. *Gend Med* 2009; **6**(Suppl 1):37–59.

35. Wise LA, Laughlin-Tommaso SK. Epidemiology of uterine fibroids: from menarche to menopause. *Clin Obstet Gynecol* 2016;**59**(1):2–24.

36. Ang WC, Farrell E, Vollenhoven B. Effect of hormone replacement therapies and selective oestrogen receptor modulators in postmenopausal women with uterine leiomyomas: a literature review. *Climacteric* 2001;**4**(4):284–92.

37. Chang IJ, Hong GY, Oh YL, et al. Effects of menopausal hormone therapy on uterine myoma in menopausal women. *J Menopausal Med* 2013;**19**(3):123–9.

38. Yang CH, Lee JN, Hsu SC, Kuo CH, Tsai EM. Effect of hormone replacement therapy on uterine fibroids in postmenopausal women – a 3-year study. *Maturitas* 2002; **43**(1):35–9.

39. Furness S, Roberts H, Marjoribanks J, Lethaby A. Hormone therapy in postmenopausal women and risk of endometrial hyperplasia. *Cochrane Database Syst Rev* 2012; (8):CD000402.

40. Palomba S, Sena T, Morelli M, et al. Effect of different doses of progestin on uterine leiomyomas in postmenopausal women. *Eur J Obstet Gynecol Reprod Biol* 2002;**102**(2):199–201.

41. Simsek T, Karakus C, Trak B. Impact of different hormone replacement therapy regimens on the size of myoma uteri in postmenopausal period: tibolone versus transdermal hormonal replacement system. *Maturitas* 2002;**42**(3):243–6.

42. Fedele L, Bianchi S, Raffaelli R, Zanconato G. A randomized study of the effects of tibolone and transdermal oestrogen replacement therapy in postmenopausal women with uterine myomas. *Eur J Obstet Gynecol Reprod Biol* 2000;**88**(1):91–4.

43. Cramer SF, Marchetti C, Freedman J, Padela A. Relationship of myoma cell size and menopausal status in small uterine leiomyomas. *Arch Pathol Lab Med* 2000;**124**(10):1448–53.

44. Palomba S, Sammartino A, Di Carlo C, et al. Effects of raloxifene treatment on uterine leiomyomas in postmenopausal women. *Fertil Steril* 2001;**76**(1):38–43.

45. Chrisman HB, Minocha J, Ryu RK, et al. Uterine artery embolization: a treatment option for symptomatic fibroids in postmenopausal women. *J Vasc Interv Radiol* 2007;**18**(3):451–4.

Appendix: Video Captions

The video files specified below are available to view at www.cambridge.org/metwally

Video 8.1 Application of bulldog clamps to uterine arteries via a robotic approach 71

Video 9.1 Initial assessment and argipressin injection 81

Video 9.2 Uterine incision and enucleation of the fibroid 82

Video 9.3 Suturing of the myometrial defect 83

Video 9.4 Morcellation of the fibroid in a containment bag 84

Video 9.5 Application of barrier anti-adhesion measure (Interceed®) 84

Video 14.1 Resection of fundal submucosal fibroid: TruClear™ Tissue Removal System using the Dense Tissue Shaver Mini 140

Video 14.2 Resection of posterior wall submucosal fibroid: MyoSure Tissue Removal System 141

Index